Margaret Warner

Public Health and the State

Changing Views in Massachusetts, 1842–1936

Barbara Gutmann Rosenkrantz

Harvard University Press
Cambridge, Massachusetts
1972

For Louise, Judith, and Debby

Acknowledgments

Often in the past three years I have imagined how pleasant it would be to thank the many people who have made it possible for me to do this work. About two years ago I began to realize how illusory and inadequate these words of gratitude would be. Practically everyone I have talked to over these months has made some comment or offered some insight which became incorporated into my work as it progressed.

In the beginning Dr. Alfred L. Frechette, Commissioner of Public Health for the Commonwealth of Massachusetts, looked for an appropriate way to commemorate one hundred years of state responsibility for public health. I was fortunate to have been selected to write this history, and since then I have benefited immeasurably from his advice and assistance. His patience and cooperation have known no bounds. Through his suggestions I came to know other people currently working in the Department of Public Health. Mrs. Marie F. Gately, Dr. Leon Sternfeld, Dr. Nicholas J. Fiumara, Dr. Geoffrey Edsall, Dr. M. Grace Hussey, Dr. A. Daniel Rubenstein, Dr. Jerome S. Peterson, Dr. Robert A. MacCready, and Dr. Morton A. Madoff were among those who spent hours talking with me. From all of them I learned not only about the Department as it is today, but also about its past.

They led me to some of the fascinating men and women whose lives had been long and intimately associated with the Department of Public Health. Miss Florence L. Wall, Miss Genevieve O. Stuart, and the late Dr. Alton S. Pope all spent time and effort to give me a better picture of that past.

In particular, four men who have now retired from public service devoted much interest and energy toward acquainting me both with their own work and the lives and contributions of others no longer living. My study could

Acknowledgments

not have been completed without Dr. Robert E. Archibald, Dr. James A. McComb, Dr. Harold L. Lombard, and Dr. Harold W. Stevens; the opportunity to know these distinguished men has been one of the most exciting experiences in my life.

Durying my first year of research Dr. Jean A. Curran took time from his own work on the history of the Harvard School of Public Health to begin my education in the history of public health. Information about the Harvard-Massachusetts Institute of Technology School for Health Officers was unearthed for me by Mrs. Margaret G. Barnaby at the School of Public Health, and Mr. Terrence Keenan of the Commonwealth Fund made it possible for me to study the correspondence connected with the programs supported by that fund in Massachusetts during the 1930's.

Five busy people who had no direct connection with the Department of Public Health talked to me about their own experiences with key figures in Massachusetts public affairs and showed me papers and personal letters which illuminated the lives of people I could not interview. Miss Helen J. Almy talked to me about early social work programs. Dr. Paul Withington told me warm stories about his close friend, Dr. George H. Bigelow, and Dr. Bigelow's daughter, Mrs. Joseph Allen, lent me papers and enlarged my picture of her father's outstanding contribution. Mrs. Henry M. Keyes made it possible for me to read some unpublished papers belonging to her grandfather, Dr. Henry P. Walcott, and told me about his life after he had retired from office. Mrs. LaRue Brown filled me with information and admiration for the men and women who worked for improved child and maternal health care in the two decades following World War I, both in Massachusetts and in Washington, D.C.

Working in any area of Massachusetts history one is struck not only by the wealth of material, but even more by the extraordinary library facilities which make so many published and manuscript resources available to the student. Like others I am indebted to the librarians and staff at the Massachusetts State Library, the Massachusetts Historical Society, the Widener Library of Harvard University, the Schlesinger Library of Radcliffe College, the Dinand Library of the College of the Holy Cross, the American Antiquarian Society, the Worcester State Hospital, and the Clendening Medical Library of the University of Kansas. This study would have been much less comprehensive and much less enjoyable to pursue without the generous and enthusiastic assistance of Mr. Richard Wolfe of the Francis A. Countway Library at the Harvard Medical School and Mr. Tilton M. Barron and Miss Marion Henderson of the Robert H. Goddard Library at Clark University.

Acknowledgments

Two fellow students, Kenneth J. Moynihan and Cynthia Briggs, helped me survey newspapers and journals. Mrs. Zelda Wilkins and Miss Madeline Bousquet typed earlier and final drafts.

I have been helped by the willingness of experienced scholars; Professors George A. Billias, Daniel R. Borg, Robert H. Bremner, Joel R. Cohen, Tamara K. Hareven, and William A. Koelsch read my manuscript at various stages and gave invaluable advice. This study would have been neither begun nor completed in its present form without the guidance of Professor Gerald N. Grob, who has been quite literally my mentor and friend since the fall of 1964.

In addition, Mrs. Angela D. Dorenkamp spent many hours carefully reading my manuscript. It would be difficult to find a single paragraph that has not benefited from her judgment. Ann Orlov gave not only the patient editorial guidance which the manuscript required, but, far more important, she provided the professional and personal encouragement that assured its completion. Revisions were made while I held a Research Fellowship (No. LM 47687) from the National Library of Medicine of the National Institutes of Health.

I have saved my most important debts for the end. The two years, 1967–1969, that I spent at the Radcliffe Institute provided the time, the financial aid, and, above all, the confidence that a student needs. There is no adequate way to acknowledge the kind of sustenance given by other members of the Institute, both staff and Scholars. Above all others, the late Constance E. Smith was responsible for an environment that is surely unique and will continue to influence my work.

Finally, any woman who has the support from her family which enables her to take on serious study is fortunate indeed. In this respect my work has been undertaken under optimal conditions. My father, James Gutmann, and my husband, Paul, have listened and read, criticized and encouraged over more months than I care to recall. Last, but in many ways most important, my work bears the imprint of my three daughters' varied expectations. They will understand the gratitude and love with which this study is dedicated to them.

Contents

Contents

Public Health and the State

Changing Views in Massachusetts, 1842–1936

Abbreviations

AJPH	*American Journal of Public Health*
BMSJ	*Boston Medical and Surgical Journal*
BHM	*Bulletin of the History of Medicine*
JAMA	*Journal of the American Medical Association*
JHMAS	*Journal of the History of Medicine and Allied Sciences*
MHS	Massachusetts Historical Society
MMFQ	*Milbank Memorial Fund Quarterly*
NEJM	*New England Journal of Medicine*

Introduction

Americans have tended to respond to disease and disorder as though they were corruptions imported to this uncontaminated continent from foreign sources. Reflected clearly in the historical scholarship and popular oratory of the last half of the nineteenth century is a heroic tradition that celebrates the purity of our air and waters, the health and brawn of our people, and the vigor of our native institutions. In this light, health is regarded as indigenous to our soil; disease, as an odious alien.

These same assumptions supported the men who worked for sanitary reform in Massachusetts during the two decades before the Civil War, and these premises led, in 1869, to the establishment of a State Board of Health, the first in the United States to be based on a comprehensive program to prevent unnecessary mortality from all causes.[1] In succeeding years, as the etiology of contagious

1. Massachusetts and Louisiana share honors for pioneer public health legislation. Louisiana was the first state to establish a general Bureau of Statistics, but, according to the Superintendent of that Bureau in 1849, Massachusetts was the first state to establish a successful system of recording births, deaths, and marriages; see Lemuel Shattuck, *Appendix to the Report of the Sanitary Commission of Massachusetts* (Boston, 1850), pp. 411-415. A Louisiana Board of Health was established in 1855 and, like its Massachusetts counterpart organized fourteen years later, it was largely limited to an advisory capacity. Public health measures in Louisiana, unlike those in Massachusetts, were almost entirely concerned with the state's largest port, New Orleans, and limited to the control of a single disease, yellow fever. Consequently, in 1861 the Louisiana Board's Health Officer, Dr. G. A. Nott, reported to the legislature "that the Board of Health from want of power has tended to dwindle to a mere 'Board of Quarantine,' void of other functions"; quoted in Gordon E. Gillson, *Louisiana State Board of Health: The Formative Years* (privately printed by Louisiana State Board of Health, n.p.: n.d.), p. 100. The Louisiana Board has a history of continuous operation except for the years following General Benjamin F. Butler's occupation, 1862-1866. Since the Board's reputation was closely linked to the success of measures to control yellow fever and since prevention awaited the discovery of the etiology of this

disease was rigorously defined and prevention became more specifically the duty of the epidemiologist and the physician, a meliorist foundation formed the seed-bed for the development of public health policy, so that sanitary science remained the partner of social reform well into the twentieth century. After World War I, when mortality from contagious disease was no longer the main obstacle to longevity, the assignment of public, professional, and personal liability for the failure to prevent disease was subjected to constant re-evaluation. Nevertheless, the perfectionist inference that a healthy populace guaranteed a sound society remained intact as a symbol of our unique inheritance. Today, well-nourished, relatively immune from the hazards of epidemic disease, and rejecting the infirmities of old age as inconsistent with our youthful image, we offer ourselves as proof of the salubrity of our climate, the decency of our values, and the efficacy of our scientific and social institutions.

There has been a consensus in this century that the state is responsible for controlling disease, grounded on the normative view that public and personal health are, and of right ought to be, the birthright of Americans, and that whatever or whoever violates this trust is external and repugnant. Sources of weakness leading to susceptibility, causes of specific endemic and epidemic disease, have been identified by a variety of social and scientific criteria. Hygienic measures for prevention of illness and medical therapy reflect these judgments, but in the nineteenth and twentieth centuries it has been and still is taken for granted that there is an ideal correlation between health and obedience to the laws of nature. The Massachusetts State Board of Health and its successors have undertaken to bring society into conformity with these laws, transforming moral and scientific knowledge into public policy. What follows is an account of events occurring within a limited period when good and evil seemed embodied in specific form — in personal behavior, in pathogenic micro-organisms, in social mores and public institutions — which could be combated when they were dangerous or assimilated to rational and orderly systems of corporate and individual obligation when they were beneficial.

This identification of health with a conformity to the harmonious rational order grew largely out of experience and contradicted an earlier belief that disease and disaster were visitations of a just God upon a frail and erring people. Englishmen settling the Plymouth and Massachusetts Bay colonies in the early seventeenth century accepted smallpox and a large number of less clearly identified fevers and plagues as part of the human condition. Attempts during the eighteenth century to reduce the spread of smallpox through isolation and inocu-

---

disease in the twentieth century, public support of state regulation was inconsistent, and the success of the Board's sanitary program was proportionately uneven.

lation, or to restrict the importation of disease through the quarantine of immigrants and the disinfection of cargo, signified not only new ideas about the etiology of disease but also, and even more important, new attitudes toward the meaning of disease itself.

Having weathered the hazards of initial settlement, the colonists suffered less often and less severely from smallpox, and more seriously from septic sore throat, dysentery, and malaria than they had anticipated. Fewer women died as a result of childbirth, and the whole population enjoyed better health and longer lives than their relatives who had remained in England.[2] By the end of the century, church and state joined prayers for the protection of a virtuous people with cautious advice on cleanliness, moderation, and isolation of the sick in an effort to keep pestilence far from these shores. Endemic disease may have taken a large annual toll, but Boston counted itself a healthy city, and after 1799 the Selectmen and General Court took increasingly elaborate precautions to prevent disease from being brought ashore.[3]

By the beginning of the nineteenth century contagionist and anticontagionist theories were debated among physicians and laymen. When it was alleged that yellow fever had been imported to New York City by Irish immigrants, Noah Webster indignantly countered that these were "vulgar tales that disgrace this age of science and philosophy . . . Not that diseases of a certain kind are not infectious . . . But," he continued, "what I would severely reprobate is, the disposition of men to trace all evils of life to a foreign source, when the sources are in their own country, their own homes, and their own bosoms."[4]

In the first decades of the nineteenth century such arguments took place

2. Carl Bridenbaugh, *Cities In the Wilderness: The First Century of Urban Life in America, 1625-1742* (New York: Ronald Press, 1938), p. 88, was among the first to suggest that New England turned out to be an unexpectedly healthy environment. Recent studies of town and family life confirm this view; see, for instance, John Demos, "Notes on Life in Plymouth," *William and Mary Quarterly,* ser. 3, 22:270-271 (April 1965); Robert Higgs and H. Louis Settler, III, "New England Demography," *William and Mary Quarterly,* ser. 3, 27:286-288 (April 1970). See also John Duffy, *Epidemics in Colonial America* (Baton Rouge: Louisiana State University Press, 1953). Duffy suggests that in New England the absence of endemic smallpox and the restriction of the disease through variolation was partly responsible for low infant and child mortality rates. This eventually resulted in an unusually large population of older children who succumbed to diphtheria and scarlet fever (septic sore throat), accounting for the elevation of morbidity and mortality from these diseases.

3. For a summary of Massachusetts public health legislation in the colonial period, see Lemuel Shattuck and others, *Report of the Sanitary Commission of Massachusetts 1850,* facsimile ed. (Cambridge, Mass.: Harvard University Press, 1948), pp. 48-53. For a full discussion, see John B. Blake, *Public Health in the Town of Boston, 1630-1822* (Cambridge, Mass.: Harvard University Press, 1959).

4. Noah Webster, *A Brief History of Epidemic and Pestilential Diseases and the Principal Phenomona of the Physical World Which Precede and Accompany Them and Observations From the Facts Stated,* 2 vols. (London, 1800), I, 389.

against a background that defined public health as freedom from epidemic disease. Consequently public health measures were almost entirely restricted to the specific disastrous episode that had called them into being. The failure to develop long-range programs for the prevention of epidemic illness was only partly related to the deliberately nihilistic nature of much contemporary medical theory. Charles Rosenberg's important study of three nineteenth-century cholera epidemics not only shows that in 1832 cholera was considered a direct consequence of undesirable behavior; it also indicates that the failure to institute permanent sanitary reform was not the result of an absence of humanitarian concern, but actually a reflection of the contemporary belief that Americans were naturally healthy.[5] If the poor and the sinful in the Old World were susceptible to disease, our countrymen asserted that they themselves had little to fear since this was a land where opportunity beckoned the industrious and the virtuous.

Indeed, Massachusetts was unusually well off. Boston was completely free of deaths from smallpox between 1816 and 1824, and yellow fever never reached the proportions experienced in other seaboard cities.[6] Social responsibility for public health in Massachusetts followed successful experience with the control of epidemic disease and the reification of health as a desirable social and personal goal. The Commonwealth escaped lightly from the cholera epidemic of 1832. Yet, without a major crisis, Boston appropriated a larger sum to clean the streets and alleys and care for the sick than any other American city, and it was similarly prepared to meet the next threatened cholera epidemic in 1849.[7] In addition, the legislature in the spring of that year established a commission to prepare a sanitary survey of the state. Registration of vital statistics indicated that mortality from other sources was increasing, and a subsequent investigation showed a correlation between fatal illness and density of population. While the specific source of disease remained the subject of controversy, a new attitude toward health was revealed in the *Report of the Sanitary Commission:* "WE

5. Charles E. Rosenberg, *The Cholera Years: The United States in 1832, 1849 and 1866* (Chicago: University of Chicago Press, 1962), pp. 55-64, 92-98.

6. There were no cases of yellow fever in Boston between 1693 and 1790; between 1793 and 1805, when the disease swept other northern cities, there were only a few isolated cases in Boston. However, the need for sanitary precautions against the possible appearance of yellow fever in 1799 was in large measure responsible for the establishment of the Boston Board of Health: see Blake, *Public Health in Boston,* pp. 151-176, 191.

7. Rosenberg, *Cholera Years,* pp. 91-92, 117. Fortunately all of Massachusetts was spared in 1849 and again in 1866. Although it is difficult to account for this in any conclusive way, municipal pride and responsibility, reflected in the relative orderliness of city government and in the 1845 inauguration of a public water supply drawn from Cochituate, outside the city limits, must certainly be assigned an important role.

BELIEVE," wrote Lemuel Shattuck in 1850, *"that the conditions of perfect health, either public or personal, are seldom or never attained, though attainable."*[8]

Others have commented on the breadth of the Commission's recommendations, which stemmed from the document and the modern tone set by Shattuck's call for state responsibility.[9] In an increasingly heterogeneous society, impersonal secular law was substituted for exhortation to individual reform. Reliance on external constraints resulted from a New World view of the orderly relationship between nature and society, rather than a germ theory of disease. In Massachusetts, health had, by 1850, become a reason for pride, a wholesome and necessary condition to be defended from those whose habits or values made them ignorant of custom and regulation. The Sanitary Commission's report, written more than fifty years before a microbial etiology of contagious disease became the foundation of preventive medicine, assumed that the danger to health came as much from the corruption of morals as from the contamination of the environment. But, because society had already achieved a measure of stability and because health had become a desirable attribute linked to the inherent virtues of the native population, public health could now be protected and enhanced by statute.

For the next seventy years, as knowledge about the etiology and transmission of disease became more specific, the sources of danger to health were variously described. Two decades after the Civil War the State Board of Health depended less upon its ability to influence individual conduct than upon the ability of engineers, chemists, and physicians to circumvent deviant behavior. By the end of the century the science of bacteriology virtually dictated public health prophylaxis and therapy. The laboratory scientist and the physician tended to describe disease in biological terms, and, as public health became a science, its methods and objectives became professional rather than broadly reformist. Until the third decade of the twentieth century, however, medical prevention and treatment presented minimal conflicts with social values; it was thought that health could be purchased if society were willing to pay the price.[10] In Massachusetts,

8. Shattuck and others, *Report of the Sanitary Commission,* p. 10.

9. *Ibid.,* introduction by Charles-Edward Amory Winslow. The facsimile edition of the *Report of the Sanitary Commission* was published in commemoration of the centennial of the original edition.

10. The words "Public health is purchasable. Within natural limitations a community can determine its own death rate," are associated with Hermann M. Biggs, Chief Medical Officer of the New York City Health Department, 1902-1913, and Commissioner of Public Health for the state of New York from 1914 until his death in 1923. The motto appeared originally in the *Monthly Bulletin* (October 1911) issued by that Department.

the history of state responsibility for public health records not only that mortality rates were reduced, but also that the quality of life was immeasurably improved by the work of able men whose scientific skill and devotion to public service led them to positions of immense authority.

The last chapter of this study suggests that the goal of perfect health, new in Shattuck's day and still implicit in our rhetoric, may no longer be a viable objective. Massachusetts public health policy in the past has consistently reflected this ideal concept. Since 1869 the dangers to life and health have been identified and countered according to the social and scientific assumptions of the day. Immoral habits, impure air, contaminated water and food, and contagious individuals have not been lightly tolerated, at least in principle; filth and corruption have been swept aside as unwelcome intruders. Health has had social and scientific components, but only rarely has there been a need to choose between them. And when demands placed on the state and the medical profession have conflicted, as in programs for cancer control or for maternal and child welfare, it appeared that "science" could help make the choice because the scientific meaning of perfect health seemed to hold firm.

This study begins at a time when the definition of "health" implied that it could be achieved, and the rules for success were modified by social experience and scientific knowledge. In Massachusetts, despite the diverse expectations of a heterogeneous population and despite environmental hazards accompanying the growth of cities and industry, an unusual set of circumstances and men fashioned a flexible institution which responded to change without violating the pattern imposed by a concept of health originating in the mid-nineteenth century.

This concept of health now belongs to the past, for it is founded on the supposition that there is a perfect fit between social and sanitary reform. Such a concept was not able to fully accommodate the indigent mother in 1922, nor the chronically diseased in 1926; nor does it do justice to the problems of the youthful drug addict in 1971. The heterodoxy of the contemporary society does not permit a single definition of health, and these ambiguities cannot be resolved, as our parents thought, by assigning them to the scientists and to the professionals. The urgent public health problems of today, posed by such hazards as drug abuse and pollution of the environment, cannot be assessed and solved exclusively by reference to scientific principles.

At the same time, goodwill and conformity to simple ethical and social precepts do not establish the criteria for choosing between individual and corporate priorities when good and evil are enmeshed in every alternative. Both the locus of authority and the limits of health have altered radically in the twentieth century. Contradiction between public expectation and personal commitment, between affluence and poverty, between laws of society and laws of nature, involve shady areas where customary standards are no longer appropriate.

This is a story of the years that preceded these dilemmas. The history of the Massachusetts State Board of Health is an account of a time when social and scientific expectations came together, fused by the idea that perfect health was an attainable goal, exceptional in its virtue, and equally available to all who subscribed to the maxims of an orderly, harmonious life. It is the story of a successful endeavor that can never be re-enacted.

1 From Records to Reform, 1842-1850

When a committee of the Massachusetts legislature confidently asserted, on May 22, 1869, that all governments since the time of Moses had made provision to protect the life and health of their people, the legislators affirmed a tradition of corporate responsibility for the welfare of their people.[1] This sentiment was shared by men of substance and goodwill throughout the Commonwealth; men were convinced that a healthy community would reflect their commitment to virtue and order and assumed that these values could be taught through example and persuasion. The pursuit of health needed no justification and was supported, moreover, by a common experience. Yet in the four preceding decades this experience had been threatened by profound changes in the social and economic life of Massachusetts citizens.

As the society began shifting from a rural to an urban setting, the standards and traditions of many families within the state were challenged. Newly established mill towns along the Merrimac River offered opportunities for wealth and adventure to young men and women who left the western hills and central Massachusetts farmlands in unprecedented numbers. The cities of Lowell, Lawrence, and Fall River came to life with the growth of textile manufacture. Although

---

1. "Report of the Joint Special Committee . . . to Consider the Expediency of Establishing a State Board of Health," *Massachusetts Senate Documents 1869, No. 340* (May 22, 1869). Despite this statement by the legislature and despite the fact that public responsibility for the sick was a traditional concern, public responsibility for the prevention of disease became one of the distinctive characteristics accompanying social and economic change in the mid-nineteenth century. For an enlightening discussion of this development, particularly in England and Europe, see George Rosen, "What is Social Medicine? A Genetic Analysis of the Concept," *BHM,* 21:674-733 (Sept.-Oct. 1947), and "Approaches to a Concept of Social Medicine, A Historical Survey," *MMFQ,* 26:7-21 (Jan. 1948).

Boston remained the hub of commerce and culture rather than a center for new industry, it also expanded in wealth and population. Even before the huge foreign immigration which followed the Irish potato famine of 1846, native Americans had started to leave the countryside, so that the ratio of city dwellers rose from 11 percent of the population in 1820, to 17 percent twenty years later. As immigrants by the thousands continued to arrive and cluster together, the cities grew in number and size; by 1855 there were 13 urban centers in the Bay State with more than 12,000 residents. At the close of the Civil War 21 percent of Massachusetts' population was foreign-born and almost 40 percent of the people in the state lived in cities.[2]

While these cities were being established and growing rapidly, morbidity and mortality rates increased faster than the population. But it was the character of the people who swept into the seaboard towns and flocked to the factory cities, as much as their numbers, which frustrated traditional methods of protecting health. The new urban dwellers, native-born Americans as well as recently arrived immigrants, adopted habits that seemed to contradict all acceptable standards of cleanliness and morality. Crowded together in tenements, they resisted influences that would otherwise have guided them. All persons appeared to be unusually susceptible to disease and immorality when subjected to the corrupting atmosphere of urban life.

Among medical men, the prevailing view associated disease with filth and improper living conditions. Bad air, putrefaction of animal and vegetable matter, and the noxious odors which arose from the streets and waterways were all seen

2. Massachusetts population more than doubled between 1820 and 1860, with an increasing rate of growth: 1820 − 523,287; 1840 − 737,699; 1850 − 994,514; 1860 − 1,231,066 (*Statistical History of the United States from Colonial Times to the Present*, rev. ed. [Stamford, Conn.: Fairfield Publishing, 1965]). For urban data, see two articles in *Quarterly Publications of the American Statistical Association*: Horace G. Wadlin, "The Growth of American Cities," n.s., 2:159-162 (March 1891); Percy Wells Bidwell, "Population Growth in Southern New England, 1810-1860," n.s., 120:813-835 (Dec. 1917). For a recent and more sophisticated interpretation, see Jeffrey G. Williamson, "Antebellum Urbanization in the American Northeast," *Journal of Economic History*, 25:592-614 (Dec. 1965). In general, the use of census data on population growth in antebellum Massachusetts has been documented so thoroughly and economically, beginning with Oscar Handlin, *Boston's Immigrants, 1790-1864: A Study in Acculturation*, rev. ed. (Cambridge, Mass.: Harvard University Press, 1959), that it seems almost unnecessary to do more than refer to this work and its tables. See also Stephan Thernstrom, *Poverty and Progress: Social Mobility in a Nineteenth Century City* (Cambridge, Mass.: Harvard University Press, 1964) and Donald B. Cole, *Immigrant City: Lawrence, Massachusetts, 1845-1921* (Chapel Hill: University of North Carolina Press, 1963). A more recent study by Michael B. Katz, *The Irony of Early School Reform: Educational Innovation in Mid-Nineteenth Century Massachusetts* (Cambridge, Mass.: Harvard University Press, 1968) describes this movement and its social implications quite precisely, esp. pp. 5-11, 221-223.

as potentially hazardous to health. In the absence of specific etiological concepts, the social and physical conditions which accompanied urbanization were
considered equally responsible for the impairment of vital bodily functions and
premature death. Although a more selective view of the relationship between
filth and disease gradually gained favor, this did not negate the belief that personal health could only be achieved through the harmonious functioning of all
human organs and that public health was threatened by disturbances which followed in the wake of social change.

In the years before the Civil War reformers were primarily concerned with prevention rather than cure. Deeply disturbed by the apparent deterioration of
health and morality, they sought to reverse the trend. In 1850 — nineteen years
before the meeting of the first State Board of Health — a special legislative commission delivered a report on the sanitary condition of the Commonwealth.[3]

Prepared by Lemuel Shattuck, bookseller and publisher, authority on statistics,
and Whig member of the legislature from Boston, the *Report of the Sanitary
Commission* was destined to emerge as the single most important document in
Massachusetts public health legislation. The *Report* followed eight years of gathering increasingly complete birth and mortality data from the cities and towns,
a movement in which Shattuck had played a key role. The accurate recording
and analysis of vital statistics served as the foundation of Shattuck's postulate
that "Could we see clearly the operation of cause and effect, we should see laws
wisely administered in every event that takes place in the universe."[4]

Shattuck shared with his contemporaries an expanded confidence in the lawfulness of the physical environment. Derived from a religious framework, this
assumption led Shattuck to formulate a plan so comprehensive that it has served
as a guide to later generations living in a far different social and physical environment. "The character of man as a social being," Shattuck stated, "is modified by
the circumstances of his existence, and varies as these circumstances vary in their
development in different places and different periods: and it is desirable for a
social and *scientific* purpose that such characteristics may be ascertained as will
exhibit the varieties of differences."[5] Written in 1850, this thesis remains the
underlying imperative of the public health movement to this day.

---

3. John L. Thomas, "Romantic Reform in America, 1815-1865," *American Quarterly,*
17:656-681 (Winter 1965). Lemuel Shattuck and others, *Report of the Sanitary Commission of Massachusetts 1850,* facsimile ed. (Cambridge, Mass.: Harvard University Press,
1948).
4. *Ibid.,* p. 291.
5. *Ibid.,* p. 127.

As far back as the colonial period, the burden of caring for the sick and the threat of smallpox and yellow fever epidemics had led to the creation of provincial laws to supplement town and city ordinances.[6] Smallpox was the only disease universally recognized as contagious through contact with the sick individual, and for this scourge specific prophylaxis was available. Despite widespread distrust of the medical profession, inoculation with material from smallpox scabs after 1721 and vaccination with cowpox following 1800 were increasingly accepted as effective means of controlling smallpox epidemics.[7] However, even after the success of vaccination, responsibility for this practice was left to physicians in most cases. Publicly enforced measures for control were largely limited to isolation and quarantine during the first two decades of the nineteenth century.[8]

Only in response to the threat of an epidemic was the government called upon to take steps for prevention as well as relief. When yellow fever threatened, the belief that filth and disease were linked was sufficiently accepted to require protective measures. In February 1799 the Massachusetts legislature responded to a petition from concerned citizens and ordered Boston to organize a Board of Health in an effort to prevent the recurrence of yellow fever. Headed by Paul Revere, this Board called upon the citizens to clean their streets and houses; it acted on the assumption that freedom from disease depended on everyone accepting the moral obligation for public hygiene and personal moderation. Acknowledging public power and responsibility on the one hand, and relying on

6. Organized community aid to the sick-poor had grown up as a pragmatic adaptation of the Elizabethan Poor Law; see Albert Deutsch, "The Sick Poor in Colonial Times," *American Historical Review,* 46:560-579 (April 1941). See also Shattuck and others, *Report of the Sanitary Commission,* pp. 50-51: "Legislation principally with reference to smallpox, has been frequent in the history of the State. As early as 1701, 'an act providing in case of sickness,' was passed, 'for better preventing the spread of infection' . . . to remove such infected persons to separate houses, and to provide 'nurses, tendance, and other assistance and necessaries for them at the charge of the parties themselves, their parents or masters (if able,) or otherwise at the charge of the town or place whereto they belong' . . . This has been the foundation of all the sanitary laws passed since that time. Its provisions were retained and much extended in the Great Act of June 22, 1797 . . . and incorporated into the Revised Statutes in 1836."

7. For a detailed narrative of smallpox immunization following 1721, see Francis R. Packard, *History of Medicine in the United States,* rev. ed., 2 vols. (New York: P. B. Hoeber, 1931), II, 76-94. For a general discussion of attitudes toward medicine in this period, see Richard H. Shryock, *The Development of Modern Medicine: An Interpretation of the Social and Scientific Factors Involved,* rev. ed. (New York: Alfred A. Knopf, 1947), Chap. xiii, "Public Confidence Lost," and below, n. 12.

8. Shattuck and others, *Report of the Sanitary Commission,* pp. 64-65, 180; John B. Blake, *Public Health in the Town of Boston, 1630-1822* (Cambridge, Mass.: Harvard University Press, 1959), pp. 180-191.

individual action on the other, these contradictory responses were brought to bear on yellow fever which was considered contagious under certain conditions.[9]

Cholera, feared above all diseases because of its swift and unaccountable onset and high mortality rate, was not considered a contagious disease. Whenever cholera appeared in Europe, it was generally acknowledged that, within a matter of months, the disease would descend on the cities of the New World. When threatened with cholera in 1832, Boston's leading citizens formed a committee which raised money to aid the afflicted and to clean the streets and alleys. No one could fail to note that, like other diseases, cholera was most likely to strike families living in squalor or those whose personal intemperance predisposed them to weakness. The specific etiology of the sickness was unclear. Physicians were far from certain whether this was one disease or whether other, less deadly illnesses took on a fatal character under the combined influence of summer heat and an "epidemic constitution." If little was known about the cause of cholera, still less was known about its cure. Although the 1832 epidemic passed lightly over Boston as compared with New York and New Orleans, no one even suggested that this situation might have been the result of any distinctive medical treatment.[10]

One reason why such an explanation was not forthcoming was the poor reputation of the medical profession. The Massachusetts Medical Society had been established in 1781, and the Harvard Medical School began to hold classes the following year. Physicians did not yet, however, enjoy an esteem that would have permitted them a decisive role in either the prevention or treatment of disease. A wide range of nonorthodox practitioners flourished, encouraged by the vagaries of medical education and theory.[11] Since it was generally believed that cholera was engendered by foul atmospheric conditions, public preventive meas-

9. Blake, *Public Health in Boston,* pp. 167-169; Oscar and Mary F. Handlin, *Commonwealth: A Study of the Role of Government in the American Economy, 1774-1861,* rev. ed. (Cambridge, Mass.: Harvard University Press, 1969), p. 248. Phyllis Allen, "Etiological Theory in America Prior to the Civil War," *JHMAS,* 2:492-498 (Autumn 1947). In the absence of a clear-cut distinction between contagious and noncontagious etiology, it was believed that all diseases became contagious under certain conditions. Thus the importance of personal and environmental variables was accentuated as determinants of individual susceptibility. Shattuck and others, *Report of the Sanitary Commission,* pp. 52-53, records that boards of health were also established in Salem (1799), Marblehead (1802), Plymouth (1810), Charlestown (1818), Lynn (1821), and Cambridge (1828), based on provisions of the Act of 1797.

10. For a most rewarding treatment of the relation between social thought and attitudes toward disease see Charles E. Rosenberg, *The Cholera Years: The United States in 1832, 1849 and 1866* (Chicago: University of Chicago Press, 1962), esp. pp. 80-81, 91, 93.

11. Henry R. Viets, *A Brief History of Medicine in Massachusetts* (Boston: Houghton, Mifflin, 1930), pp. 130-135; Walter L. Burrage, *A History of the Massachusetts Medical*

ures involved the removal of filth and all other sources of foulness. The best defense against susceptibility to cholera, however, was considered to be a mode of life consonant with the maintenance of physical and moral integrity, rather than reliance on medical advice.[12]

This attitude toward the medical profession was in part the reflection of a much broader mood prevailing in American society at the time. The search for effective methods to guide and, where necessary, to reform the course of the republic during these years led to tensions that were frequently expressed in political language. While Andrew Jackson's presidency served to sharpen ideological positions in the 1830's, the appearance of new class and sectional interests were viewed as an unwelcome departure from the past when differences presumably had given way to solutions based on a moral posture. Ideals and rhetoric which had been almost unanimously accepted in a predominantly agrarian society were still viable, but the old words carried new meaning under the pressure of working and living in an increasingly industrial society. In Massachusetts the rapid growth of manufacturing fostered elements which seemed threatening to the unique social and political institutions of the Commonwealth.

Those who feared that the old standards might be forgotten when subjected to the extremes of wealth and poverty which accompanied city life, looked for ways to assure continuity with past humanitarian practices. Services formerly exercised by the individual or by the joint effort of self-appointed groups were assumed by the government. During the 1830's the nonlicensed medical practitioner, the consumer, and the worker in the mill turned to the Massachusetts legislature to protect their interests. Men were elected to political office who,

---

Society, 1781-1922 (Norwood, Mass., privately printed, Plimpton Press, 1923), pp. 9–23, 63-104; Charles E. Rosenberg, "The American Medical Profession: Mid-Nineteenth Century," *Mid-America,* 44:163-171 (July 1962); Richard H. Shryock, *Medical Licensing in America, 1650-1965* (Baltimore: Johns Hopkins Press, 1967), pp. 27-33; Joseph F. Kett, *The Formation of The American Medical Profession: The Role of Institutions, 1780-1860* (New Haven, Conn.: Yale University Press, 1968), pp. 5-16, 24-31. For an interesting contemporary comment by the medical profession see Zadok Howe, "On Quackery," *Medical Communications of the Massachusetts Medical Society,* 5:308 (1830-1836): "A law which would deprive a citizen of the privilege of tampering with the lives of his fellow citizens, might be deemed an infringement upon the rights of the people, and incompatible with the spirit of our free institutions . . . . The remedy — for this evil — second to none but the evil of intemperance — is a change in public opinion." See also Jacob Bigelow, "On Self Limited Diseases," *Medical Communications of the Massachusetts Medical Society,* 5:319-346 (1830-1836).

12. Rosenberg, *Cholera Years,* pp. 165-166. By the time of the next threatened cholera epidemic in 1849, although most physicians agreed that the disease was probably caused by a specific poison, a letter in the *BMSJ,* 41:298 (Nov. 14, 1849), noted that Americans had been largely spared while foreigners had been ready victims, due largely to the crowded, unventilated condition of their houses.

twenty years before, would have been rejected because of the tradition of deference to class and established social status. It was a time of stress, when the desire for social harmony often conflicted with the demand for reform. In the
search for ways to integrate divergent interests and new citizens, traditional sym-
bols of order competed with utopian schemes. Among those who looked first
to the past as the guide to lawful change was Lemuel Shattuck, who returned to
New England from the West in 1823 and rapidly found his way to service and
recognition.[13]

Lemuel Shattuck was born in 1793, the fifth child of John and Betsy (Miles)
Shattuck.[14] Before he was a year old the family moved from Ashby, Massachusetts, to New Ipswich, New Hampshire, a small farming community where his
father struggled to make a living as a shoemaker and a farmer. His mother died
of tuberculosis when he was five, and his father soon married a widow with
children of her own. Opportunities for formal education were limited to a common school and a local academy. A combination of cold winters, illness, and
the struggle to keep the family intact, however, prevented regular attendance
at school.

In Shattuck's eyes, the religious and moral atmosphere in which he matured
was more important than any formal education.[15] Primary among his concerns
were his two sisters, about whom he later wrote: "Just as they were maturing
into womanhood, and about to take their stations as heads of families, and as
useful members of society, their career was arrested, and they were numbered
with that great multitude of similar cases, in which Providence seems mysteri-

13. Handlin and Handlin, *Commonwealth*, chaps. ix and x, describe the complexity of
government functions and the underlying objectives of changes in legislation during this
period. For a concise and persuasive description of two contemporary views, see the positions of Samuel C. Allen and Orestes A. Brownson as defined in Arthur M. Schlesinger, Jr.,
Orestes A. Brownson: A Pilgrim's Progress (Boston: Little, Brown, 1939), pp. 39-41. I see
Shattuck's position as very similar to Brownson's in the early 1830's. Both men believed
that an improved moral posture was the prerequisite to solid reform. For further material
on the background and mood of political thought in the 1830's, see the opening chapters
of Arthur M. Schlesinger, Jr., *The Age of Jackson* (Boston: Little, Brown, 1945), and
also Louis Hartz, "The Rise of the Democratic Idea," pp. 37-51, in Arthur M. Schlesinger,
Jr., and Morton White, eds., *Paths of American Thought* (Boston: Houghton, Mifflin,
1963).
14. Biographical material on Shattuck is from the following sources: Lemuel Shattuck,
*Memorials of the Descendents of William Shattuck, the Progenitor of the Families in
America that have Borne his Name* (Boston, 1855); Lemuel Shattuck Papers, *MHS*; John
Ward Dean, "Lemuel Shattuck," *Memorial Biographies of the New England Historical
Genealogical Society*, 3:290-321 (1883).
15. Shattuck, *Memorials*, p. 302, states that his formal education ended with two quar-
ters at the academy.

ously to select the most meritorious, and those of greatest promise of usefulness in this world for another sphere of existence. And yet we trust they did not live entirely in vain; and that even their short lives were not useless lives."[16]

Their lives and his had been touched by the Second Great Awakening, a great religious rededication which came to New Ipswich in the winter and spring of 1812. Shattuck was moved to begin teaching school in nearby communities during the winter, returning home at other seasons to farm and to school himself in Latin. "I did not however think of making it a profession for life," he recalled later. "To benefit my fellow beings as well as myself was then and ever has been considered a part of my duty."

Duty also beckoned him to make a better living, but unfortunately this was far more difficult. A trip to Boston in May 1814 sent him packing back to New Hampshire, for no one had a place for a "raw country boy."[17] A year later he sought to enter manufacturing, an experience more dignified in memory than in actual success. Ten months after this sobering experience, reflecting on the unhappy state of the world and his own bleak future following his father's death, he decided to leave New Ipswich and take a position teaching school in upstate New York.

In Troy, where he was to stay for almost two years, from December 1816 to October 1818, he wrote his first "Journal" entry in a miniscule hand "Oh Lord forgive and [sic] unworthy rebellious worm."[18] Little in his early years indicated the possibility of achievement in worldly affairs, but the thread of personal commitment and dedication to pious concern remained with him throughout his life. "I have received several invitations," he wrote to his wife twenty years later while in Washington on a business trip, "but have been to but two or three — but enough to see the society in Washington — enough to shew me that one who makes it a point to attend generally will become a slave to society and expose himself to habits of dissipation which must be ruinous to indulge in."[19]

Even after he had achieved a degree of success and comfort, Shattuck retained that sense of his own duty and dedication, and the world around him was often not so much a challenge as a threat and a temptation. In the winter of 1843–1844 he wrote his daughter Rebecca to "fortify your mind by sound, right, and consistent, moral and religious principles, that your

16. *Ibid*., appendix, pp. 382-383.
17. Shattuck "Autobiography" for the years 1793-1821, written in 1844, Shattuck Papers, MHS.
18. Shattuck "Journal," Dec. 31, 1816, Shattuck Papers, MHS.
19. Shattuck to Clarissa Shattuck, Feb. 18, 1837, Shattuck Papers, MHS.

mind — your soul — might be preserved in health as well as your body. You are destined, if you live, to live in a wicked world, surrounded by temptations, and to resist this influence, will require soundest principles, great caution and watchfulness, and constant prayer to your maker to aid you." Shattuck expected much of himself and of his offspring, and he reminded Rebecca that "You will be *looked* at more than some girls of your age for an example . . . and great care and circumspection, on your part, will be necessary to do as you ought and preserve consistency of character. I wish to have you cheerful and happy — to have you mingle in the enjoyment of your associates, and not to appear singular in any of those amusements wherein strict morals are preserved, but when anything is done, or proposed to be done, inconsistent with your moral or religious *duty*, you ought to have independence enough to do what your conscience dictates you to say a [*sic*] do, when that conscience is guided by right notions of right and wrong."[20]

Shattuck's religious views stemmed from quite different experience than that typical of the leading citizens of the busy eastern Massachusetts communities in which he spent his most productive years. Unlike Boston businessmen whose wealth and station complemented a comfortable appreciation of their role and a commanding stewardship for those less fortunate, Shattuck acquired his moral sense as a result of being exposed to the precarious character of life. If Amos Lawrence and Nathaniel Appleton, two of Boston's most successful founders of industry, envisaged themselves as intermediaries in God's plan, Shattuck assumed the place of translator.[21] Never in a position to assume the guise of patron, he was not specifically concerned for the individual — the poor, the abused, or the ignorant. He sought instead to establish the grand plan of nature by collecting records which would demonstrate irrefutable laws. For Shattuck, this organic moral view, linking order and virtue, grew from a pietistic faith in God rather than man. It prevented him from becoming a simple genealogist and turned him to the social science of statistics.

He achieved recognition beyond the small community of Concord, where he had lived for the ten years after 1823, as a result of writing the town's anniversary history. His work included a thorough statistical analysis derived from church and town records. Three years of diligent effort along these lines revealed to him the possibility of giving order and meaning to facts of the past,

20. Shattuck to Rebecca Shattuck, Dec. 16, 1843, and Feb. 26, 1844, Shattuck Papers, MHS.
21. Paul Goodman, "Ethics and Enterprise: The Values of a Boston Elite, 1800-1860," *American Quarterly*, 8:437-451 (Fall 1966).

and, at the same time, directed his attention to the inadequacies of existing vital statistics.[22]

During these same years he published a new code of school regulations. Looking back, Shattuck felt that his first effort to bring order to this exercise of community responsibility had been the precursor of his later proposals for the registration of vital statistics and sanitary regulation. Records, for Shattuck, provided the necessary foundation of reform since they established the facts from which all social order and progress could be derived. A master plan would be no better than the discrete segments from which it was drawn. Thus, in 1850 Shattuck attested to the merit of his proposed sanitary survey by recalling his success in working with school records.

Bound books were provided each teacher to record the progress of every pupil. Aided by these compiled records, the school committee prepared a written report for the annual town meeting. Shattuck was entirely responsible for the preparation and publication of the first Concord report in 1831. In 1838, when Shattuck was a member of the Massachusetts legislature, he was able to have this plan adopted for all schools throughout the Commonwealth. With pride he claimed "that no one measure, aside from the establishment of the Board of Education, has done so much good."[23] This was the first of Shattuck's numerous efforts to provide individuals and institutions with standard forms to organize and record the data of their lives. The school registers were not the germ of a later insight, but rather the complete conception executed in miniature.

In 1835 Shattuck moved to Boston, where he established a partnership for book publishing and distribution and extended his contacts as a recognized genealogist. Invited to join the Massachusetts Historical Society in 1830, and the American Antiquarian Society in 1831, he was now a well-known figure in scholarly circles. No longer an obscure teacher, he was elected to the Boston City Council in 1837;[24] three years later he was asked to compile an analysis of the vital statistics of Boston for the period of 1810 to 1841.

Published in 1841, Shattuck's study of vital statistics was a provocative demonstration of deteriorating health in Boston as reflected by mortality rates. Shat-

22. Lemuel Shattuck, *A History of the Town of Concord, Middlesex County, Massachusetts, from its Earliest Settlement to 1832; and of the Adjoining Towns of Bedford, Acton, Lincoln, and Carlisle: Containing Various Notices of County and State History Not Before Published* (Boston, 1835).
23. Shattuck and others. *Report of the Sanitary Commission*, pp. 124-125.
24. Shattuck served on the Boston City Council from 1837 to 1842, when he declined renomination. He was elected to the General Court in 1838 and 1849.

tuck pointed out that although longevity had greatly increased during an earlier period, the past twenty years had seen a reversal of the trend. He particularly emphasized the poor chances for life of children under five who accounted for just under 34 percent of all mortality in the second decade of the century, and over 43 percent of all deaths in the past ten years. Following guidelines established for similar studies in England, Shattuck showed that increased mortality in Boston was due to the proportional increase of "zymotic," or epidemic disease, as compared to sickness of "sporadic," or constitutional causes.[25]

Although he criticized the inadequacy of a nomenclature in which "a disease is often returned one year under a name differing from that of the same disease contained in the return of another year," he directed his main attention in this study to the apparent difference in morbidity and mortality rates from different localities. He ascribed this imbalance both to environmental changes which accompanied urbanization, and to changes in the style of life. "More luxury and effeminacy in both sexes prevail now than formerly," he noted with disapproval, "and this may have had some influence in producing constitutional disability, and the consequent feeble health of children. The nursing and feeding of children with improper food is another cause. The influence of bad air in confined, badly located, and filthy houses is another and perhaps the greatest."[26]

As time went on Shattuck continued to believe that disease was the inexorable penalty for deviation from moral behavior. Sickness and death could be repelled by adherence to a code available to men of all stations and mediated through Godliness and cleanliness. At the same time it was primarily the dangers released by a changing society which denied individuals the health they would have enjoyed living under simpler and more natural conditions.[27] In 1845, at the request of the Boston City Council, he compiled a city census. This project called

25. Lemuel Shattuck, "The Vital Statistics of Boston from 1810-1841," *American Journal of Medical Sciences*, n.s., 1:369-400 (April 1841). Republished in *Bills of Mortality 1810-1849, City of Boston* (Boston, 1893), p. xxiv. In this essay Shattuck simply groups diseases into these two major divisions, a procedure commonly accepted by the medical profession at the time. There was a third category of "accidental deaths." He complained that in both the United States and Great Britain physicians neglected to specify the exact causes of death, listing only "Rupture," "Infantile Disorder," etc. He included a tabulation of deaths from 1811-1839 in which he designated the proper category for each disease, pp. xxxviii-xli. Six years later, in 1847, Shattuck helped prepare a new nosology for the National Medical Convention, and at this date the similarity of divisions suggests that a common body of assumptions about the nature of disease continued to exist; see Appendix IV.

26. Shattuck, "Vital Statistics of Boston," pp. xxv, xxx.

27. Shattuck and others, *Report of the Sanitary Commission*, pp. 9-10, 277.

attention to a total population increase of 35 percent since 1840. Of particular interest was the fact that a third of Boston's 114,366 residents were foreign-born, or the children of foreign-born. "The influence of unacclimated foreign immigrants," he reminded the city fathers, "and the great number of families crowded into the houses in Broad Street, Ann Street, and other densely popula-ted parts of the city, render the air very impure, and expose the lives of infants, who are compelled to breathe it, to disease and death."[28]

Shattuck showed that the conditions under which the immigrants lived threat-ened the community at large. Even those persons who attempted to maintain clean and decent homes were foiled in their efforts to resist disease if the be-havior of others invited the visitation of epidemics; the need for a public au-thority to promote health was created by special causes springing, somewhat ambiguously, from the changed mode of life in the city. The report stressed, therefore, the obligation of municipal government to assume supervision over the necessities of life which in rural areas could properly be left to the individual. But private and corporate responsibility were so enmeshed in his report as to leave it unclear wherein ultimate authority resided.

It behooves the city authorities — it behooves every individual citizen, to seek out and remove every removeable cause of disease and death, in whatever sec-tion of the city, under whatever circumstances, and among whatever class of citizens, it may appear. An increase in the number and density of population in-creases the liability to disease. Greater caution should therefore be taken in the structure of our dwelling houses, our school houses and our work shops, to se-cure better ventilation, that we may better enjoy that indispensible element of life — *pure air*. More strict attention should be given to internal and external cleanliness. Pure water should be introduced into every dwelling house. All vegetable and other offal should be removed before it decays and poisons the atmosphere. Our excellent system of sewerage and drainage should be further extended. A more strict supervision should be exercised over cesspools, privies and all other noxious agencies to the public health. And especially should every individual take care of his own health, and strive, as far as possible, *to live with-out being sick.*[29]

Shattuck's report adopted a generally optimistic view, which coincided with the outlook of native Bostonians in the early 1840's. With time and proper in-

---

28. Lemuel Shattuck, *Report to the Committee of the City Council Appointed to Obtain the Census of Boston for the Year 1845, Embracing Collateral Facts and Statistical Researches Illustrating the History and Conditions of the Population, and their Means of Progress and Prosperity* (Boston, 1846), pp. 26, 37, 156.
29. *Ibid.*, pp. 176-177.

fluence, Shattuck believed the immigrants would accept the clearly superior standards and customs of native residents. "We may safely say that few cities of the same extent of territory can present stronger hopes for future progress," he wrote, acknowledging his position of responsibility. "In the benevolent operations of our citizens, the poor and unfortunate, the foreigner and the native, and even the criminal, are not neglected. Inducements are offered to the vicious to reform; and to the reformed to persevere in their course."[30] In 1845 Shattuck was certain that steps to counteract deteriorating trends could be successfully undertaken; it was a question of identifying the flaw and applying simple and logical corrective measures.

Much as Shattuck had written his daughter two years earlier to take upon herself a special role of personal responsibility, he stood apart from much contemporary reform which he considered unsound and visionary. While he greeted the establishment of the Department of Education as an important advance, he joined with other Whigs in public office to restrain the function of state and city government in the name of economy. At the same time that he recommended that pure water should be introduced into every dwelling, he argued against municipal control and expansion of the public water supply. He believed that the population of Boston would not continue to increase, and he feared that the assumption of municipal responsibility would lead to private negligence and political corruption.[31] Unlike other reformers of the antebellum period whose advocacy of good causes encompassed a wide scope of activities to regenerate American society, Shattuck continued to call attention to the practical and traditional nature of the measures he advocated. "These are not the speculations of a visionary theorist," he reminded his readers, "but the legitimate deductions from sober facts. We are not a theorist — an experimentalist. We have no sympathy with the opinions of some modern reformers, who seem to be governed

30. *Ibid.*, p. 179. Shattuck took pains in this report that his data on the Irish should not be misinterpreted. For example, see p. 155: "In speaking of this class separately, we do not wish to foster prejudice; their peculiar condition should rather excite our sympathy. They are the only persons, unfortunately, who can be selected as a class. They are mentioned separately only to show the influence of circumstances. It is presumed that other classes similarly situated would show the same results." For the ambivalent attitude of other native Bostonians toward foreign immigrants, see Handlin, *Boston's Immigrants*, esp. chaps. v and vii.

31. *Letter from Lemuel Shattuck, in Answer to Interrogatories of J. Preston, in Relation to the Introduction of Water into the City of Boston* (Boston, 1845); *How Shall we Vote on the Water Act?* (Boston, 1845), anonymous pamphlet acknowledged by Shattuck in *Memorials*. See also John B. Blake, "Lemuel Shattuck and the Boston Water Supply," *BHM*, 24:554-562 (Nov.-Dec. 1955).

by theories founded on uncertain and partial data, or vague conjecture. We are a statist — a dealer in facts. We wish to ascertain the laws of human life, developed by the natural constitution of our bodies, as they actually exist under the influences that surround them, and to learn how far they may be modified and improved. This can only be done by an accurate knowledge of the facts that are daily occurring among us."[32]

His interest in accumulating accurate data led him to call a small meeting in 1839, which led to the establishment of the American Statistical Association. As a leading member of this organization and its secretary, Shattuck was responsible for an extensive exchange of documents with like-minded individuals and organizations in this country and abroad. In particular, he corresponded with the Statistical Society of London and the office of the Registrar General of England, where civil registration had begun in 1837.[33] During the two years following its organization, the American Statistical Association, with Shattuck as its spokesman, added its influence to petitions of the Massachusetts Medical Society and the American Academy of Arts and Sciences in pressing the General Court to enact a more effective code for annual registration of births, marriages, and deaths. The memorialists proposed that town clerks be assigned the responsibility for collecting reports, which would be turned over to the Secretary of State to compile annually and to present to the legislature. It was agreed that such an accumulation of information would aid public health, morals, and the advancement of science and medicine by making available large numbers of observations on conditions that accompanied changes in health in different localities.[34] Shattuck's initial contribution to the Registration Act of 1842 was extended in the next seven years as inadequacies of data collection were corrected.

Registration returns at the outset were viewed primarily as aids in establishing settlement (residence) and matters of probate. Therefore, improvements were guided mostly by the influential legal profession.[35] Shattuck's concern for im-

32. Lemuel Shattuck, letter in *Fourth Annual Report to the Legislature Relating to the Registry and Returns of Births, Marriages and Deaths in Massachusetts, for the year ending April 30, 1845* [hereafter cited as *Registry Report*] (Boston, 1845), p. 99.

33. Shattuck Papers, MHS. Also John Koren, "The American Statistical Association 1839-1914" in John Koren, ed., *The History of Statistics: Their Development and Progress in Many Countries* (New York: Macmillan, 1918). The ASA was interested in all problems related to statistics. Each member was obliged to submit one paper annually to be read at the quarterly meetings. The first recorded paper was by Lemuel Shattuck on statistics of Saxony.

34. For the memorials of the AAAS and the MMS, see Appendix IV.

35. Robert Gutman, "Birth and Death Registration in Massachusetts: II, The Inaugura-

proving the accuracy and scope of registration was motivated by different concerns. He believed in a casual relation between moral and physical laws and that such laws could be understood through the accumulation of discrete data. As the leading statistician in the Commonwealth, he helped analyze the annual reports of 1843 and 1845 and submitted an extensive memorial on procedure to the General Court in 1848.[36] In his analysis Shattuck pointed out that Massachusetts was already collecting statistics describing pauperism, crime, insanity, agriculture, banks and insurance companies, as well as conducting scientific surveys on topography, geology, mineralogy, botany, ornithology, entomology, and icthyology. He noted that it was inconsistent "with the present state of enlightened public opinion" to fail to collect facts on the condition of human life as it was influenced "by seasons, locality, disease and other circumstances which may exist." Incomplete facts, he contended, made it impossible to ascertain what forces pressed most heavily upon the people.

Although Shattuck drew upon England's experience to establish census schedules and analytic procedure, he was apparently little influenced, at first, by English and continental findings which related disease specifically to poverty. Concentrating on the dangers inherent in urbanization, Shattuck showed a concern for the debilitation of American character and society as a whole, rather than focusing on the poor class. Instead, he voiced his fear that the old values had been lost and that "the universal thirst for wealth in America, the reckless speculations of some, the hap-hazard mode of living and the disregard to health of others, the luxury and extravagance of certain classes and other practices of modern society — tend to check the progress of the population, increase disease, and weaken the race."[37]

---

tion of a Modern System, 1800-1849," *MMFQ*, 36: 381 (Jan. 1958). This is the second in a series of three interesting articles on registration in Massachusetts from 1639 to 1869. See also John B. Blake, "The Early History of Vital Statistics in Massachusetts," *BHM*, 29:46-68 (Nov.-Dec. 1955).

36. Shattuck, letters in *Second Registry Report* (1843), pp. 61-73, and *Fourth Registry Report* (1845), pp. 67-106. Commenting on the *First Registry Report* (1843) the *Boston Medical and Surgical Journal*, 28:146 (March 22, 1843) suggested that Shattuck was the logical person for the Secretary of State to select to edit the reports. As an indication of the inadequacy of returns during the early years, Boston, with one-seventh of the state's population, failed to file from 1846 to 1848, but resumed in 1849. Twenty-eight towns did not file at all from 1846 to 1848, and thirty more did not file death records. This number was reduced to fourteen in 1849. See Gutman, cited above, and *Fifth* through *Eighth Registry Reports* (1846-1849). See also Shattuck, "Memorial for a Revision of the Laws in relation to the Registration of Births, Marriages and Deaths," *Documents of the Senate of the Commonwealth of Massachusetts during the Session of the General Court for 1848, No. 24* (Jan. 21, 1848).

37. Shattuck, letter in *Fourth Registry Report* (1845), p. 92.

When Shattuck was elected to the General Court for a second time in 1849, he became the leading spokesman for the view which linked the initial aims of registration to the conviction that the state must intervene to protect the health of the people. Supported by reports from England and France which associated better health with improved sanitary conditions, Shattuck began showing a more explicit interest in the possibility of action to prevent unnecessary disease and death.[38] As chairman of the legislative committee responsible for substantial improvements in the registration law, he described the effect of improved records on the extension of life. "Health is a possession capable of increase, or diminution, of growth or decay," he wrote. "It and even death itself, are, in some measure, within the control of men. The laws of nature, applicable to the life and health of man, are framed by a beneficial hand. When they are fully understood and obeyed, mankind will almost reach that degree of power which will enable them to say to disease and death, thus far shalt thou go, and no further, until 'a ripe old age.'"[39] With the widespread acceptance of registration procedures, Shattuck, along with representatives from the Massachusetts Medical Society and others in the American Statistical Association, turned his attention to improving the accuracy of information on the causes of death.

The American Statistical Association had only a handful of members, but largely through the initiative of Shattuck and Dr. Edward Jarvis, a physician and statistician from Dorchester, its library became a storehouse of information on disease and mortality rates.[40] At a meeting of the Association in 1848, it was

38. In 1849 Dr. John Snow of London published a pamphlet *On the Mode of Communication of Cholera*. In 1855 an elaboration of this original thesis was reprinted as *Snow on Cholera Being a Reprint of Two Papers by John Snow M.D. . . .* (New York: Commonwealth Fund, 1936). He stated that there was a specific contagious element in cholera found in the excreta of patients and spread through contaminated water supplies. Despite a general belief in England and the United States that cholera was spread as the result of improper sanitary facilities, Snow's thesis of specificity was not widely accepted until the epidemic of 1866; see Rosenberg, *Cholera*, p. 193, and Bernard Stern, *Society and Medical Progress* (Princeton, N.J.: Princeton University Press, 1941), p. 211.

39. "Report of the Joint Special Committee . . . to consider the expediency of modifying the laws relating to the registration of births, marriages and deaths," *Massachusetts House Documents 1849, No. 65* (March 3, 1849), pp. 8-9. Gutman, "Registration in Massachusetts, II," concludes that, with the revisions of 1849, Massachusetts procedures for recording vital statistics were comparable with the best European practice, a feat which had been accomplished within a seven year period.

40. Dr. Edward Jarvis (1830-1884) was a Dorchester physician and an authority in the fields of insanity and vital statistics. As the most consistently active member of the American Statistical Association, he served as its president from 1852 to 1882. See Edward Jarvis, MS "Autobiography" (1873), Houghton Library, Harvard University, pp. 238-239. For a more extended discussion of Jarvis' contribution to Massachusetts sanitary reform, see chap. ii.

agreed that Jarvis should petition the Massachusetts legislature for a sanitary survey of the state which could determine, through accurate observation, what the major diseases were and to what degree they were preventable.

The memorial emphasized that Massachusetts was becoming a manufacturing center, but that no one had examined the effect of new occupations upon the health of the population. "The cost in material goods and labor is carefully computed by both private and public interest," it stated. "But what is the cost in life and health, — what is the waste of human life and power, — caused by the different employments, has not yet been inquired into and ascertained." A sanitary survey would not necessarily lead to the imposition of new regulations, but rather through "negative principles of legislation" it would warn against unhealthful conditions and, where necessary, enforce existing laws. The memorial, although written by Jarvis, clearly bore the influence of Shattuck's earlier work by pointing out that the difference between the life expectancy of those in comfortable circumstances and the poor was growing wider. Jarvis reminded the legislature that the reputation Americans enjoyed for unusually good health was no longer supported by fact. A sanitary survey modeled on the English plan, he suggested, might lead to constructive competition between the nations for better health. The legislature, however, felt that such a survey was a departure from previously exercised authority and postponed further action until the following year.[41]

The Massachusetts Medical Society added its petition for a sanitary survey to that of the Statistical Association in the next legislative session. This action reflected not only local concern, but also the interest of the newly formed American Medical Association. Two years earlier when a meeting had been called in Philadelphia to organize the first national body of physicians, Shattuck was asked to serve as the only lay member of a committee on medical nomenclature. The report of this committee to the National Medical Convention in 1847 called for the adoption of the categories for disease assigned by William Farr, who since 1841 had compiled the annual statistical reports published by the Registrar General of England. Shattuck's earlier work on Boston had shown that the variety of names under which diseases were reported represented a substantial obstacle to the useful interpretation of statistical information on the causes of death. It is very likely that Shattuck was responsible for introducing Farr's nosology from the *Eighth Report of the Registrar General* (1846) to the Philadelphia

41. *Massachusetts House Documents 1845, No. 16* (Feb. 9, 1848), pp. 2-3, 8-11, 13, 18-19.

meeting. Shattuck had recently corresponded with Farr and received from him a copy of this new refinement of an earlier nomenclature. Farr's letter closed with encouraging words urging Shattuck to continue his able work on the health question. The Medical Convention asked all physicians to adopt these standard names for diseases and recommended public registration of disease and mortality as the first step in the prevention of unnecessary illness.[42]

At the first regular meeting of the American Medical Association, held in Baltimore in 1848, a Committee on Public Hygiene was appointed to report to the second convention on the sanitary condition of ten principal cities throughout the United States. The results of these investigations were publicized in May 1849, when the Association met in Boston and revealed a common body of information in this "unexplored region of medical inquiry." As had been suspected but never before established on a wide scale, mortality rates throughout the nation were higher in the cities than in the surrounding countryside. The committee concluded that "certain causes were invariably in operation . . . among these, deficient drainage, street cleaning, supply of water and ventilation; together with improperly constructed houses and the various nuisances incident to populous places."[43] On the whole, responsibility for the elevated disease and mortality rates which accompanied city life was placed on conditions that could be prevented.

A similar relationship between sanitation and health was posited by Dr. Josiah Curtis, who reported on the cities of Lowell and Boston at the same convention.[44] Although death rates in both cities were substantially higher than those

42. William Farr to Shattuck, Nov. 5, 1846, Shattuck Papers, MHS. *Proceedings of the National Medical Conventions* (Philadelphia, 1847): "Report of the Committee on the Organization of the National Medical Association," pp. 55-62; "Report of the Committee for the Registration . . . of Births, Marriages, and Deaths," pp. 125-131; "Report of the Committee to Prepare a Nomenclature of Diseases Adapted to the United States having Reference to a General Registration of Deaths," pp. 144-175. For selections from this report see Appendix IV. Included was a list of the causes of death used in official records compiled in Boston, Baltimore, Charleston, and New York City for the preceding twenty-five years. In addition to Shattuck, the committee included Dr. Edward Jarvis and three members from New York including Dr. John Griscom, author of an 1845 report on the sanitary condition of New York City.

43. *Transactions of the American Medical Association*, 2:431-432 (1849).

44. *Ibid.*, pp. 487-554. Other reports were from Portland, Maine; Concord, New Hampshire; New York City; Philadelphia; Baltimore; Charleston, South Carolina; New Orleans; and Louisville, Kentucky. Josiah Curtis (1816-1883), the Lowell physician who wrote this report, continued his interest in public health as he supervised the Massachusetts registration reports from 1849 to 1851, and again from 1857 to 1859. He visited Europe to study sanitary conditions abroad and later prepared a *Report of the Joint Special Committee on the Census of Boston, May, 1855* (Boston, 1856). In the early 1860's he was secretary to the Boston Sanitary Association (see chap. ii), and he also

for the rest of the state, Dr. Curtis discovered that the situation in Lowell was far worse than in Boston. The difference occurred because "zymotic" diseases, particularly dysentery and typhoid, were more prevalent in Lowell, and Curtis suggested further examination of the connection between the manufacturing occupations of Lowell residents and their susceptibility to this type of epidemic.[45]

Lowell was barely a quarter of a century old, but its rapid growth as a textile center had attracted a large and transient population, including many recent immigrants and a high proportion of women and younger men. Although Curtis believed that the character of work in the mills and the regularity of hours were conducive to good health, he found that many of the workers lived in crowded, filthy, poorly ventilated homes. The Middlesex District Medical Society had called the attention of the city government to these unfavorable conditions, but no remedial action had been taken.[46] Unfortunately, Curtis said, this matter had been dealt with too long by "politicians and partialists" who were more concerned with avoiding responsibility than with revealing the true state of affairs. On the other hand, he was encouraged to find that "the high-minded and humane gentlemen" who had charge of the manufacturing establishments were interested in discovering the cause of poor health among their employees.

In preparing his report, Curtis consulted a number of the most concerned local citizens, and he found at least one who disputed the position which ascribed responsibility for poor health and morals to the inherent character of the population. Reverend Wood, "minister at large" to Lowell, asked if it was "not true that many of these morbid appetites and unnatural desires that seek to assuage

---

assisted in the preparation of the 1860 federal census. During the Civil War he moved to Washington and later to Knoxville, Tennessee, where he remained and became chief officer of the Indian Service in 1873. Biographical material on Curtis is in part from *Cosmos Club Bulletin* (May 1964).

45. Although William W. Gerhard (1809-1872), a Philadelphia physician who had studied under P.C.A. Louis in Paris in 1831, differentiated typhoid from typhus fever in 1837 as a result of combining clinical observation with the study of pathological anatomy, Josiah Curtis and most American doctors continued to lump both diseases together through diagnosis based on symptomology. See Allen, "Etiological Theory Prior to the Civil War," p. 489, and Shyrock, *Development of Modern Medicine*, pp. 170–185.

46. *Transactions of the American Medical Association*, 2:519 (1849). The Massachusetts Medical Society began the reorganization of district medical societies in 1849, and there were sixteen organized districts by 1851. As a result, physicians outside of Boston not only had a greater voice in state affairs, but they were also able to make their views known on local issues; see Burrage, *Massachusetts Medical Society*, pp. 121-123. Concern over whether the factory system was inherently unhealthy was the subject of considerable debate. There was greater optimism during the relatively prosperous years of 1830-1837 than in the economically depressed years which followed; see George Rosen, "The Medical Aspects of the Controversy over Factory Conditions in New England 1840-1850," *BHM*, 15:483-497 (May 1944).

their longings by indulgence and excess, have their origin in the action of a distempered body upon the mind, rather than of the mind upon the body?"[47] Curtis apparently thought there was merit in this question and included Reverend Wood's entire letter in his report. Although he believed, with his fellow physicians, that disease and death were surely the outcome when physical laws were violated, Curtis noted that the "diseases which are most fatal among us, are those that are most easily prevented by hygienic prophylaxis." Curtis closed his report by stating unequivocally that responsibility for public health rested first with the medical profession. He believed that ignorant individuals, burdened by living conditions beyond their means to correct, should be able to look to physicians for help before they suffered from disease. Wise governments also should heed the advice of physicians whose skill and knowledge were available to prevent disease as well as treat it. By 1849, therefore, the American Medical Association had gone on record in affirming its responsibility to serve as the guardian of public health.[48]

When the Massachusetts Medical Society memorialized the legislature on the need for a sanitary survey in 1849, it anticipated sentiments expressed later at the meeting of the American Medical Association.[49] The movement to standardize medical names for diseases lent further impetus to the growing authority of the physician since his skill was needed to perfect the uniformity of diagnosis. In Massachusetts the Secretary of State had recognized the special interest of the medical profession and in this same year appointed a member of the Medical Society to interpret the annual registration reports. Dr. Curtis, who first held this post, and Dr. Nathaniel B. Shurtleff, who followed him, worked to have the Farr nomenclature adopted for both local and state reports.[50] Many physicians and laymen expected that this procedure would lead to better records, which, in turn, would allow delineation of the laws of illness by a kind of medical calculus. Sanitary regulations would thus be derived from factual data and quite reasonably disseminated through education.

Further extension of these assumptions to include an active concept of prevention was stimulated in Massachusetts by improved registration returns per-

47. *Transations of the American Medical Association*, 2:521-524 (1849).

48. *Ibid.*, pp. 441-442, 515-516, 530-534.

49. The AMA congratulated Massachusetts for being the first state to undertake a sanitary survey. "Report of the Joint Special Committee . . . for a Sanitary Survey of the State," *Massachusetts House Documents, No. 66* (March 3, 1849), pp. 4-19. The earlier memorial of the American Statistical Association was included in this report, pp. 20-39.

50. The Farr nosology was finally used in the *Fourteenth Registry Report* (1855), pp. ix, 259-265.

mitting statistical comparison of urban and rural health. The registration report for 1849 showed that if Boston mortality rates had been as low as the average for the state in the twenty months preceding December 31, ten lives a day might have been saved. Curtis, who edited this report in the same year as he presented his report on Lowell and Boston to the American Medical Association, again identified overcrowding and the accompanying poor sanitary conditions as the major factors predisposing the individual to disease and premature death. Contamination of water supplies, failure to remove refuse, and improper ventilation in factories and homes characterized those communities in which mortality rates had soared. As attention focused on the deteriorating physical environment, the concept of "preventable disease" took on a new dimension.[51]

Widespread interest in registration was the inspiration for a state sanitary survey. By the late 1840's pressure for a broad study of state sanitation in Massachusetts was mounting rapidly. Shattuck introduced the Medical Society and Statistical Association memorials for a sanitary survey with the statement that "many of the facts and arguments . . . in favor of registration may be considered as applicable to a sanitary survey."[52] Further prodded by public concern over the threat of an impending cholera epidemic, the legislature directed, on May 2 that local boards of health be established in towns where they had not previously existed. This extension of the 1797 Board of Health Act specified a general procedure for the identification of sanitary hazards by either individual citizens, local health officers, or boards of health, and provided a legal apparatus to permit the cities and towns to remove "any nuisance, source of filth, or cause of sickness" on private property.[53]

On the same day, while the American Medical Association was meeting in Boston, a joint resolution from both houses of the legislature authorized the appointment of a commission to make a state sanitary survey. In July Governor Briggs appointed three members to serve on it: Jehiel Abbott, a Democrat from Westfield; Nathaniel P. Banks, a Free-Soil member from Waltham; and as chairman, Shattuck, a Whig from Boston.[54] Since neither Abbott nor Banks had any spe-

51. *Eighth Registry Report . . . for the Period August 31, 1847 to December 31, 1849* (1850), p. 120. It should be noted that Curtis emphasized environmental hazards, while Shattuck and Jarvis continued to stress the failure of individuals to observe the laws of health.

52. *Massachusetts House Documents, No. 66*, p. 1.

53. "An Act in Relation to Public Health," *Acts and Resolves of the Commonwealth of Massachusetts for the Year 1849* [hereafter cited as *Acts and Resolves*] (May 2, 1849), pp. 150-152.

54. *Acts and Resolves 1849, Chapter 110* (May 2, 1849), p. 232. Abbott was a physician, although apparently not a member of the Massachusetts Medical Society. Banks, a

cial qualifications for the job, they were glad to leave the responsibility to Shattuck, who conducted the investigation and wrote the lengthy report which he presented to the legislature on April 25, 1850.

Shattuck's new study of sanitary conditions throughout the state supported three assumptions that had gained popularity through registration reports: first, that deteriorating health had been accompanied by changes in the environment; second, that social factors had led to these changes; and third, that responsibility for identifying and abating the effects of dangerous surroundings upon the populace rested primarily with the public authority.[55] The extent of Shattuck's statistical sophistication prompted him to show the limitation of comparative mortality figures which ignored the age distribution of the total population. Guided by his belief in the lawfulness of nature, he accepted as a settled principle that "a uniform law of mortality exists, which destroys more persons at one age than at another, in all other circumstances exactly similar; and that this law is modified in its operation in a healthy or in an unhealthy locality, only by its being less stringently regulated in the one than in the other." Far more subtle in his analysis of data than he had been five years earlier, he also showed that "the average age at death, as well as the aggregate number of a population out of the whole of which one dies annually, though interesting as a characteristic of the population, is a fallacious test of its sanitary condition; and cannot be employed alone, for that purpose, without leading to serious errors."[56]

Shattuck had a grasp of his material which a mere accumulation of vital statistics would fail to impart. His analysis of the relation between births and deaths indicated that, contrary to popular belief, an increased birth rate was a cause rather than a consequence of high mortality. In an effort to take stock,

---

lawyer and a politician who later served as governor, was connected with the Boston Customs House. He was serving his first term in the legislature. The three commissioners were to be paid at the same rate as legislators, with additional compensation for travel. There was also an allowance for postage and other supplies, and a special allotment of not more than fifty dollars for books. For Shattuck's appointment, see Governor Briggs to Shattuck, July 4, 1849, and Jehiel Abbott to Shattuck, July 7, 1849, in which Abbott states that he does not expect to be of much help on the commission, Shattuck Papers, MHS.

55. Shattuck and others, *Report of the Sanitary Commission*, pp. 10-11.

56. *Ibid.*, pp. 141-142. It is interest that recent population studies suggest that the rise in birth rates rather than the fall in death rates was responsible for the population increase in England during the late eighteenth and early nineteenth centuries. Also, of the three factors assigned responsibility for decline in mortality, i.e., medical therapy, changes in the relation between the infectious organism and the host, and the general improvement in standard of living, the last is considered the most significant; see Thomas McKeown and R. G. Brown, "Medical Evidence Related to Population Changes in the Eighteenth Century," *Population Studies* (London), 9:119-141 (1955-1956).

he appraised the great accumulation of two centuries of legislation related to health and concluded that it was either obsolete or redundant and should be repealed. Shattuck recommended the establishment of a general board of health which could maintain the constant vigilance necessary in changing times.

A major factor confounding the enforcement of health regulations was the large influx of immigrants. Even as late as 1845 the assimilation of the foreign-born to the dominant culture had seemed only a matter of time and goodwill. Changes wrought by the influx of an additional 125,000 newcomers to the state in the next four years, however, shattered that expectation for Shattuck. He showed that the death rate in Boston in those years had risen sharply at the same time that the total population was increased by 23,000. The foreign-born and their children accounted for most of the increase. Of 5,031 children born in Boston during 1849, 62 percent were first-generation Americans. "Appalled and astounded" at the consequences this had already produced, Shattuck concluded that it was the immigrants — the poor and unwanted from England and Ireland — who were primarily responsible for bringing disease and impoverishment to an otherwise predominantly healthy and productive native stock: "Our own native inhabitants, who mingle with these recipients of their bounty, often themselves become contaminated with diseases, and sicken and die; and the physical and moral power of living is depreciated, and the healthy, social and moral character we once enjoyed is liable to be forever lost. Pauperism, crime, disease and death, stare us in the face." Sanitary reform, of course, was not the only corrective. In the city of Boston in 1845 approximately eleven persons lived in a single dwelling; by 1850 there were sections in which the number had risen to thirty-seven. There was no possibility of alleviating with alms and education conditions inherently disease producing.[57]

Unlike English sanitary reformers, very few Americans at this time suggested that poverty might be the cause of increased morbidity and mortality rates. Dr. Josiah Curtis and Dr. John H. Griscom of New York City were among the exceptions; Shattuck made only passing reference to the possibility that poverty itself might be preventable. In 1850 Shattuck shared with most Americans a

57. Shattuck's figure of 125,000 arrivals by sea was broken down to show:

1846	15,504
1847	24,245
1848	25,042
1849	34,873

This makes a total of 99,658, to which he added an estimated 25,342 arrivals from other states or Canada by land. He does not account for those who left Massachusetts for other areas. Shattuck and others, *Report of the Sanitary Commission*, pp. 201-206, 280-282.

lack of compassion for the conditions which poverty engendered and tended to assume that being poor was no excuse for neglect of cleanliness of person or surroundings.[58] Shattuck believed that what he saw as the complacent attitude of the poor indicated a lack of moral fiber; he failed to recognize that impoverishment of the new immigrant was more profound and permanent than it had been twenty years earlier. His first fear was the effect this degrading atmosphere might have on the health and virtue of Americans. He found that his countrymen tended to ignore endemic diseases which, a decade before, would have caused community alarm and received concerted attention.[59]

Contemporary medical theory likewise supported the belief that increased morbidity in urban slums was the result of the abnormal character of city life. As the new critical spirit of medical investigation moved toward the concept of specificity in disease, it continued to identify a broad range of personal and environmental causes as predisposing factors responsible for the susceptibility of particular victims.[60] In 1850, when Shattuck charged the government with responsibility to provide pure water and to take on authority which five years earlier he had urged be left to individual initiative, it was not the result of any changed concept of the etiology of disease; rather, it was because he faced the hard fact that the character of the population had changed. An accumulation of statistical information reinforced the assumption that disease was most likely to affect those who, through poverty, ignorance, or lack of concern, failed to heed the accepted warnings. With a large proportion of the population unable or unwilling to take on personal responsibility to conduct their lives in accord with recommended sanitary principles, the state could properly play the role of guardian to society and policeman to the uninitiated.

The statistics spoke for themselves. In the 1849 cholera epidemic 81 percent of the more than 700 deaths in the metropolitan area were among the foreign

58. For a study of public health reformers with a different background, see Charles E. and Carroll S. Rosenberg, "Pietism and the Origins of the American Public Health Movement: A Note on John H. Griscom and Robert H. Hartley," *JHMAS*, 23:16-35 (Jan. 1968). It is interesting that Shattuck fails to include Griscom's pioneering *Sanitary Condition of the Laboring Population of New York* . . . (New York, 1845) in his appendix to the *Report of the Sanitary Commission*, when he lists suggestions to local boards for a sanitary library. For general reaction to poverty and disease, see Rosenberg, *Cholera Years*, pp. 135, 150. See also a letter from Shattuck to his brother, May 8, 1849, following a visit to New Ipswich, in which he found conditions in the country had also deteriorated: "The fact is that the race of men who formerly lived here were *strong men*, the present are not so" (Shattuck Papers, MHS). For Shattuck's reaction to English thought, see *Report of the Sanitary Commission*, p. 30.

59. Shattuck and others, *Report of the Sanitary Commission*, p. 81.

60. Rosenberg, *Cholera Years*, pp. 159-160.

population. In the thirty years prior to 1837, smallpox claimed the lives of 37 persons in Boston; in the first six months of 1850, with vaccination not compulsory since 1836, the death toll reached 146. Consumption, the greatest destroyer of life and health throughout the Commonwealth, took 7 lives each day. Figures showed a progressive decline of deaths from "phthisis" in Boston from 1810 to 1840, but between 1840 and 1849 there was a reversal toward higher mortality rates. Although the private individual had the primary responsibility to see that he was properly protected — particularly in regard to vaccination — Shattuck believed that the city or the state had to assume responsibility if the person failed to do so.[61] Upright citizens could no longer assume that mere exposure to the opportunity for a wholesome and healthy life was sufficient incentive to change the damaging habits which the foreign immigrant brought with him, thereby endangering the moral and physical integrity of the native community.

Shattuck's recommendations were detailed. They included the design of new census schedules and a decennial state census to ascertain the changing character of populations. A general board of health was prescribed to recommend legislation for the prevention of disease and the promotion of health, to advise the state as to sanitary arrangements for public buildings and installations, and to make a cumulative annual report to the legislature. Regular surveys of local health conditions to identify public nuisances were advised, along with the supervision of water supplies and waste disposal. Shattuck urged the organization of "libraries of health," the training of nurses to care for the sick, and the establishment of voluntary health agencies to aid local and state boards.

The major threat to health came from the increased density of population. Shattuck's observation that cities were not necessarily unhealthy but that conditions were permitted to exist which made them so represented a major adjustment. Five years earlier, Shattuck had not expected Boston to grow any larger. City life was at best a temporary evil, fraught with dangers to be constantly resisted at every turn. By 1850 Shattuck acknowledged that the population of Boston had both grown and changed its character. He proposed a program of sanitary control based on a foundation of municipal and state rather than individual responsibility. The plan was practical and provident, and he repeatedly emphasized that this was "no transcendentalism, or other ism or ology."[62]

Many of the specific proposals suggested by Shattuck became standard public health practice during the next century under vastly different conditions. In

61. Shattuck and others, *Report of the Sanitary Commission*, pp. 204, 180-181, 90-99.
62. *Ibid.*, pp. 108-112, 151, 154, 301-302.

1850, however, they were a triumph of innovation in response to the futility of lesser measures. Shattuck had demonstrated how disaster took place; now he directed attention to the possibility of avoiding it.

This was a new age in which the laws of nature and science were to be revealed. The critical question was how should new laws be ascertained? Shattuck's answer was in tune with the perfectionist mood of antebellum reform; the rules of sanitary hygiene could be readily extrapolated from the moral and orderly laws of nature. Disease was preventable: "Pain, suffering, and the various physical evils to which we are exposed," wrote Shattuck, "may not seem to be a necessary part of the scheme of nature, but only as incidental to it . . . It is easy to perceive that the sources of many, even a vast majority of these evils, may be removed by those who suffer from them; and that they do not lie so deep that human agency cannot discover and destroy them. Man has power to wield over and destroy disease."[63]

The report combined dire warnings of imminent danger with reassurance of the simplicity with which apparent disorder could be reassembled into a rational plan. For twenty years Shattuck had proposed that complete records would reveal the inherent order of human life. He was widely known already as the author of *A Complete System of Family Registration* (1841), *The Domestic Bookkeeper and Practical Economist* (1843), and *The Scholar's Daily Journal* (1843), in addition to his work on the registration of vital statistics. His plan for the promotion of public and personal health was still another blank book to be filled in by the proper agency — the state.[64]

The *Report of the Sanitary Commission* was accepted by the legislature in April 1850, and two thousand copies were ready for distribution by January 1851.[65] He saw to it that the document was circulated widely, both in this country and in Europe, among physicians and public officials concerned with

---

63. *Ibid.*, pp. 272, 292-293.

64. I have interpreted Shattuck's position in relation to other *social reformist* thought of the period. It is certainly possible to see an analogous outlook in some contemporary *medical* thought, particularly as expressed by Dr. Elisha Bartlett (1804-1855), *An Essay on the Philosophy of Medical Science* (Philadelphia, 1844). However, I found no evidence that Shattuck was acquainted with Bartlett's work or interested in theoretical medical-scientific debate.

65. Boston *Daily Advertiser*, Jan. 25, 1850, noted that the *Report of the Sanitary Commission* had been sent to the clerk of every Massachusetts city and town, boards of health throughout the United States, various federal agencies, and the editors of one hundred newspapers. See also Edward Jarvis, "Review of the Report of the Sanitary Commission of Massachusetts made by the Legislature in 1850," *American Journal of the Medical Sciences*, n.s., 21:391-409 (April 1851).

vital statistics and sanitation. Within the United States the *Report* was received favorably in medical journals and among those who traditionally shouldered responsibility to enlighten and aid the less fortunate. The reviewer in the long-established *North American Review* wrote that the "sanitary movement does not merely relate to the lives and health of the community; it is also a means of moral reform . . . The ultimate connection between filth and vice has been noted by all writers upon this subject. Outward impurity goes hand in hand with inward pollution, and the removal of one leads to the extirpation of the other. Cleansing the body is not more a symbol, than it is a means and condition of inward purity."[66] For those who accepted the identification of cleanliness with virtue, Shattuck's *Report* was the confirmation of old wisdom.

While Shattuck was moving from obscurity to recognition, developments in political and social affairs were destined to undermine the reforms he was advocating. The influx of immigrants had been accompanied by a substantial growth in political power for various dissident groups, and the two old parties of Whigs and Democrats, already divided by local internal struggles, were further fragmented by the slavery issue, especially after 1848. The emergence of the Free-Soil party and other political movements dedicated to specific local issues, such as greater legislative representation for the less populous towns, reform of the judiciary, and more stringent liquor laws, challenged Whig domination of Massachusetts politics. The 1850's were turbulent years in Massachusetts, marked by the growth of a vocal nativist movement, demands for a new state constitution, and the successful, though uneasy, alliance of antislavery, anti-immigrant, and agrarian sentiment. The coalition of Locofoco Democrats and Free-Soil and Know-Nothing elements was able to control the state political machinery from 1854 to 1856, and it remained a vigorous force for another two years. The Whigs, who had traditionally represented the established interests of the commercial and manufacturing classes and important elements from Boston's oldest families, were forced into an "unnatural" alliance with the city Irish. This temporary alliance successfully defeated radical reforms only to founder with the emergence of a national Republican party at the end of the decade. This was a decade of sharpened antipathies; urban-rural, nativist-immigrant, and conservative-reform differences were all finally overwhelmed by the slavery issue which eventually reassembled all previous political alignments.[67]

66. Attributed to E. H. Clarke, *North American Review,* 73:117-135 (July 1851).
67. Handlin, *Boston's Immigrants*, pp. 190-212; Handlin and Handlin, *Commonwealth*, pp. 214-217; George H. Haynes, "The Cause of Know-Nothing Success in Massachusetts," *American Historical Review*, 3:67-82 (Oct. 1897); William G. Bean, "Party Transformation

Before the outbreak of the Civil War in 1861, therefore, the reform movement in Massachusetts had changed its character. Reform became largely the object of political argument rather than the ideal of an ethical social movement. With this shift in orientation, Shattuck's proposals for sanitary reform suffered the same fate as other crusades fundamentally directed toward transforming society by redeeming individual morality.[68]

The religio-moral implications of the Shattuck *Report* were lost on Massachusetts politicians more concerned with the voting behavior of the immigrant and the urban poor than with their hygienic habits. The *Report* drew its strength from old assumptions about the relation between filth and sickness and defined health as the perfect balance of physical functions achieved by adherence to old-time virtues of cleanliness and morality. In the 1850's, however, the institutional forms which could give authority to this view were more contested than relied upon. Along with the increasing secularization of daily life, a large section of the population fell outside traditional Protestant influence within the state because so many immigrants were Catholic. The Roman Catholic Church tended to be more accepting of man's frailty; while by no means condoning those conditions which led to the weakening of man's spirit and body, the Church was less likely to seek salvation in improvement of the earthly environment.[69]

There was no recognized cohesive group to lead the mission for sanitary reform. Although individual physicians continued to point to the connection between urban living conditions and excessively high mortality rates, the prestige of the medical profession remained rather low in the decade preceding the Civil War. Registration practices were improved to conform with standards assigned by medical science, but there was no well-publicized attempt to introduce legislation for general sanitary reform until 1861.[70] In these politically tempestuous

in Massachusetts with Special Reference to the Antecedents of Republicanism, 1848-1860," unpub. diss., Harvard University (1922), and "Puritan versus Celt, 1850-1860," *New England Quarterly*, 7:70-89 (March 1934); Martin B. Duberman, "Friends Divided: Debate on the Massachusetts Constitutional Convention of 1853," *Mid-America*, 45:50-55 (Jan. 1963); Samuel Shapiro, "The Conservative Dilemma: The Massachusetts Constitutional Convention of 1853," *New England Quarterly*, 33:207-224 (June 1960).

68. Thomas, "Romantic Reform," p. 679.

69. Robert H. Bremner, *From the Depths, The Discovery of Poverty in the United States* (New York: New York University Press, 1956), p. 28. For a further discussion of social controls see Thernstrom, *Poverty and Progress*, pp. 49-56.

70. Richard H. Shryock, "The Origins and Significance of the Public Health Movement in the United States," *Annals of Medical History*, n.s., 1:644-665 (Nov. 1929), see esp. pp. 650-651 and 658-659, n. 25, in which Shryock suggests that Shattuck's influence has been exaggerated; Shryock, "Public Relations of the Medical Profession in Great Britain and the United States, 1600-1870," *Annals of Medical History*, n.s., 2:308-339, esp. pp. 319, 324, 329. Attention to public health continued to revolve around improvements in

years, moreover, no major epidemic of disease threatened Massachusetts, a situation that doubtless contributed to the feeling that public health measures were not particularly urgent.

Although Shattuck continued to live in Boston until his death in 1859, there is no record that he pressed for legislation directly connected with public hygiene. He continued to pursue his twin interests in statistics and genealogy: in 1850 he was called to Washington to aid in the analysis of census returns, and, by 1855, he was able to publish his *Memorials of the Descendants of William Shattuck*. There is no indication that he participated in the political struggles which surrounded him, for he never again held elected office. Apparently Shattuck remained aloof from the controversies that culminated in the Civil War and was unmoved by the issues that would divide and reshape American life.

Ironically, Shattuck's *Report* was laid aside, not because it was visionary, which he had feared, but because it was irrelevant. The seed of Shattuck's plan was the pietistic tradition which identified health with cleanliness and virtue. His investigations eventually led him to acknowledge the corrupting influence of the social and physical environment, but his proposals, while practical, were not compelling in a period when disease and poverty were looked upon, even by him, as retribution for sin.

---

registration. On rare occasions legislative inquiries were made on the expediency of organizing a general board of health, with negative results; see, for example, Boston *Semi-Weekly Advertiser*, Feb. 5, 1853.

2 The State Board of Health Becomes a Reality, 1861–1879

Twentieth-century American historians have seen the Civil War as the critical turning point in the social and economic development of the United States. The war not only tested the material resources of the nation; it also revealed the aspirations and ideological conflicts of a changing culture. Although historians have agreed that the war profoundly altered contemporary attitudes toward reform, they have differed in their assessment of the relative importance of antebellum concern with individual immorality and fear of social change as a means by which institutions could control undesirable conduct. Similarly, the humanitarian impulse which aroused sympathy with the slave, with the wounded soldier, and with the destitute at home, was exemplified by individual and organized response which has been variously interpreted.

Efforts to relieve suffering during the war and to rededicate the nation to humane and moral behavior reflected both despair over materialist values which seemed to have warped the fiber of personal virtue and hope that the bloody struggle would inspire a new social morality. There was little disagreement among contemporary reformers that the war was the crucible in which the viability of all progress would be tested. On the one hand, disobedience to man's and God's law was seen as the sign of personal depravity, to be countered by philanthropy, education, and persuasion; on the other hand, the sourse of disobedience was found in the corrupting influence of society, to be remedied by discipline exercised by the knowledgeable through social institutions. Conflicting assumptions not only guided the hands of the participants; they have also tempered the historian's account. The outpouring of money and volunteers to aid the sick and wounded and even the formation of the much-troubled United States Sanitary Commission were both expressions of humanitarian benevolence and the first successful applications of scientific principles to social problems.[1]

The generation of sanitary reformers who came of age in Massachusetts during the decades preceding the Civil War saw the battle against slavery as intimately connected with issues of personal and public health. However, this commitment did not necessarily involve a departure from earlier beliefs as to the cause and nature of personal and social ills. Immorality, intemperance, poverty, and disease, had all been seen as evidence of individual weakness, and slavery was the most blatant example of an evil which poisoned all society. In the three decades before the war, efforts to restrict the spread of disease and poverty rested largely on the assumption that these misfortunes were caused by the failure of individuals to follow the essentially moral laws of nature.[2] Even though Shattuck and other concerned citizens pointed to the perverting influence of both affluence and poverty, the onus of resistance to corruption lay with the afflicted. Prevention of disease depended on determining the effect of different conditions upon the laws of nature, and interception was largely limited to making the proper information available.

The experience of war added a new element to the methods and goals of reform endeavor. A continued increase in the number of dependent poor despite wartime prosperity, the high toll of sickness and death among the troops, the deprivations suffered by their families — all evoked an unprecedented response. In the course of the attempt to meet these emergencies, the layman and the professional alike became aware of the nonpersonal factors involved in poverty and disease. Skills which had helped to alleviate war-borne misery and illness became part of the syllabus of prevention, and there was new hope of actively combating social ills through curbing destructive influences. The belief that health and well-being depended on individual integrity did not disappear entirely. But, along with an increasing awareness that the individual was often the victim of social circumstances, there was also a growing confidence that these circumstances could be manipulated. In Massachusetts, even as a functioning State Board of Health elaborated the scope and objectives of sanitary reform, men of the same generation voiced profound differences in their social and po-

1. George M. Fredrickson, *The Inner Civil War: Northern Intellectuals and the Crisis of the Union* (New York: Harper and Row, 1956), pp. 79-112; Robert H. Bremner, "The Impact of the Civil War on Philanthropy and Social Welfare," *Civil War History*, 12:293-303 (Dec. 1966).

2. For a discussion of American attitudes toward poverty in the first half of the nineteenth century, see Samuel Mencher, *Poor Law to Poverty Program: Economic Security Policy in Britain and the United States* (Pittsburgh, Pa.: University of Pittsburgh Press, 1967), pp. 144-153, 243-244; Robert Bremner, *From the Depths: The Discovery of Poverty in the United States* (New York: New York University Press, 1956).

litical ideologies. Restraint remained the watchword of prevention, but what was to be restrained, how the restraint was exercised, and to what end restraint was to be imposed shifted perceptibly between 1861 and 1876. The change was exemplified by the difference between Edward Jarvis' memorial in 1861 for a state board of health and vital statistics and Henry Bowditch's speech fifteen years later predicting the advent of state preventive medicine.

In the years immediately preceding the Civil War, citizens of Massachusetts had some reason to believe that their state had made commendable progress in sanitary affairs. Although urban mortality rates continued to be a cause for concern, there had been no major incidence of epidemic disease since 1849. Certainly there was need for continued vigilance since the rapid and unregulated growth of cities had led to overcrowded tenements, and the conditions which characterized the dwellings of the less fortunate were generally conceded to be conducive to illness. The intemperate and unwholesome life which this situation encouraged made the poor particularly susceptible to disease, as well as subjecting the surrounding neighborhoods to risks from impure air and disease-carrying "effluvia." However, Massachusetts, and the city of Boston, had a reputation for generally good health, and a New York medical journal praised the Commonwealth for its attention to the special problems of urban sanitation.[3] When the National Quarantine and Sanitary Convention held its fourth annual meeting in Boston early in June of 1860, representatives from city and state governments and members of the medical profession were congratulated upon the character of public institutions in Massachusetts and told of the prospect for further advances in the application of "sanitary science" to the health of the population.[4]

The convention met in an optimistic mood. The first meeting of this group had been called in 1857 to reform and standardize quarantine regulations. The meeting that convened in 1860, on the other hand, singled out "internal hygiene" as its central concern. The cities sending representatives to the convention were all busy, commercial centers whose further growth and prosperity were dependent on assuring the health and activity of a large and heterogeneous population.

3. For instance, the *BMSJ*, 60:504-505 (July 21, 1859) questioned whether even smallpox could be effectively controlled while unvaccinated immigrants continued to arrive in Boston, while encouragement was given by the *American Medical Times*, 1:46-47 (July 21, 1860).

4. *Fourth National Quarantine and Sanitary Convention* (Boston, 1860), pp. 105-118, speeches delivered when the convention visited Deer Island, the site of the House of Industry, the House of Reformation, and the Quarantine Station.

Speakers cited the crowded and filthy tenements which disgraced all urban areas as the major source of disease. Although there was no resolution specifically dealing with housing, city governments were urged to take on full responsibility for sewerage and public water. There were 109 delegates from Massachusetts, largely from the greater Boston area, attending the convention. Many of the 65 local physicians represented medical organizations, and they spoke about the contributions that scientific medicine was prepared to make toward the prevention of disease.[5]

The importance of sanitary regulation for urban health had received public recognition. Dr. Jacob Bigelow, consulting physician for the city of Boston, enthusiastically suggested that "we are still standing in the vestibule of reform, — one of the greatest reforms that this country has ever entered upon, the great reform of the age . . . The day is rapidly approaching," he said, "when clinical doctors will scarcely be needed, and when sanitarians will take their places, and when we shall not so much attend to the health of the human body as to the condition of the body politic."[6] The Sanitary Convention made only passing reference to the sharp political and social antagonisms which divided the country. It looked forward instead to a period of agreement and progress, particularly in the areas of quarantine regulation, registration of vital statistics, and civic cleanliness.

Although the great national issue of slavery increasingly absorbed the attention of individuals committed to various special appeals for the moral and material regeneration of society, the central arguments for sanitary reform remained within the framework defined by the earlier registration movement. In Massachusetts, Dr. Edward Jarvis, the best-known proponent of improved registration and sanitary measures, steadfastly held to the collection of vital statistics as the critical determinant of harmonious social order. Jarvis, echoing the words that Shattuck had written a decade before, emphasized that social reform was dependent on individual acquiescence to the properly established laws of life. As the Civil War took on the character of a great moral crusade through

5. *Ibid.*, pp. 54-64, 241-267, 277-279. See also, E. B. Elliot, *Instructions Concerning the Registration of Births, Deaths and Marriages in Massachusetts* (Boston, 1860), p. 231: "The character of the members of the Medical Profession, and the interest which they are led by their present pursuits to take in information of this nature, authorizes the confident belief that they will afford ready and important cooperation in rendering the registration of deaths as complete as possible."

6. *Fourth Sanitary Convention*, pp. 123, 126. Jacob Bigelow (1786-1879), a botanist and physician of distinction, had been a member of the committee credited with protecting Boston from a major cholera epidemic in 1832, see Walter L. Burrage, *A Brief History of the Massachusetts Medical Society, 1791-1922* (Norwood, Mass.: privately published, Plimpton Press, 1923), pp. 116-117.

which many saw the opportunity to transform all corrupt aspects of behavior, Jarvis continued to argue for the more traditional road to reform. While most of his fellow physicians left Boston to care for the sick and wounded either through the army or the civilian-based Sanitary Commission, Jarvis remained in Massachusetts and became the recognized spokesman for medical and lay organizations devoted to sanitary reform.[7]

Jarvis addressed a public meeting of the Boston Sanitary Association early in 1861 and called attention to the economic and social inequities which made the poor victims of disease while the rich escaped "by virtue of cleanliness, exercise, wholesome food, and other advantages derived from their position." A few months later, he joined with Dr. Josiah Curtis and former mayor Josiah Quincy to present a memorial to the legislature from the Sanitary Association, urging the establishment of a state board of health and vital statistics. The reasoning of these men rested on the simple, philosophical premise that the vital force of life was determined by a universal law which varied as the external circumstances were favorable or detrimental. The memorial proposed no extensive program of sanitary reform; nor did it call upon the medical profession to aid in the identification and prevention of disease. Instead, it again asked the legislature to influence those "tendencies among the people, the motive of which is gain or position," which cause them to crowd together in cities.[8] In 1861 Jarvis was still looking for the means of returning civilization to the better ways of the past. Although he spoke in general about correcting the external circumstances which deprived the poor of their opportunity for health, his underlying objective was to restore a normalcy best described by the quality of life he had known as he grew up in the town of Concord, a few miles west of Boston.

When Edward Jarvis was born in 1803, Concord was a small, reasonably prosperous farming town of 1,500. Its essentially homogeneous population was

7. The war was also believed to advance the principles of hygiene; see *American Medical Times*, 3:89-90 (Aug. 22, 1863). The Massachusetts Medical Society almost ceased to function during the war, see Burrage, *Massachusetts Medical Society*, p. 134. On Jarvis' role see Josiah Curtis to Jarvis, March 8, 1855; March 21, 1855; March 8, 1861; Sept. 22, 1865, Jarvis Letters, Holmes Hall, Countway Library, Harvard Medical School, Boston, Mass.

8. *BMSJ*, 63:525-526 (Jan. 24, 1861); "Memorial of the Boston Sanitary Association," *Massachusetts House Documents 1861, No. 112* (Feb. 15, 1861). p. 26. The Boston Sanitary Association was formed in April 1861 to improve the sanitary condition of the people "By promoting the investigation of facts and principles relating to personal, domestic and public Hygiene . . . by diffusing information on the laws of health and life, and the best means for their practical application." John Ware, former president of the Massachusetts Medical Society, was the president. A call for members was included with the above information in a pamphlet publicizing the legislative memorial.

growing more slowly than the relatively high ratio of births to deaths would indicate, and although opportunities for economic success were limited, there was ample reason for pride in the practical accomplishments of the community. A vigorous local government with a notable historic tradition was guided by an unusually active group of educated men who joined together in the "Social Circle." This esteemed society of twenty-five devoted itself to improving the political and cultural life of all the town's citizens. The success of these efforts was reflected in a fine local school system, the town library, and numerous public lectures which supplemented weekly sermons delivered by the Reverend Ezra Ripley in the single church which all attended.[9]

Edward Jarvis was the fourth of seven children born to Francis and Melicent Jarvis. His father was a baker and storekeeper whose interest in books and learning belied his limited education and contributed to his respected position in the community.[10] Edward went to the local schools. Because of meager family finances, he did not follow his older brother to Harvard; instead, he was sent off to learn the woolen business. Despite his decided mechanical aptitude it soon became clear that the boy's frail health and absorption in books would better suit him to another career. Thus, after a year of additional study he went to Harvard and graduated in 1826. He planned to become a minister at first, but was dissuaded because of a speech defect. He then turned to medicine, possibly because of the influence of his brother, a young doctor who had died a short time before. By 1830 Edward Jarvis had completed his training, and with grave doubts as to the efficacy of medical therapy — doubts which were to remain with him throughout his long life — he set out to earn his living as a physician.

After two years of diligent although not wholly successful effort to establish a practice in Northfield, a small town in western Massachusetts, Jarvis was pleased

9. Ruth R. Wheeler, *Concord, Climate for Freedom* (Concord, Mass.: Concord Antiquarian Society, 1967), pp. 141, 146-147, 160, 174. Concord had a population of 1,633 in 1810, and 2,021 twenty years later. The ratio of births to deaths was three to one, which meant that a sizable number of young men and women emigrated in search of greater economic opportunity. In 1829 there were only nine unnaturalized residents. See Lemuel Shattuck, *The History of the Town of Concord, Middlesex County, Massachusetts, from its Earliest Settlement to 1832* (Boston, 1835), pp. 210-211.

10. Biographical material on Francis Jarvis from Edward Jarvis, "Memoir of Francis Jarvis," in *Memoirs of the Members of the Social Circle in Concord*, 2nd ser., 1795-1840 (Cambridge, Mass., 1888), pp. 30-40. Biographical material from Edward Jarvis, MS "Autobiography," Houghton Library, Harvard University; John S. Keyes, "Memoir of Edward Jarvis," in *Memoirs of the Social Circle* (Cambridge, Mass., 1888), pp. 317-355, which supplements the autobiography with material from 1873-1884, and Robert W. Wood, "Memorial of Edward Jarvis, M.D.," a paper presented at the annual meeting of the American Statistical Association, Jan. 16, 1885.

when the departure of an older physician from his native Concord made it practical for him to return there in 1832. For the next five years he was often more occupied with town affairs than with medicine. Like Shattuck, he taught Sunday school and was elected to the School Committee.[11] Deeply concerned with the development of moral character in young and old alike, he delivered a series of lectures on "First Steps Toward Intemperance." Forty years later he recalled a bazaar to benefit the blind and noted, with disapproval, that although the cause had been good "yet the measures were not in accordance with the principles of private and political economy." What was more, the goods sold were not well made or useful and "The motive of purchase was, in many cases, the fear of public or social disapprobation."

While in Concord he successfully treated an insane patient, and after this experience made the first of numerous unsuccessful attempts to find a position as superintendent of an asylum. But his search for professional advancement seemed futile, and in 1837, in hopes of a more remunerative practice, he moved to Louisville, Kentucky, where many Yankees had settled as a result of hard times at home.

The unstable life in this rapidly growing community displeased Jarvis. Despite every effort to impose the standards and customs he associated with civilized life, Louisville remained a frontier town to him. In addition, slavery was "hateful" and Jarvis found it impossible "to live there without, in some measure, using the services of bondsmen."[12] By 1842, almost in despair as a result of his repeated failures, he decided to return to New England.

While in Kentucky Jarvis had continued to care for a few insane patients. His interest in this field caused him to stop on the trip north to visit the Philadelphia Insane Hospital and the Bloomingdale Asylum in New York. Fascinated by what he saw, and encouraged by Drs. Thomas Kirkbride and Pliny Earle, he again looked for a job as superintendent at a hospital for the insane. He applied for a number of positions, but each time was rejected in favor of another candidate. Jarvis finally resolved to settle outside Boston in Dorchester, where his father had been born, and to pursue private practice specializing in care of the insane. Much to his surprise and pleasure he found that new patients came to his office, and, what was more important, they promptly paid for his services.

11. Although George C. Whipple, *State Sanitation: A Review of the Work of the Massachusetts State Board of Health*, 2 vols., (Cambridge, Mass.: Harvard University Press, 1917), I, 189, writes of Shattuck's influence on Jarvis, it is difficult to determine how important this was. In the Jarvis "Autobiography" Shattuck is mentioned only in 1849, when he consulted Jarvis concerning the Sanitary Commission report (see n. 15).
12. Jarvis, "Autobiography," pp. 74, 122.

Jarvis, however, remained minimally interested in the treatment of disease; he continued to read and investigate areas which he believed would reveal the common laws governing all of life.

He was attracted especially to the study of physiology and vital statistics. By 1848 he had published two books and numerous articles on these subjects, along with an extensive and appreciative review of Chadwick's work on sanitary reform in England.[13] Having been invited to join the American Statistical Association, he was soon its most devoted member and public spokesman. In 1852 he was elected its president and held this responsibility until 1883, the year before his death.

Collection and analysis of statistical data was the hub of Jarvis' work, for he saw this as the source of all useful knowledge. Throughout his long and productive life Jarvis was bound to a mechanical conception of the relation between disease and social organization; moral and physical order were interchangeable parts of an organic scheme, and personal health and morality were indissoluble. The laws of this relationship could be exactly determined through careful observation and statistical analysis.

Jarvis was even more specific than Shattuck in describing the prerequisites for health. Responsibility for abiding by these laws rested with the individual since the "vital essence" could be snuffed out or sparked to life by the moral character and energy of the properly informed and directed person. In Jarvis' writings there was always a tie between nature's moral law as the basis for social and political power and individual morality, or adherence to this law, as the foundation for personal health. The responsibility of the state to protect and promote public health was "advisory, instructive and encouraging." The state had an obligation to "teach the people their best interest," and to mitigate those evils, which under the abnormal conditions epitomized by city life, could reduce the vital spirit.[14]

---

13. Edward Jarvis, *Practical Physiology; for the Use of Schools and Families* (Philadelphia, 1847), and *Primary Physiology for Schools* (Philadelphia, 1848). See also review for the *Philadelphia Medical Journal* (1848), included in his "Autobiography," p. 186.

14. In the 1870's Jarvis wrote two major articles for the State Board of Health, and both included a full statement of his matured philosphy. See "Infant Mortality," Massachusetts State Board of Health, *Fourth Annual Report* (1873), pp. 194-233, and "Political Economy of Health," *Fifth Annual Report* (1874), pp. 335-390. For a contemporary evaluation of Jarvis' position, see Reverend Andrew P. Peabody, "Memoir of Edward Jarvis, M.D.," *New England Historical and Genealogical Register*, 39:5 (July 1885) which states that "He [Jarvis] justly regarded the tabulated results of actual enumeration as the only proper basis for sanitary regulations, for the specific mode of treat-

During the decade preceding the Civil War, Jarvis critically analyzed the annual registration reports in Massachusetts, made recommendations for their improvement, and wrote a Code of Health for the town of Dorchester. As a statistical expert his advice was sought by federal officials in the preparation of census schedules from 1850 through 1870. Ill-compensated for this work, he found evidence of political maneuvers and special interests which frustrated all his efforts. With each new experience Jarvis accumulated additional proof of the corruption and inherent immorality of American life. In particular, he saw the growth of urban populations as productive of disastrous consequences. Shattuck's *Report* in 1850 suggested the possibility of reducing the hazards of the city, but Jarvis found this conclusion illusory.

His best-known public achievement, the 1854 *Report on Insanity and Idiocy in Massachusetts*, despite its important recommendations for the extension of state responsibility in the institutional care of the insane, clung to previous methods of care and treatment in the face of enormous social and financial obstacles.[15] Throughout the Civil War Jarvis continued to look backward for his standards. Asked by the *Atlantic Monthly* to write an article on sanitary conditions in the army, Jarvis sharply criticized the government for its failure to provide adequately for the nutrition and housing of soldiers.

Army life, he wrote, should as nearly as possible approximate conditions at home. Health deteriorated when men assumed domestic duties for which they were untrained. Drawing on British experiences in the Crimean War, Jarvis argued for good records as the first deterrent to slovenly conditions. He stated flatly that the high rate of sickness was preventable. Such was the case, he argued, because certain common laws were operating, and, "Nature keeps an exact account with all her children, and gives power in proportion to their fulfillment

---

ment in certain forms of disease, physical and mental, and for conclusions in very many cases of the mutual relation and interaction of physical and moral causes and effects."

15. Jarvis describes his attitude toward the Shattuck *Report* in his "Autobiography," pp. 188–189; "He [Jarvis] did not agree with him [Shattuck] in all of his recommendations for he feared that Mr. Shattuck's plan would prove impracticable and useless . . . Although Dr. J. thought his propositions were all good yet it seemed to him that they could not be put into operation until the state and the people should be cultivated and have grown to it by many years of trial and experience. The result was that the whole terminated in nothing. The Report was made, printed, distributed, and there was an end of this movement. The Legislature took ño action." For a full discussion of Jarvis' contribution to the study and institutional care of the insane, see Gerald N. Grob, *The State and the Mentally Ill: A History of the Worcester State Hospital in Massachusetts, 1830-1920* (Chapel Hill: University of North Carolina Press, 1966), pp. 156-174. Professor Grob finds that Jarvis retained a social philosphy characteristic of "agrarian assumptions" appropriate to an earlier, more homogeneous society and rejected "radical solutions" which would have

of her conditions."[16] Although he likened the barracks to "the crowded and filthy lanes and alleys of cities," he avoided designating any specifically dangerous diseases or possible sanitary prophylaxis. He did suggest, however, that the location and administration of camps should be supervised by medical and sanitary officers.

Jarvis' proposals for improving sanitary conditions at home were couched in the same terms. After 1860, as a result of his wife's poor health, Jarvis could no longer care for insane patients in his home. Unable to secure a position in a state or private asylum, he devoted his attention to the proposal of the Boston Sanitary Association and the Massachusetts Medical Society for a state board of health and vital statistics. Although this proposition received the endorsement of Governor Andrew, the legislature consistently rejected as inexpedient all motions to extend registration of vital statistics under the general authority of a board of health.[17]

The arguments which Jarvis presented in support of such a board were limited to the advantages which could be gained from uniform and complete statistical information and the need for more efficient supervision of public institutions.[18] The failure of the legislature to establish this board did not reflect any abrogation of state responsibility for the health of the Commonwealth but, rather, the absence of any compelling arguments to link a new authority for registration with the prevention of disease.[19] Although failing to establish a general board

---

necessitated recognizing that the individualistic moral therapy that had been successful in the past did not conform to present social needs.

16. Jarvis, "The Sanitary Condition of the Army," *Atlantic Monthly* 10: 463-497: (Oct. 1862).

17. Edward Jarvis to Governor John A. Andrew, Feb. 11, 1861, in Andrew Papers, MHS; John Ware to Edward Jarvis, Dec. 13, 1861, Jarvis Letters. Although proposals for a state board were regularly brought before the legislature from 1861 to 1868, it is impossible to follow legislative response through any single series of official documents; "Report of the Joint Special Committee to whom were Referred the Petitions of the Massachusetts Medical Society, Boston Sanitary Association and the American Statistical Association Asking for the Establishment of a Board of Health and Vital Statistics," *Massachusetts Senate Documents 1861, No. 127* (March 27, 1861), supported the proposal. See also "Report of Joint Special Committee to Inquire into the Expediency of Establishing a Supervisory Board of Control of Public Institutions and a Board of Health and Vital Statistics," *Massachusetts Senate Documents 1862, No. 82* (March 12, 1862), in which the majority report rejected the proposal. The Boston *Semi-Weekly Advertiser*, Jan. 20, 31, March 21, 24, and 28, 1866, reported a special legislative hearing on sanitary necessities and proposals for a board of health, which were rejected. The *Journal of the House of Representatives of the Commonwealth of Massachusetts for the Year 1868* (Feb. 18, March 10, 19, 24, 25), pp. 137, 216, 255, 269, 276, shows that the proposals were again considered and rejected.

18. "Boston Sanitary Association Memorial," p. 31.

19. Jarvis believed that opposition came from the Secretary of State's office, for

of health until 1869, the legislature continued to amend Chapter 26 of the General Statutes to prevent the sale of contaminated and adulterated food, to facilitate the abatement of nuisances, and to restrict the operation of offensive trades.[20]

Throughout the 1860's Jarvis fought all proposals for sanitary reform which were not directly tied to ascertaining general laws derived from statistical information.[21] He continued to insist on individual reform as the prerequisite for change, but the pressure of accumulated experiences with the sick and the poor, both at home and on the battlefield, caused others to look for new methods to cure the ills of society. State, city, and town governments were already taking practical steps in that direction.

Along with the increase in urban mortality noted in the annual registration reports, the growth of pauperism caused widespread alarm in the 1850's. However, most Massachusetts citizens, like other native Americans, saw little reason to examine the causes of indigency. Poverty, they believed, was the unfortunate and perhaps irremediable price paid when the state became host to the foreign immigrant. Although the early years of the Civil War were unusually prosperous, the number of state-supported paupers increased, and the resulting financial burden on state and local governments was real cause for concern. Following the usual Massachusetts custom, in March 1863 the legislature appointed yet another committee to investigate the possibility of reducing welfare expenses. Within six weeks, as a result of the committee's report, the Board of State Chari-

---

although the clerks were "conscientious and capable," they viewed all changes in routine work as "meddlesome interferences" and feared they would lose their jobs if registration was transferred to a new authority. See Jarvis, "Autobiography," p. 200.

20. "An Act . . . to Punish Fraud by the Sale of Adulterated Milk," *Acts and Resolves 1859, Chapter 206* (April 6, 1859), pp. 364-365; "An Act to Provide for the Abatement of Nuisances," *Acts and Resolves 1866, Chapter 211* (May 3, 1866), p. 164; "An Act Concerning Offences Against the Public Health," *Acts and Resolves 1866, Chapter 253* (May 23, 1866), p. 242; "An Act in Relation to Boards of Health," *Acts and Resolves 1866, Chapter 271* (May 28, 1866), p. 252; "An Act for the Regulation of Tenement and Lodging Houses in the City of Boston," *Acts and Resolves 1868, Chapter 281* June 4, 1868), pp. 200-206.

21. See Henry I. Bowditch to Edward Jarvis, May 18, 1869, Jarvis Letters: "I cannot tell you how sorry I am that you take such a determined position about the *necessity* of Registration being *connected* with a Board of Health. There are many ways that a State Board of Health might do good without having one word to say of Registration — why then fly in the face of the state officials and excite their determined opposition as you have already done by suggesting that idea. I was in hope that by trying to carry the *simple* idea of such a Board we would get what we have both long waited for. Now I fear we are to be foiled again. I write plainly because I really think you have hurt a cause we both have at heart, by claiming too much at once."

ties was established to oversee administration of all public aid to the indigent.[22]

The Board consisted of five unpaid members, a salaried general agent, and a secretary. Although the Board was established to function in a purely advisory capacity, it had broad powers of investigation. Consequently, from the outset the members concerned themselves with the prevention as well as the alleviation of indigency. Under the guidance of its first chairman, Dr. Samuel Gridley Howe, the Board took on the task of examining the causes of poverty.[23]

Poverty was for Howe what disease and premature death were for Shattuck and Jarvis — the consequence of failure to obey the natural laws of humanity. Unlike Jarvis, Howe directed his attention primarily to specific measures for social reform which he confidently believed would restore the harmony of natural law. In the Board's *Second Annual Report* Howe described the social forces which could be utilized as "remedial agencies": "Foremost among the measures for social reform must be those which improve the material condition and daily habits of persons . . . Improvement of dwellings; encouragement to ownership of homesteads; increased facility for buying clothing and wholesome food; decreased facility for buying rum and unwholesome food; restriction of exhausting labor; cleanliness in every street, lane and yard . . . "[24] While giving a nod in the direction of hereditary predisposition, Howe stressed the social conditions rather than the personal inadequacies which led to dependency. He optimistically proposed that the creation of a physically and morally healthy environment would result in the return of the degenerate individual to an independent, healthful, and socially useful life. This shift in emphasis resulted from a determination to manipulate the conditions which permitted degradation and a confidence in the possibility of reducing the incidence of preventable poverty.[25]

22. *Acts and Resolves 1863, Chapter 240* (April 29, 1863), pp. 540-543. For a review of Massachusetts welfare policies and the changes which led to the Board of State Charities, see Grob, *The State and the Mentally Ill*, pp. 180-189.

23. For a recent biography of Howe, whose lifelong activity in behalf of the needy is best remembered through his work as founder and director of the Perkins Institution and Massachusetts School for the Blind, see Harold Schwartz, *Samuel Gridley Howe, Social Reformer, 1801-1876* (Cambridge, Mass.: Harvard University Press, 1956). Jarvis was appointed physician to Perkins, 1849-1860, serving without salary. In Howe's absence, Jarvis took charge of the institution, and was generally relied on for aid and support.

24. Massachusetts Board of State Charities, *Second Annual Report* (1866), pp. xliv-xlv, xxxvi-xxxvii. Although F. B. Sanborn was secretary of the Board from 1863 to 1868, according to Sanborn, Howe wrote the *Annual Report*.

25. For a discussion of public and private programs designed to reduce the burden of poverty in the years following the Civil War, see Mencher, *Poor Law to Poverty Program*, pp. 279-309. For a concise description of the changing ideology supporting these programs, see Robert H. Bremner, " 'Scientific Philanthrophy,' 1873-1893," *Social Science Review*, 30:168-173 (June 1956).

The relationship between poverty and disease was recognized by Howe and others, but it was by no means certain that the remedies for both were identical. Poverty, on the one hand, could be alleviated or eliminated by a change in character and outlook on the part of the lower classes. Disease, on the other hand, was less amenable to restraint by reformation of character and morality. What was required for the prevention or eradication of disease was the application of far more complex solutions.

Although city life was associated with the deplorable increase in mortality rates, physicians noted that certain diseases required specific medical attention. Speaking at the annual meeting of the Massachusetts Medical Society in 1863, Dr. Morrill Wyman called attention to the responsibility and achievement of medical science. In a frank attack on therapeutic nihilism, Wyman stated that there were illnesses and injuries in which human intervention was necessary. He spoke of scientific hygiene as "the highest branch of medicine," and singled out General Benjamin Butler, the Massachusetts politician and soldier who had directed the occupation of New Orleans, for special praise. Butler's scrupulous insistence on cleanliness and quarantine had been responsible, Wyman believed, for the prevention of a yellow fever epidemic in New Orleans during the summer of 1862.[26]

During the Civil War, belief that susceptibility to disease could be diminished by specific intervention suggested a new role for medical authority. Evidence that personal hygiene could be guided and supplemented by scientific knowledge was reinforced by the efforts to improve health in the army camps and hospitals. Beneficial effects were observed following the practice of boiling contaminated water, the prescription of sunlight and ventilation as a source of health, and the assignment of physicians to responsible army and hospital posts, all of which contributed to the recognition that it was possible to curtail disease.[27] Although the filth theory of disease continued to be the basis for etiolo-

26. Morrill Wyman, "The Reality and Certainty of Medicine," *Medical Communications of the Massachusetts Medical Society*, 5:227-228, 239 (1863).
27. Although there are studies of the medical profession in America from the colonial period to 1860, relatively little has been written on the changes in medical practice and status which accompanied and followed the Civil War. For an examination of the Sanitary Commission, see Elisha Harris, *The United States Sanitary Commission* (Boston, 1864); William Quentin Maxwell, *Lincoln's Fifth Wheel: A Political History of the U.S. Sanitary Commission* (New York: Longmans, Green, 1956); William Y. Thompson, "The U.S. Sanitary Commission," *Civil War History*, 2:41-63 (June 1956); Fredrickson, *Inner Civil War*, 98-112. For a more general discussion, see *ibid.*, pp. 183-216; Howard D. Kramer, "Effect of the Civil War Upon the Public Health Movement," *Mississippi Valley Historical Review*, 35:449-462 (1948-1949).

gical concepts, public hygiene and personal health required the application of social as well as individual controls.

As support grew for a general sanitary program based on scientific principles, the medical profession gained a measure of public favor. The extraordinary devotion and skill of physicians during the war removed some of the suspicion that had characterized popular attitudes in the antebellum period. Following the war a concerted effort to improve medical training, together with demands from within the profession for greater attention to the principles of hygiene, also contributed to the expectation that sanitary reform could improve public health.[28] Although registration reports were an unending source of informative statistics on the relation between conditions of life and disease, the time had come for reinterpretation. The principles which analysis of these reports revealed suggested a possible basis for a program of remedial intervention.

The first year of peace after the Civil War marked a quarter-century of continuous registration of vital statistics in Massachusetts. Dr. George Derby, who had been appointed to edit the reports, looked forward to new progress as the medical profession and the state shared the responsibility of preventing disease. "Physicians gain through registration the invaluable guide to judicious treatment," he wrote, "based upon the epidemic constitution of the season or the year, — a doctrine taught by Sydenham, but which in his day was very difficult to apply, for the want of certain knowledge what the drift of the period really was . . . It has always been the reproach of medicine that its rules of practice are vague. This is the result of the complex organism with which it deals; but vital statistics are taking a more comprehensive view of disease . . . extinguishes many errors, and shows us the influences which effect [sic] public health in such a manner that we can claim to be exact about our conclusions."[29] The magnitude of the problem left plenty of room for contradictory attitudes. Although the etiology of disease remained unclear and the gospel of self-help was no less appropriate to the pursuit of health than to the pursuit of wealth, clearly the proper interpretation of registration returns could supplement individual virtue with scientific skill.

Derby, who became the first secretary to the State Board of Health three

28. John Richardson Bronson, "A Review of Medicine — Its Worth and Work," *Medical Communications of the Massachusetts Medical Society*, 12:111-117, 122-124 (1877); Richard H. Shryock, "Public Relations of the Medical Profession in Great Britain and the United States: 1600-1870 — A Chapter in the Social History of Medicine," *Annals of Medical History*, n.s., 2:318-325 (1930); Henry R. Viets, *A Brief History of Medicine in Massachusetts* (Boston: Houghton, Mifflin, 1930), pp. 171-173.

29. *Twenty-fifth Registry Report for the year ending Dec. 31, 1866* (1868), p. 2.

years later, continued to edit the registration reports until his death in 1874. Unlike earlier advocates of sanitary reform, Derby looked to medical science as the catalyst for preventive practice. Born in 1819, he graduated from Harvard in 1838 and went on to receive his medical degree in 1843. He left his Boston practice for service with the 23rd Massachusetts Volunteers during the Civil War. When he returned after the war to resume his work, his activity was severely limited by poor health. In 1866 he accepted an appointment at the Harvard Medical School as a lecturer in hygiene and earned a reputation as an authority on sanitary science.

Derby delivered an important address on the prevention of disease to the Boston Social Science Association in 1868. He argued for an active interventionist medical ideology which would utilize statistical information as a proof of effective action rather than as a principal weapon for control. In analyzing mortality and morbidity statistics, he said that it was necessary to consider the effect of specific diseases. He noted, in particular, the reduction in deaths from consumption between 1853 and 1868 and asserted that it was of no value merely to accept this improvement without question. The reason for this change had to be found, and he felt that the answer might lie in the course of the disease itself; "but here statistics fail us," he noted, "and we are left to conjecture. Our own belief is that they [the explanations] are to be found in the *advance of medical science*, which has given to physicians a better knowledge of the nature of disease, derived from careful observation of cases, and from modern discoveries in chemistry and physiology; and a greatly improved acquaintance with the means by which consumption can be avoided by those predisposed to it by inheritance, derived from all these sources combined."[30] In contrast to the skepticism of Jarvis, Derby stated that knowledge of the nature of disease was the critical determinant of prevention. The descriptive character of statistical information failed, in Derby's judgment, to establish causes, which the promotion of health required. Derby's words implied two important points: that susceptibility could be circumvented by scientific knowledge, and that disease was not the inevitable outcome of individual weakness.

Although Derby spoke for a more direct program of medical intervention, it

30. Biographical material on George Derby from Harvard Archives, Widener Library, and eulogy in Massachusetts State Board of Health, *Sixth Annual Report* (1875), pp. 3–4. The quotation from Derby, "The Prevention of Diseases," was reprinted in *First Annual Report* (1870), p. 48. For a summary of the relation of "regular" medical practice to the "irregular" theories of Thompsonian and homeopathic medicine at this time, see Joseph F. Kett, *The Formation of the American Medical Profession: The Role of Institutions, 1780-1860* (New Haven, Conn.: Yale University Press, 1968), pp. 163-164, 179.

is not apparent that this position was shared by the Massachusetts legislature or by laymen. As already indicated, responsibility for the control of local nuisances, polluted water, and contaminated food was accepted as the legitimate business of town and city governments. Complaints depended upon the conscience and scruples of local citizens. Restraints differed with each community and were more dependent on the character of the board of selectmen or, where it existed, the board of health than on any established sanitary code.

The establishment of the first State Board of Health, as a result, did not stem from any medical or sanitary justification, but rather from an effort by the Massachusetts legislature to reorganize and strengthen the administrative apparatus of government. During and following the Civil War the need to guard the state's resources and to regulate the demands of expanding private enterprise required the assignment of new supervisory authorities, such as the Board of State Charities in 1864 and the Railroad Commission in 1869. State government still operated under the Constitution of 1790, which guaranteed equal representation to all towns regardless of size and hedged the office of governor with restrictions; at every turn there were obstacles to any simple centralization of government.[31] When Thomas Plunkett, representative from Pittsfield, moved to set up a State Board of Health, it was in line with the trend toward setting up new supervisory agencies to handle specific problems.

Plunkett, who served only a single legislative term, may have been inspired to make this motion by his wife's interest in the control of epidemic disease.[32] The joint committee of the legislature, however, did not refer to any new scientific knowledge or theory of prevention to support his motion. Instead, the well-known discrepancy between death rates in rural Barnstable and urban Suffolk counties was cited again to indicate that much illness was probably preventable. Without benefit of added rhetoric, the committee urged that a State Board of Health and Vital Statistics be established, "with such powers as will enable them thoroughly to investigate matters relating to public health, and with a view

31. Wellington Wells, "Political and Governmental Readjustments (1865-1889)," in Albert Bushnell Hart, ed., *Commonwealth History of Massachusetts: Nineteenth Century Massachusetts, 1820-1889,* 4 vols., (New York: States History Co., 1930), IV, 613-614. The problems faced in legislative regulation of private and quasi-public business suggest that similar solutions seemed appropriate in the restriction of "public nuisances." See Leonard D. White, "The Origin of Utility Commissions in Massachusetts," *Journal of Political Economy*, 29:177-197 (March 1921).

32. *Journal of the Senate of Massachusetts for the year 1869* (March 17, 20), pp. 198, 209. Henry I. Bowditch, "Report on the Proposition for a National Sanitary Bureau, and the Organization and Practical Working of the Massachusetts State Board of Health," *Transactions of the American Medical Association*, 25:397 (1874).

to advise concerning it; but without any authoritative control or right of active interference."[33]

The proposed bill had its first reading on May 22 and was favorably acted upon. Amended only to include specific powers to investigate the use and effects of liquor and passed without further debate, the bill was sent to Governor Claflin, who signed it on June 21 to make it law. The Act provided that the Governor appoint a board of seven men who would choose from among themselves a secretary at an annual salary of $2,500. Despite the fact that since 1850 advocates of a state board had consistently linked sanitary reform with the analysis of mortality and morbidity data, the board was assigned no specific responsibility for the registration of vital statistics. Aside from the instructions concerning intoxicating beverages, and an injunction to make an annual report to the legislature, the scope of the Board's activities was left undefined.[34]

Coming at the close of legislative session, the creation of the Board attracted favorable comment but no special enthusiasm. Twenty-nine years had elapsed since Shattuck's original proposal, but no one looked back to trace the circuitous road of state responsibility for the people's health. The *Boston Medical and Surgical Journal* noted that the motion for a State Board "was initiated, strictly speaking, in the legislature . . . and without the interposition of medical men."[35] The Republican Boston *Advertiser* stated that the Act creating the Board was the most constructive accomplishment of the legislative session; the Board would "encourage and stimulate local authorities to exercise power already in their hands . . . and make evident the positive right which everybody may claim from public authority to the enjoyment of air and water and soil unpolluted by their neighbor's negligence." Providing wise and capable men were appointed without regard to political considerations, the editorial said, the effectiveness of the Board was assured.[36]

33. "Report of the Joint Special Committee . . . to consider the expediency of establishing a State Board of Health," *Massachusetts Senate Documents 1869, No. 340* (May 22, 1869).

34. *Journal of the Massachusetts Senate 1869* (May 22, 25, 26, 28, June 2, 16, 19), pp. 430, 438, 442, 450, 463, 515, 520; "An Act to Establish a State Board of Health," *Acts and Resolves 1869, Chapter 420* (June 21, 1869), pp. 738-739.

35. *BMSJ*, 81:177-178 (Oct. 7, 1869).

36. Boston *Daily Advertiser*, June 15, 1869; Boston *Semi-Weekly Advertiser*, June 23, 1869; Governor Alexander H. Bullock, "Valedictory Address," *Massachusetts Senate Documents 1869, No. 1* (Jan. 7, 1869), pp. 36-37: "But when faith in humanity is combined, in its executive and advisory officers, with intelligence and high culture, with matured judgment, strong will, and resolute fidelity of performance, we can confidently look for an abatement of some immediate evils, and for a further solution of many difficult problems in the treatment of the pauper, the lunatic, and the criminal."

The question of *who* would be responsible for the Board's work was critical. It was colored by contemporary attitudes toward public service as much as by any question of competence in the broad area of the Board's authority. Since the Republicans in Massachusetts held every major elective office, the party also controlled appointments to the state's regulatory commissions and boards. Selection of responsible and capable leadership was not seen as a contest between men of differing political and social outlooks, and it was, therefore, not to be resolved at the polls. On the contrary, the duty of guiding state health policy should not be subjected to the coarsening consequences of running for office; it should be assigned to men whose private lives were above reproach, men whose civic responsibility was independent of the whims of the electorate.[37]

Postwar disillusionment with the morality of politics, a sentiment which would dominate public debate in the next two decades, was magnified in Massachusetts by the emergence of the Irish as a political force. Although the Republican party still easily won national and local elections within the state, the Democrats gained strength in the Berkshire region as well as in Boston, and the political unity of the war years was already a thing of the past. Even within the Republican party charges of corruption threatened to split the organization. Lack of confidence in the traditional forms of organization were heard on all levels, and the surest safeguard for conservative and reformer alike was in the leadership of responsible and reliable men.[38]

The gentlemen appointed to the first State Board of Health reflected this tradition which joined commercial and financial interests in Massachusetts with those patrician families long distinguished for their philanthropic and social concerns.[39] Two members, Dr. Henry Ingersoll Bowditch and Richard Frothingham, historian and journalist, had grown up with a legacy of service to the Commonwealth and the nation. Two others, William C. Chapin and Warren Sawyer, were business men: the first, a cotton manufacturer from Lawrence; the second, a wholesale leather dealer from Boston. P. Emory Aldrich, a lawyer,

37. See, for instance, Charles Francis Adams, *Individuality in Politics* (New York, 1880), pp. 11-13. Adams was a member of the Massachusetts Board of Railroad Commissioners from its establishment in 1869, and its chairman from 1872 to 1879.

38. Wells, "Political Readjustments," pp. 588-596; Edith Ellen Ware, *Political Opinion in Massachusetts During the Civil War and Reconstruction* (New York: Columbia University, 1916), pp. 162-178; Gamaliel Bradford, "The Reform of our State Governments," *Annals of the American Academy of Political and Social Science*, 4:895 (May 1894).

39. For a discussion of this tradition in a western Massachusetts city, see Michael H. Frisch, "The Community Elite and the Emergence of Urban Politics: Springfield, Massachusetts, 1840-1880," pp. 277-296, in Stephan Thernstrom and Richard Sennett, eds., *Nineteenth Century Cities: Essays in the New Urban History* (New Haven, Conn.: Yale University Press, 1969).

came from the rapidly growing central Massachusetts city of Worcester. Only one member, Dr. Robert T. Davis of Fall River, was foreign-born, but he had received his medical education at Harvard.[40] The seventh member, Dr. George Derby, was a logical choice because of his work with the annual state registration reports. The three physicians were leading members of the Massachusetts Medical Society, and they combined their private practices with participation in the political and social life of their communities. Every member of the Board merited public confidence, and all were drawn from that class of citizens which could be counted upon to maintain high standards of personal responsibility in the midst of charges that public morality was deteriorating.

The Board met for the first time on September 15, 1869, and named Dr. Derby as secretary, and Dr. Bowditch as chairman.[41] The elaboration of a state program for public health would depend largely on their vision and determination, for the legislature had defined the area of responsibility in all-inclusive terms. At the same time the power of the Board was limited to investigation and advice. Its budget was limited to five thousand dollars, there were no trained persons to carry on the work, and no similar bodies in other states upon which to draw for experience. At the very first meeting Bowditch indicated that this would be a new venture, dedicated to improving the intellectual, moral, and physical condition of the population. Recognizing that "these various powers and qualities of man act upon each other," it was the physical condition of the people which had been most neglected in the past. "State Medicine," the term

40. Biographical material on Robert Thompson Davis (1823-1906) suggests that, although he came from a different background, he held medical and social views compatible with those of Bowditch at the time of his appointment to the Board of Health. Born in northern Ireland of Quaker-Presbyterian parents, Davis came to Amesbury, Massachusetts, as a small child, when his father became superintendent of a woolen mill. Robert Davis' medical training began with his apprenticeship under a Fall River physician and was completed at Harvard Medical School in 1847. A strong abolitionist, Davis worked with Bowditch as early as 1851, both as a doctor and as a defendant of the fugitive slave. Elected to the Constitutional Convention in 1853, he later served two terms in the State Senate (1858, 1860), and three terms as a congressman (1883-1887). He remained loyal to the Republican party throughout his life, attending three national conventions (1860, 1876, 1904). His closest ties were with the cotton and woolen industry of Fall River, and in the latter part of his life, as a major stockholder in a number of companies, he was an outspoken advocate of a strong protective tariff. As a result of his chairmanship of the Massachusetts Senate Committee on Charitable Institutions, he was appointed to the Board of State Charities when it was formed and to the State Board of Health in 1869. He continued as an active physician, recognized as a bold advocate of new methods of treatment and a supporter of preventive sanitary reform. See the *Protectionist* (Boston), 18:410-411 (Dec. 1906); Fall River *News*, Oct. 30, 1906.

41. MS "Minutes of the State Board of Health," (1869-1879), p. 7, Massachusetts Department of Public Health.

used by Bowditch from the start to describe the power of the state linked to the skill of the physician, would reverse the older emphasis on individual compliance with natural law and stress the larger environment which the state and the physician could manipulate.[42] Bowditch, long a defender of the victims of social injustice, was well prepared to lead a movement to protect the victims of preventable disease.

Henry Ingersoll Bowditch was sixty-one years old in 1869, but the years had not diminished his vigor. He was known as a man of strong enthusiasms, whose passion for justice had led him to speak for unpopular causes and to act decisively when others had counseled moderation. In public affairs and in medicine he had advocated bold intervention, whether it was to challenge slavery by thwarting the extradition of runaway slaves or to relieve the critically ill by the application of new surgical techniques. His work on consumption had received recognition nationally and in England, and a small book published in 1846, *The Young Stethoscopist*, was favored as a textbook by students and young doctors in every part of the country. Bowditch brought to the State Board of Health, in addition, experience accumulated in years of medical investigation based on clinical observation. Henry Bowditch was one of those fortunate men born into a family where the expectation of success was enlarged by opportunity.[43]

Bowditch spent his early years in Salem. His father, Nathaniel, well-known mathematician and author of several books on navigation, moved his family to Boston in 1823 when he accepted a position as actuary to the Massachusetts Hospital Life Insurance Company. Two years later Henry entered Harvard, and by 1832 he had completed his medical training.

Medical education in the United States at the time was often supplemented, for the sons of the affluent, with further study abroad. Bowditch accordingly was sent to Paris to join Dr. James Jackson, Jr., and Dr. Oliver Wendell Holmes. These young physicians were tutored by the famous clinician and teacher, Pierre Charles Alexandre Louis, in a new method which combined observation at the patient's bedside with postmortem study of pathological anatomy.[44]

42. Massachusetts State Board of Health, *First Annual Report* (1870), pp. 1-2.
43. Biographical material from Vincent Y. Bowditch, *Life and Correspondence of Henry Ingersoll Bowditch*, 2 vols. (Boston: Houghton, Mifflin, 1902); Charles F. Folsom, "Henry Ingersoll Bowditch," *Proceedings of the American Academy of Arts and Sciences*, n.s., 22:310-331.
44. V. Y. Bowditch, *Life of H. I. Bowditch*, I, 1, 10, 18-21, 337; H. I. Bowditch, *Brief Memories of Louis and Some of his Contemporaries in the Parisian School of Medicine Forty Years Ago* (Boston, 1872).

Besides his rewarding hospital experiences at La Pitie', Bowditch was introduced to a stimulating social milieu quite different from the purposefully simple life at his father's comfortable house. As a result of Nathaniel Bowditch's earlier friendship with the eminent mathematician Leplace, his son was welcomed into French homes alive with intellectual and political activity. Greatly moved by the egalitarian atmosphere he felt in France, Bowditch saw himself returning to America in the role of young reformer, to extend the freedom and opportunity which his father's generation had originally secured. "I want to see everything more free than it is now," he wrote home, "libraries thrown open, at least at certain times to the whole public. That is what is done here, and ought to be done in America. On the contrary, we are rather inclined to follow the example of Old England, and make men pay for everything. A slight affair often alters the whole course of a man's life. The difference produced in Boston by having the libraries open or not may not be very manifest immediately, but who can say that many a young man would not be excited to tread in the paths of learning by being invited to enter them . . . I will express my determination that on my return, and when in the course of time I shall perhaps fill some of the places which are now occupied by those older, my grand aim shall be to give to everybody the opportunity to study, and in this way repay to humanity at large the immense debt of gratitude I owe to France."[45]

Bowditch spent two years abroad, and, when he returned to open a private practice in Boston, he looked for ways to make good his promise. He soon began teaching the children of the poor in the afternoons and Sundays at the Warren Street Chapel. This was the kind of benevolent work which was expected of him as a matter of course, but Bowditch was already concerned with more controversial issues. Even prior to his trip to Europe he had been an opponent of slavery, in part as a result of reading the works of William Wilberforce, the British abolitionist.[46]

Within a few months of Bowditch's return to America, events close to home committed him deeply and permanently to the abolitionist cause. "On the afternoon of October 21, 1835," he recollected later, "having finished most of my professional work, I walked down Washington Street, and at the corner of Court Street found a large and noisy, excited crowd . . . I asked the reason of the mob, as it evidently was. 'They are trying to snake out Garrison and Thomp-

45. H. I. Bowditch to Nathaniel Bowditch, May 12, 1833, in V. Y. Bowditch, *Life of H. I. Bowditch*, I, 50.
46. "Henry Ingersoll Bowditch," *Dictionary of American Biography* (New York: Charles Scribner's, 1929).

son to tar and feather them' 'What have they done?' I asked. 'The Abolitionists have been holding a meeting in opposition to slavery.' 'Then it has come to this,' I said, 'that a man cannot speak on slavery within sight of Faneuil Hall and almost at the foot of Bunker Hill? If this is so, it is time for me to become an Abolitionist.'"[47]

For the next fifteen years Bowditch subordinated his career to participation in the struggle against slavery. Often ostracized by his colleagues and friends, he believed that he had forever turned his back on a successful medical practice. In 1842, while Shattuck as spokesman for the American Statistical Association joined with the Medical Society to secure the first unified registration of vital statistics in Massachusetts, Bowditch was fighting the extradition of George Latimer, a runaway slave from Virginia. There is no evidence that Bowditch was interested in early efforts at health reform; the legislation which concerned him most that year was a bill to forbid the use of state and town jails to retain fugitive slaves.[48] Years later he wrote about the antislavery movement with un-abated fervor: "It was a good moral tonic which even now, after the lapse of thirty-seven years, yet tingles in my veins. God bless the hour [in which], under the great leadership of Garrison, I became an Abolitionist."[49]

Bowditch was not the only young Bostonian of good family and tradition who felt compelled to lead militant antislavery agitation in these early years of resis-tance. Wendell Phillips, the son of Boston's first mayor, and Dr. Samuel Gridley Howe were among those who took this stand fifteen years before the federal Fugitive Slave Act provoked Massachusetts citizens to broader opposition.[50] Bowditch, however, was one of the few from his social class to support William Lloyd Garrison; Phillips and Howe more typically eschewed the "fanaticism"

47. From "Thirty Years' War of Anti-Slavery," written at the request of L. Vernon Briggs, and quoted in V. Y. Bowditch, *Life of H. I. Bowditch*, I, 99-100. In Bowditch's "Journal," Aug. 1889, this note accompanies a clipping about John Greenleaf Whittier: "What a blessing the 'Garrison Mob' has been to me all my life long, because by it I was led to take a stand for liberty and justice, and at a time, too, when friends advised to the contrary, and my professional success was, in their minds, bound up in my following the crowd and damning or sneering at Abolitionists and their 'isms.' I have found all through life that the vigor given me by the earlier anti-slavery work has been of immense service in the various struggles for woman and liberality of thought in the profession, etc." (V. Y. Bowditch, *Life of H. I. Bowditch*, II, 339).

48. "An Act Further to Protect Personal Liberty," *Acts and Resolves 1843, Chapter 69* (March 24, 1843), p. 331.

49. V. Y. Bowditch, *Life of H. I. Bowditch*, I, 137. For an extended account of Bowditch's abolitionist activities, see pp. 98-229, or his MS "Journal" beginning Oct. 18, 1842, Holmes Hall, Countway Library.

50. Harold Schwartz, "Fugitive Slave Days in Boston," *New England Quarterly*, 27:191-212 (June 1954).

which they believed did harm to the cause.[51] Unwilling to soften his voice, Bowditch denounced any compromise as an immoral alliance with evil. Concern for his professional reputation seemed unworthy in the face of mortal dangers faced by escaping slaves, and even in the last decade before the war, when he felt rewarded by the change in public sentiment, Bowditch continued to advocate an even more determined opposition to slavery.[52]

Although his early commitment to abolitionism presented enormous obstacles to successful medical practice, Bowditch kept his Washington Street office open in the years after that crucial incident in October 1835. He was also appointed three years later to the house staff of Massachusetts General Hospital. By the summer of 1838 he was sufficiently established to marry Olivia Yardley, a young Englishwoman whom he had met while studying in Europe.[53] In the early years of his marriage his future must have looked bleak as wealthy patients who would have ordinarily sought his advice were reluctant to consult a man of his political notoriety. His casebooks indicate, however, that he saw many who knew that they would never be turned away because of failure to pay a fee.[54] Even as an admitting physician at the hospital, he found that his convictions would be a matter of controversy. In 1841 he resigned his post after a rule was passed excluding Negroes from admission. Apparently his action forced the trustees to reconsider their position, and Bowditch remained at the hospital, where his skill at percussion and auscultation earned him a reputation, especially among younger physicians.[55]

51. Three recent biographies of Garrison recount the tribulations he faced in Massachusetts: Russel B. Nye, *William Lloyd Garrison and the Humanitarian Reformers* (Boston: Little, Brown, 1955); John L. Thomas, *The Liberator, William Lloyd Garrison* (Boston: Little, Brown, 1963); Walter M. Merrill, *Against Wind and Tide: A Biography of William Lloyd Garrison* (Cambridge, Mass.: Harvard University Press, 1963). Bowditch remained devoted to Garrison both politically and personally, and, although Garrison generally followed "eclectics" on medical questions, he once consented to consult Bowditch; see Thomas, *The Liberator*, p. 308. In 1866 Bowditch took the leadership in raising a National Testimonial Fund for Garrison, calling sixteen leading citizens, including Governor John A. Andrew, to his home for this purpose; see Merrill, *Against Wind and Tide*, p. 309.

52. After 1850 Bowditch continued his radical stance, and in 1854 supported the Anti-Man Hunting League as contrasted with the more passively defensive League of Freedom organized by James Freeman Clarke, see V. Y. Bowditch, *Life of H. I. Bowditch*, I, 263-283.

53. V. Y. Bowditch, *Life of H. I. Bowditch*, I, 97–98; Folsom, "Bowditch," pp. 315–316.

54. Henry I. Bowditch's "Medical Records," March 1839-April 1891, Holmes Hall, Countway Library, show the gradual growth of his practice. Although he did not indicate receipt of fees, he noted the symptoms and circumstances of each patient, as well as diagnosis, prognosis, and remedies prescribed. A rough count of his patients at intervals between 1839 and 1861 indicates that his practice showed no growth between the first date and 1846; it doubled by 1852 and trebled by 1861.

55. V. Y. Bowditch, *Life of H. I. Bowditch*, I, 130-132.

In medicine, as in politics, Bowditch was an innovator and an advocate of active intervention. His training under Louis in France led him to reject what he believed was the unwarranted therapeutic skepticism expressed by many of his seniors. He was certain that much could be done to cure as well as relieve the sick, provided that treatment began with "strict deductions from facts actually studied out with the utmost care at the bedside." In later years Bowditch appreciated the fact that the nihilistic attitude of older physicians was a reaction to the theorizing and heroic medicine of a still earlier period. At the time, however, he was eager to bring the new "scientific deductive" methods of Louis into the hospital.[56]

Together with Dr. Morrill Wyman he developed a procedure to relieve patients suffering from pleurisy. *Thoracis paracentesis* involved the insertion of a small trocar or hollow needle into the pleural cavity so that excessive fluid could be aspirated. Despite opposition from the majority of the medical profession, including the much-respected Dr. James Jackson, Bowditch and Wyman continued the succesful practice of this method. Ten years after their first case in 1850, the technique was in wide use both in this country and abroad.[57] Within a few years, Dr. Bowditch was a recognized authority on all diseases of the chest.

Consumption was generally recognized as the greatest killer and crippler of men, women, and children at all ages. But there was little agreement on how the disease could be cured, and still less on specific steps for prevention. Mortality from phthisis, as consumption was often called, was not as clearly correlated with urban crowding as was death from other diseases; physicians believed that it was almost equally endemic throughout New England.[58] Although the term

56. H. I. Bowditch, *Louis*, p. 30. Bowditch was a staunch advocate of clinical experience and observation as opposed to "speculation" in medical training; see his "Medical Records" and H. I. Bowditch to Charles W. Eliot, Dec. 2, 1874, Eliot Letters, Harvard Archives, Widener Library, Cambridge, Mass.; also Henry I. Bowditch, *Centennial Discourse on Public Hygiene in America* (Boston, 1877), pp. 7-29.

57. V. Y. Bowditch, *Life of H. I. Bowditch* I, 230-235, 310; Henry I. Bowditch, *On Paracentesis Thoracis, with an Analysis of Cases* (Philadelphia, 1852), and *Treatise on Diaphragmatic Hernia* (Buffalo, 1853). Bowditch taught at the Boylston Medical School, a proprietary institution which attracted first rate students and teachers, 1852-1855. In 1859 he was appointed James Jackson Professor of Clinical Medicine at Harvard Medical School. Despite the political events which reduced attention to his own practice, he joined with other young physicians interested in directing the medical profession to vigorous scientific investigation. Bowditch and John Ware organized the short-lived Society for Medical Observation in 1835, and, with George Derby and others, the more successful Boston Society for Medical Observation in 1846.

58. *Tenth Registry Report* (1852), p. 99: "Consumption stands far above every other destroyer of human life in our climate. It has removed from the citizens of Massachusetts more than ten persons every day for the last three years . . . In Boston, in 1849, six persons died of the cholera out of every seven who had it. Not one in a hundred persons,

"tuberculosis" was occasionally used to describe the broad category of diseases characterized by the presence of tubercules in various parts of the body, consumption was not considered contagious or "zymotic." It was classified instead with diseases known as "sporadic" in which heredity or constitutional predisposition were considered primarily responsible for susceptibility.[59] Consequently, prevention of the disease lay within the power of the individual, rather than in assuring the cleanliness of the external environment or the identification of a specific infecting agency. Most physicians and laymen matched their dread of phthisis with a philosophical acceptance of its pervasiveness.

By 1854, when Dr. Bowditch decided to begin an extended study of consumption, he had had much personal and professional experience with the disease. His mother died from it while he was a student in Paris; later his office in Boston was often filled with patients in various stages of consumptive debilitation. Although he had no reason to doubt that heredity played a major part in selecting victims, his experience as a clinician seemed to contradict the belief that certain individuals were inevitably doomed to die from tuberculosis. As Bowditch studied consumption at the patient's bedside, he became convinced that it should be possible to frame general laws to guide the physician in both the treatment and prevention of this illness. Unwilling to accept the conventional view that there was little relation between the environment and the incidence of consumption, and unable to formulate a trustworthy hypothesis from the study of individual patients, Bowditch turned to the method most favored by mid-nineteenth-century science, the accumulation of statistical data.[60] He wrote to physicians throughout the state for information on the number of cases of consumption in their locality and the conditions of housing, soil, and climate. After three years of repeated inquiries, only 183 doctors had replied. Bowditch proceeded, nevertheless, to coordinate this data with the very incomplete registration returns.

---

once afflicted with pure consumption, ever recover." Oscar Handlin, *Boston's Immigrants: A Study in Acculturation*, rev. ed. (Cambridge, Mass.: Harvard University Press, 1959), Table xviii, p. 254, derived from figures in Charles E. Buckingham and others, *Sanitary Conditions of Boston* . . . (Boston, 1875); in 1865 the death rate from tuberculosis was 4.61 per thousand in Boston's least crowded district, compared to a death rate of 4.34 per thousand in next to the most crowded district; at the same time the death rate from all diseases together was 19.8 in the former and 27.9 in the latter. Henry I. Bowditch, *Consumption in New England; or Locality one of its Chief Causes* (Boston, 1862), pp. v, 11-12, reprint of his address to the Massachusetts Medical Society.

59. René and Jean Dubos, *The White Plague: Tuberculosis, Man and Society* (Boston: Little, Brown, 1952), pp. 118-120, 128.

60. John B. Blake, "The Early History of Vital Statistics in Massachusetts," *BHM*, 29: 62-68 (Jan.-Feb. 1955); George Rosen, "Problems in the Application of Statistical Analysis to Questions of Health: 1700-1880," *BHM*, 29:40-42 (Jan.-Feb. 1955).

In 1862 he announced his findings to the Massachusetts Medical Society: consumption was not equally distributed throughout the state; on the contrary, it was almost always associated with residence on or near damp soil. This was the single fact which stood out clearly from Bowditch's survey, and he concluded that here was a law which might well be applied "in a Prophylactic point of view."[61]

Bowditch told his colleagues that this new law was derived solely from the data which they had provided. This argument may well have helped pave the way for a favorable reception to his argument, but it was misleading. Bowditch looked to vital statistics to confirm rather than to inspire his study. He had learned from Louis and the "numerical method" to focus on the physiological manifestations of a specific disease, rather than the gross symptoms of disease in general. Although he, fully as much as Shattuck and Jarvis, assumed an orderly, coherent world, he believed that the prevention of disease demanded more than acquiescence to the purposeful law of nature; it required understanding the particular disease itself and intervention based on medical science.

Bowditch inferred that in his approach to one disease, consumption, lay the answer to those who clung to medical skepticism. He took a position which, nine years later at the inception of the State Board of Health, would make him impatient with Jarvis' reliance on vital statistics as the only sound foundation for sanitary reform.[62] Far from being an accomplished statistician, Bowditch asked questions calculated to support his original thesis. Unlike Jarvis, he expected figures to corroborate rather than reveal the regularity of nature. Bowditch was determined that the laws he elucidated should do more than reflect God's purpose; they should be useful instruments for change. Positive of man's power to improve the human condition, Bowditch acted where Jarvis merely observed. Eleven years later, he spoke with confidence on "Preventive Medicine and the Physician of the Future":

61. H. I. Bowditch, *Consumption in New England*, pp. 85, 76. Bowditch complained that "very little of valuable information on the topographical distribution of disease will ever be accomplished as long as the registration of vital statistics is left in the hands of men, non-professional, and who have no just appreciation of the difficulties or value of such investigations." Two years later he rejected Morgagni's finding, that consumption is a contagious disease, as a "delusion." At the same time he said that under certain very special conditions such as intimate contact, tuberculosis might be contagious, and dealt sketchily with the question of susceptibility, differentiating between consumption, cancer, and other chronic diseases; Henry I. Bowditch, *Is Consumption Even Contagious or Communicated by One Person to Another in Any Manner?* (Boston, 1864), pp. 12–15, 79. In 1859 he made a trip to Europe and presented his thesis on soil moisture to Louis, and before the International Medical Congress in Paris and the Society for Medical Observation in London (H. I. Bowditch, *Centennial Discourse*, Appendix iv, pp. 458–460).

62. See 21, above.

To submit quietly to any remedial evil, as if to the Will of Providence, is not now considered an act of piety, but an unmanly and really irreligious act. It is the part of error and stupidity which does not believe in the duty of studying the physical causes of disease, and in at least endeavoring to crush out these originators of pestilence and death.[63]

For Bowditch the practice of medicine was a deeply moral act, commiting the physician to a life of service. Addressing the Harvard Medical School graduating class in 1863, he cautioned them against complaisance and exhorted them to bring compassion as well as scientific skill to their profession.[64] During the Civil War, Bowditch asked that this dedication be directed toward the goals of freedom for the slave and preservation of the Union. After the war he believed that continued effort could remedy the social and physical ills which still plagued the nation. With such a determined spirit to direct the first State Board of Health, its work was steered rather than guided.

When the Massachusetts State Board of Health first met, only Bowditch and Derby saw their task in terms of innovation. The other members believed that they should sit as a tribunal, considering evidence presented by complainants and handing down judgments through the application of pure and disinterested reason.[65] Despite this understanding, there was the problem of how the Board would move from investigation to effective action since it possessed no executive powers. The legislature did not expect the State Board to exercise regulative functions in its own name; instead, it assumed that the Board would enunciate new principles of public hygiene which would then be adopted by local governments.

The State Board, as a result, began its work with efforts to create local boards of health and invest them with authority. On the whole, the results were discouraging. Specific measures for sanitary reform cost money and were often ignored or rejected. Even in Boston, where the city government assumed reponsibility for waste disposal and the supply of pure water, there had been no independent board of health since 1822. Responsibility for sanitary matters was delegated by the Board of Aldermen to several departments. The five consulting physicians who were supposed to guard the health of the population complained

63. Henry I. Bowditch, "Preventive Medicine and the Physician of the Future," Massachusetts State Board of Health, *Fifth Annual Report* (1874). p. 32.

64. Henry I. Bowditch, *An Apology for the Medical Profession as a Means of Developing the Whole Nature of Man* (Boston, 1863), p. 25.

65. Henry I. Bowditch, "Short History of the Massachusetts State Board of Health," *MS Monograph VIII*, pp. 17-27, Holmes Hall, Countway Library.

repeatedly that they were powerless to enforce existing regulations. No action was taken until after 1872, when public reaction following a devastating fire coupled with alarm at the failure to control a severe smallpox epidemic forced the Board of Aldermen to finally establish an autonomous Board of Health.[66]

In the smaller cities and towns, where no such dramatic disaster threatened security, few saw the justification for a permanent board of health. Freedom from disease was viewed as primarily a personal responsibility dependent on the character and habits of the individual. Although the State Board of Health did not deny this premise, it urged every citizen to recognize that, as the population grew and changed, public health needed special attention from "wise, discreet and fearless men," and that this could best be accomplished under a special board directed by a physician. Apparently such suggestions met with little success, and, to reinforce this advice, the legislature was asked, in 1876, to require a board wherever the population exceeded 4,000. The law that was passed, however, merely authorized the appointment of a board of health when and if the electorate so requested. The response was far from heartening: five cities, Fitchburg, Gloucester, Newton, Lynn, and Chelsea defeated the motion; Haverhill, Holyoke, Salem, Springfield, and Taunton failed to even take a vote.[67] If "State Medicine" was to become a reality in the 1870's, it would surely not begin at the local level.

Although Bowditch and Derby believed that sanitary policy must be implemented by local boards, they were also interested in establishing the State Board's authority to act in its own right. At the second meeting on September 27, 1869, Dr. Derby proposed two independent investigations by the members or by experts engaged for the purpose. The Board agreed to examine the con-

66. For discussion of the events leading to the formation of the Boston Board of Health, see Dorothy Therese Scanlon, "The Public Health Movement in Boston, 1870-1910," unpub. diss., Boston University Graduate School (1956), pp. 20-27, 32-48; Henry Bartlett and others, "Report of the Consulting Physicians," *Documents of the City of Boston for the Year 1870, II, No. 43* (April 14, 1870). In view of the critical attitude of the Consulting Physicians in 1870, it is interesting to read of the 1875 report of Buckingham and others, *Sanitary Condition of Boston*, pp. 5, 23-24, 35, 38. This special medical commission appointed by the Boston Board of Health found that mortality rates for the city were deceptively high and that they would not place the blame on poor sanitary conditions but, rather, on the large Irish population and the unusual epidemics which raged from 1871 to 1873.

67. Massachusetts State Board of Health, *Fourth Annual Report* (1873), p. 8, *Seventh Annual Report* (1876), p. 408, *Ninth Annual Report* (1878), p. xiv; "An Act Relating to the Boards of Health in the Several Cities of the Commonwealth," *Acts and Resolves 1877, Chapter 133* (April 17, 1877), pp. 493-495. The next year the Board suggested an amendment to assure the creation of local boards for emergencies, Massachusetts State Board of Health, *Tenth Annual Report* (1879), pp. xxxii-xxxvi.

ditions under which cattle were slaughtered. It agreed also to compare "the amount of sickness and mortality in the (so called) model lodging houses, and in the tenement houses and rookeries occupied by the poor and improvident classes."[68]

The first issue lent itself most readily to dramatic investigation as well as measurable results. "We have no room left for nuisances," declared Dr. Derby in his first report on threats to the health of the population of Boston and its surrounding towns. The situation in Brighton, where most of the slaughterhouses serving Boston were located was a clear affront to popular and scientific opinion about the dangers from water and air polluted by decomposing animal offal. Despite recommendations which followed an investigation made in 1866 by Dr. Henry Clark at the behest of the Brighton selectmen, local butchers had taken no steps to dispose of waste matter properly or to dispel offensive odors. Dr. Derby noted in 1870 that there had been no changes in slaughtering methods in the past fifty years. The situation was surely leading to disastrous consequences that would inevitably result in lowered resistance to disease and premature death. The careless procedures were, moreover, economically wasteful since meat by-products which could be utilized for farming and manufacture were left to rot. Pointing to the successful establishment of large unified slaughterhouses in New York City and Paris, the Board advised the legislature to order similar remedial action in Brighton.[69]

The attempt of the State Board to translate advice into action met with resistance at first. Derby reported that the directives of the legislature had been thwarted by opposition from the butchers. In 1871, however, the Board was given the power to enforce its recommendations and to close slaughterhouses which were found to operate in such a way as to endanger the public health. Moving with caution, the State Board called a meeting of the Brighton butchers to inform them of the need to improve slaughtering conditions and stressed the hope that they would establish a new abbatoir without further legal restraints. All through the year individual establishments, particularly the largest and most influential, continued to oppose regulation. The state's attorney general advised the Board to forego its power of direct interference and to attempt regulation through the complaints of "third parties." Continued publicity concerning offensive and dangerous practices and support from the supreme judicial court to enforce minimal restraints brought compliance from a substan-

68. MS "Minutes of the State Board of Health," pp. 7-8.
69. "Report on Slaughtering for the Boston Market," in Massachusetts State Board of Health, *First Annual Report* (1870), p. 20-22, 25, 27-28.

tial number of butchers by the end of 1872.[70] In the next spring the newly incorporated Butchers Slaughtering and Melting Association began to erect a large general abbatoir in Brighton. Thus, the Board was in a position to effectively regulate all slaughtering of meat within eight miles of the State House. By 1876 the whole operation functioned so smoothly that the legislature directed the Boston Board of Health to take over supervisory responsibilities which had originally been assumed by the State Board of Health. This entire action brought credit to the Board and established a general procedure which was acceptable for the regulation of properly identified "nuisances" in densely populated communities.[71]

Dr. Derby's second proposal, to study the relation of tenement life to the incidence of disease and death, reflected contemporary apprehension over the most serious problem facing the cities of the Commonwealth. Ever since 1842 statistical evidence had supported the popular view that urban life was inherently unhealthy and that the habits and attitudes of immigrants, especially those crowded into Boston's squalid slums, aggravated this tendency. Not only were sickness and immorality considered endemic to the North End, but its inhabitants also failed to show acceptable concern for the improvement of their lot. The situation lent itself to the impression that the dangerous environment was in many ways a reflection of the depraved character of the residents.

Although the pioneering work of the Board of State Charities suggested a new thesis — that filthy and degrading surroundings doomed the poor to immoral and unhealthy lives — the tradition of private charity and humanitarian benevolence tended to retard legislation to correct these underlying evils. Those whose social and religious concerns supported missions to the poor regarded individual pledges of virtue and cleanliness as the best inducement to effective reform. Consequently, remedial legislation, even when it existed, was easily ignored. The Tenement House Act of 1868 had provided a code of minimum sanitary stand-

70. Massachusetts State Board of Health, *Second Annual Report* (1871), p. 3; the original proposal for a Butcher's Slaughtering and Melting Association is reprinted in the *Third Annual Report* (1872), pp. 227-229; "An Act Concerning Slaughter Houses and Noxious and Offensive Trades," in *Acts and Resolves 1871, Chapter 167, Section 2, 3,* (April 8, 1871), pp. 534-535; Massachusetts State Board of Health, *Third Annual Report* (1872), pp. 2-5, 230-239.

71. Massachusetts State Board of Health, *Eighth Annual Report* (1877), pp. 3-4. In 1872 the board asked the legislature to appoint meat inspectors; see, *Fourth Annual Report* (1873), p. 10. In 1873 the regulations were extended to cover slaughtering of pork; see *Fifth Annual Report* (1874), pp. 8-21. After a long contest which was finally settled in court (*Cambridge* v. *Niles Brothers*), the Board extended its jurisdiction to Cambridge; see *Tenth Annual Report* (1879), pp. 117-227; H. I. Bowditch, *Centennial Discourse*, pp. 48-51.

ards for buildings in Boston: there must be one privy for every twenty persons in a dwelling; waste disposal should wherever possible be linked to city sewers; health officers were to inspect all slum buildings at regular intervals.[72] In the absence of a board of health in Boston, there was no attempt to enforce this law, and in the spring of 1871 Dr. George Derby and the other consulting physicians resigned, protesting the lack of cooperation from the Board of Aldermen and the owners of tenement housing.[73]

A year earlier the newly formed Massachusetts Bureau of Labor Statistics had dramatically described the net of poor housing, high prices, and low wages in which even honest workmen were caught. The Bureau concluded that "there are no places within the settled portions of the city of Boston, where the low paid toiler can find a house of decency and comfort." Among other things, the Bureau recommended that responsibility to investigate and correct these evils be delegated to the State Board of Health.[74]

No matter how widely conditions were publicized, attempts to reduce the disease and death rate were frustrated by contradictory attitudes toward the poor. The behavior of residents in the Crystal Palace, a notorious slum block, and in other tenements did not encourage much hope for rehabilitation. On the contrary, an 1875 report on the sanitary conditions of Boston cautioned that "Morborific tendencies of the foreigners" were "so marked as to outweigh, and to a great extent *mask* the conditions . . . to which we might look for the cause of endemic disease."[75] Enforcement of the Tenement Code, although desirable, could not assure the elimination of filth or the reform of behavior. As chairman of the State Board of Health, Dr. Henry Bowditch made a trip to England in 1870 to visit the London slums and investigate corrective programs there, which were reportedly successful.

A tour through the worst sections of London in the company of a police inspector confirmed his expectations; conditions in the cities of the Old World were even more depressing than those in Boston. His letters home were filled with compassion for the poor; "learn a lesson of pity rather than anger," he wrote his daughter, "at the wrong doings . . . of those whose early lives are subjected to such terrible scenes." Bowditch's religious and ethical commitments

72. "An Act for the Regulation of Tenement and Lodging Houses in the City of Boston," in *Acts and Resolves 1868, Chapter 281* (June 4, 1868), pp. 200-206.
73. *BMSJ*, 83:100-104 (Aug. 18, 1870); 84:231-238 (April 16, 1871); "Report of the Consulting Physicians, 1870."
74. *First Annual Report of the Massachusetts Bureau of Statistics of Labor* (1870), p. 182.
75. Buckingham and others, *Sanitary Condition of Boston*, p. 23.

caused him to reject what he believed was the cynical attitude of politicians — that reform was an illusion — and, instead, to look for practical remedies. Before he left England, he found a young woman whose work supported his conviction that the dependent and the diseased could be rescued.

On his return Bowditch reported enthusiastically to the State Board of Health on the success of model tenements organized and directed by Miss Octavia Hill.[76] This remarkable woman had persuaded John Ruskin to finance the purchase and rehabilitation of a number of slum houses. Certain that her tenants would adopt a more acceptable mode of life when surrounded by physical cleanliness and good example, Miss Hill personally attended to every detail in the maintenance and organization of these homes. Her approach did not deny the importance of changing the behavior of each individual; it assumed that this could be accomplished only by attention to the physical, moral, and intellectual needs of destitute people. Her goal was rehabilitation, and her method required that the poor accept her values as rapidly as possible.

Miss Hill had no illusions about the difficulty of her undertaking, but she was convinced that, given proper surroundings and direction, the "permanent poor" would adopt a provident and healthy life. A kind but firm hand would lead the way. Appeals to reform character were destined to failure, according to Octavia Hill, unless they were accompanied by scrupulous attention to all the details, beginning with the physical surroundings, which could elicit the desire to conform to acceptable behavior.[77]

Bowditch accepted her point of view and agreed that the first step in reducing morbidity and mortality among the poor was to change the environment in which they lived. His investigation of consumption had shown that unhealthy surroundings were a major factor in the incidence of this disease. He believed that the same principle could be applied to reduce susceptibility to other diseases. This proposition he presented with absolute certainty: "Health, physical and moral, are the results of the model lodging houses." The question that remained was how to speedily engage private charity and the government in preventive measures. Bowditch maintained that, whereas it was the responsibility of the government to prohibit unhealthy conditions, it was the duty of individual citizens to guarantee the construction and reconstruction of proper housing. Thus, he saw the Board of Health exerting its larger function, as an agency which

76. V. Y. Bowditch, *Life of H. I. Bowditch,* II, 153-178, esp. pp. 174, 178; Massachusetts State Board of Health, *Second Annual Report* (1871), pp. 203-218.
77. Robert H. Bremner, "An Iron Scepter Twined with Roses: The Octavia Hill System of Housing Management," *Social Science Review*, 39:222-231 (June 1965).

could appeal directly to the most responsible members of society without being constrained by the limits of the law.[78]

The call was entirely appropriate in a community where financial and philanthropic interests had frequently justified each other. The renovation of slums, both here and in London, was considered not only a charitable act, but also a business venture in which a proper return on monies invested was one measure of success. On this basis the Boston Cooperative Building Company was organized in 1871, "To cooperate, so far as possible, with the middle and lower classes of people, in providing houses for them."[79] Dr. Bowditch was one of the original corporators, and the company began its work by purchasing a building block infamous for the high rate of drunkeness, crime, and disease among its tenants.

Great improvements were registered at first, despite difficulties arising from the extremely poor condition of the property and the particularly hopeless character of the predominantly Irish tenants. Bowditch proudly reported to the State Board that the residents of this block showed many signs of improved behavior; rents were paid regularly, and thirty-four children were persuaded to make weekly deposits in the Boston Five Cents Savings Bank.[80] Five years later, the project failed. The desperate economic situation following the panic of 1873 made it clear to the incorporators that it would be foolhardy to renew the original investment. The committee, in addition, was unable to maintain that direct influence on individuals which had been so important and effective in Miss Hill's work. Notwithstanding earlier indications that the tenants had adopted a more salutary mode of life, Dr. Bowditch reluctantly admitted "that we saw some boys grow up to be thieves, and girls fall into unchaste lives, in spite of any effort we as a committee could exert."[81]

Bowditch concluded there was much for the State Board to learn from this enterprise, and the task was too great to rely on private investment. Speaking to the International Congress of Hygiene meeting in Philadelphia in 1876, he described the limitations and accomplishments of public hygiene to this date and looked forward to the future role of "State Preventive Medicine." Confidently he predicted that by the next century enlightened governments would

78. Massachusetts State Board of Health, *Second Annual Report* (1871), p. 228.

79. H. I. Bowditch, *Centennial Discourse*, p. 88.

80. Massachusetts State Board of Health, *Third Annual Report* (1872), pp. 10-12. For a discussion on the important role of savings banks, see Stephen Thernstrom, *Poverty and Progress: Social Mobility in a Nineteenth Century City* (Cambridge, Mass.: Harvard University Press, 1964), pp. 122-131.

81. H. I. Bowditch, *Centennial Discourse*, p. 88.

provide for the physical and moral well-being of the urban poor who now occupied those "purlieus of filth" which predestined their victims to a life of destitution and disease.[82]

Although Bowditch phrased his hopes for the future in terms of the state, he believed that, for the moment, reform must rely on right-thinking men who would remain independent of politics. In a very real sense this was the dilemma of "State Medicine" in Massachusetts. The State Board of Health began with no power of its own, and in many ways it remained powerless. Born out of attempts to understand and restrict the disequilibrium of social change, confined on the one hand by legislative limitations and on the other by inability to respond decisively to the threats which accompanied urbanization, the Board began its work with a narrow definition of authority and an unlimited obligation. Under the direction of Dr. Bowditch the State Board assumed responsibilities which a few decades earlier had been relegated to individuals. In the four areas where specific legislation was involved, the Board faced conflict which was only resolved when the remedy was based on the accepted definition of "public nuisance." As a result, the slaughterhouses surrounding Boston were restrained, and, even more important, by 1878 the Board was given responsibility to prevent the pollution of most of the major streams and rivers throughout the Commonwealth.[83] Meanwhile, in most cities and towns local boards of health did

82. *Ibid.*, p. 89. For other contemporary investigations of Boston's housing, see Massachusetts Bureau of Labor Statistics, *First Annual Report* (1870), pp. 164–198, and *Second Annual Report* (1871), pp. 517–531; F. W. Draper, "House Accommodations for the Poor in our Most Populous Cities," in Massachusetts State Board of Health, *Fourth Annual Report* (1873), pp. 396–441.

83. The legislature directed the Board in 1872 to investigate pollution of Miller's River in relation to Cambridge and Somerville, and further to study sewage disposal in other cities and towns; see Massachusetts State Board of Health, *Fourth Annual Report* (1873), pp. 4-7, 10-11; W. R. Nichols, "On the Present Condition of Certain Rivers of Massachusetts," in *Fifth Annual Report* (1874), pp. 63-152; "An Act to Provide for an Investigation . . . of the Use of Running Streams as Common Sewers in its Relation to the Public Health," in *Acts and Resolves 1875, Chapter 192* (May 8, 1875), pp. 785-786. Massachusetts State Board of Health, *Seventh Annual Report* (1876) dealt almost entirely with the problem of water pollution; there were a group of special reports financed by a special appropriation of $8,480: James P. Kirkwood, "The Pollution of Rivers," pp. 23-154; William Ripley Nichols, "Tables of Analyses . . . on the Waters of Different Valleys," pp. 155-174; Frederick Winsor, "The Water Supply, Drainage and Sewerage of the State, From a Sanitary Point of View," pp. 175-275; Charles F. Folsom, "The Disposal of Sewerage," pp. 276-401. In addition, there were three related reports under the regular appropriation of just under $5,000. For the next three years the Board continued specific investigations at the behest of the legislature leading to "An Act Relative to the Pollution of the Rivers, Streams and Ponds used as a Source of Water Supply," *Acts and Resolves 1878, Chapter 183* (April 26, 1878), pp. 133-135, which gave the Board responsibility to prevent pollution of all supplies, except the Merrimack, Concord, and Connecticut rivers; Massachusetts State Board of Health, *Tenth Annual Report* (1879), pp. xxiii-xxv.

not exercise authority beyond emergencies, and tenement housing remained largely unregulated.

The movement for sanitary reform in Massachusetts bore the mark of its origin in vital statistics, which gave substance to the obvious: that death and disease accompanied the filth and disorder of densely populated urban communities. For Jarvis, who described health in terms of adherence to fixed laws, the power to prevent disease lay within the individual, and the obligation of the state was instruction. Although Dr. Bowditch predicated his program of "State Medicine" on a broader concept of health, he was also obliged to describe prevention within a framework of public deterrents which were acceptable only when the individual was powerless to protect himself. Yet both his scientific and his social views persuaded him that the major determinant of physical disease and personal immorality was the environment in which the individual lived. Bowditch was satisfied that his work on consumption established this principle as a guide to the prevention and cure of disease, and he assumed that men who shared his values would extend its application. For the first ten years of its life, the State Board of Health functioned as the corporate embodiment of the scientific knowledge, social conscience, and personal commitment of those appointed to lead it. Bowditch could see no other way.

At a time when the etiology of disease was not clearly differentiated from the sources of insanity and poverty, prevention and relief could also be joined. The legislature, faced with the need to reduce expenditures, saw an easy answer in the dissolution of three separate administrative bodies, and in June 1879 it established a joint Board of Health, Lunacy, and Charity. Bowditch opposed this not only because he regarded public health problems as unique and too important to be subsumed under this hydra-headed monster, but even more because he believed the proposal resulted from narrow political considerations. He was fearful that, as a result, members of the new Board would be subject to unseemly political pressures that would subvert public health to partisan interests. Although asked to serve on the new Board, he found that little could be accomplished by so unwieldy a body with so many diverse responsibilities; by the end of the year he resigned.[84]

84. "An Act to Create a State Board of Health, Lunacy, and Charity," *Acts and Resolves 1879, Chapter 291* (April 3, 1879), pp. 615-618, to take effect July 1, 1879. The joint Board included Bowditch, Dr. Robert T. Davis, and John C. Hoadley, a civil engineer from Lawrence, from the original State Board of Health; Moses Kimball, Dr. Nathan Allen, and Charles F. Donnelly, who had served on the Board of State Charities; and Drs. Albert Wood and Ezra Parmenter, who had served neither board previously. Dr. Charles F. Folsom, who had replaced Dr. Derby on the State Board of Health since 1874, became secretary to the new body, and F. B. Sanborn, H. B. Wheelwright, and S. C. Wrightington

Bowditch believed that the State Board of Health was a victim of corrupt politics in Massachusetts, and he saw a continuity between his present refusal to join it and his earlier abolitionism. He was seventy-two years old at this time, but his energy and outlook led him to identify with those younger men who forsook their allegiance to the Republican party during the presidential campaign of 1884 in favor of the New York Democrat, Grover Cleveland. These independents, who adopted the name Mugwump, received active support from a number of older men, well established in the business and professional world. Among them was Charles Francis Adams, Jr., who had chaired the Massachusetts Railroad Commission since 1869, and who, like Bowditch, refused to support the presidential aspirations of James G. Blaine. Bowditch regretted that he had not been invited to help lead the bolt to Cleveland, but assumed that his age and poor health was the reason he had been overlooked.[85] Massachusetts state politics was also disrupted by accusations of corruption, as charges and investigations of malpractice characterized succeeding gubernatorial administrations. The Board of Health, Lunacy, and Charity, regularly embroiled in controversy over the competence of its officers, became the object of damaging publicity. By 1886 it was no longer able to carry out any of its functions satisfactorily, and it was reorganized under two separate authorities. Bowditch viewed the Board's failure as the inevitable result of political interference.[86]

When the State Board of Health was reorganized as a separate and independent body, Bowditch wrote to its chairman, Dr. Henry P. Walcott, offering his services and inquiring as to the organization of the new Board. Dr. Walcott assured Bowditch that the Board had no patronage and that vacancies in the clerical services and inspectorships for food and drugs would be filled from the Civil

---

were all transferred from the Board of State Charities to head special departments under the new arrangement; see *First Annual Report of the State Board of Health, Lunacy, and Charity of Massachusetts* (1880), p. vii. For Bowditch's resignation, see H. I. Bowditch to V. Y. Bowditch, Oct. 28, 1879, and H. I. Bowditch to Dr. A. N. Bell, Dec. 2, 1882, for publication in the *Sanitarian*, in V. Y. Bowditch, *Life of H. I. Bowditch*, II, 245-250; *BMSJ*, 102:143 (Feb. 5, 1880). The resignation of four other members of the nine-man board caused delays in the work; see Massachusetts State Board of Health, Lunacy, and Charity, *Second Annual Report* (1881), p. cvii.

85. Geoffrey Blodgett, *The Gentle Reformers: Massachusetts Democrats in the Cleveland Era* (Cambridge, Mass.: Harvard University Press, 1966), pp. 21-23; H. I. Bowditch, "Journal," Nov. 9, 1884, Holmes Hall, Countway Library.

86. Butler was the symbol of venality for Bowditch and other Massachusetts reformers. For a further discussion of reaction to Butler, see chap. iii. For other opposition to the joint Board, see Henry I. Bowditch, MS Monographs VI and VIII, Holmes Hall, Countway Library.

Service list.[87] Bowditch was satisfied that "all these pretenders to the sacred calling of 'state preventive medicine' . . . have at length been hurled from power. This sentiment may be unchristian," he wrote, "but it is human."[88]

The new Board, led by a physician who had already given proof of his independence from political storms, measured up to Bowditch's expectations. However, while the necessity for an effective and competent independent State Board of Health was generally accepted by 1886, the difficult question of determining who was qualified to lead it remained. Bowditch had presided over investigations which had partially redefined the causes of susceptibility to disease. As a result, responsibility for prevention shifted to those who claimed special eligibility and skills. A curious paradox emerged which would become characteristic of "State Preventive Medicine": as knowledge of specific agents or conditions became identified as the cause of preventable disease and personal behavior became less important as the determinant of susceptibility, the qualifications of those authorized to protect the public health gave them rights previously seen to be the responsibility of the victims of disease. Moral behavior remained indispensable to the prevention of disease, but, as sanitation and hygiene became more scientific, the privilege of establishing adequate standards of behavior became the prerogative of the knowledgeable, and possession of knowledge became the sanction of moral behavior.

87. H. P. Walcott to H. I. Bowditch, July 28, 1886, with Bowditch "Journal," Holmes Hall, Countway Library.

88. H. I. Bowditch, "History of the Massachusetts Board of Health," p. 53. In this same paper Bowditch accused Governor Thomas Talbot and the Republicans of destroying the Board of Health because they feared General Butler would come to power and spend money wastefully. Bowditch also believed that the chairman of the Board of Health, Lunacy, and Charity, Charles Francis Donnelly, sought the position in order to guarantee that his manufacturing interests would not be interfered with by regulations to prohibit the pollution of water, pp. 34, 36, 42-43.

3 Reassigning Responsibility
for Health, 1879-1888

The belief that public health was best protected by absolute isolation from the grime of politics became the hallmark of sanitary policy during the three decades following the reconstitution of an independent State Board of Health in 1886. Supporters of increased state commitment to public health blamed corrupt politicians for the controversy which had hobbled the Board of Health, Lunacy, and Charity. Henry Bowditch, who had predicted from the start that the joint Board would be ineffectual, was sure that state preventive medicine could not prosper when public affairs were in the hands of men who lacked conscience and character. After Cleveland's election in 1884, Massachusetts reformers believed there was hope of returning state government to responsible leadership. They looked about for ways of reaping the benefits of their bolt from the Republican party. The dilemma of reform, however, persisted; the defenders of clean politics sought effective power yet feared the contamination of alliances. In the gubernatorial election of 1886 Mugwump John F. Andrew, son of the Republican war governor who had supported proposals for a board of health during the Civil War, received the Democratic nomination. Despite the prospect that this arrangement would lead to victory, Andrew declined to campaign or contribute money in his own behalf, believing that it was contrary to his larger code of conduct. His defeat by Republican industrialist Oliver Ames, who received the aid of former Democrat Benjamin Butler, symbolized the difficulty facing those advocates of reform who supposed that the claim to honesty and a good name were sufficient to attract votes.[1] In this same year sanitary reform-

1. Geoffrey T. Blodgett, *The Gentle Reformers: Massachusetts Democrats in the Cleveland Era* (Cambridge, Mass.: Harvard University Press, 1966), pp. 25-26, 63-65. For a comprehensive discussion of the political and social mood of the period, see Robert H.

ers pledged to keep the new State Board of Health free from political entanglements. Proponents of public health also needed new friends, and the alliance they entered turned out to be more durable and successful than that of the Mugwumps and Democrats.

Increasingly complex concepts of environmental sanitation already sanctioned the authority of a whole new group of experts to protect the people from the evils accompanying urbanization and industrialization. Alarm over apparent deterioration of the environment under the stress of increased demands for water and sewage facilities was accentuated by the fear that private interests would manipulate prior legislative restrictions to their own ends. The growth of manufacturing and population centers in Massachusetts required constant vigilance under the Act passed in 1878 to prevent the pollution of inland waterways; the condition of three major rivers exempt from control showed the effect of purposeful negligence.

Meanwhile, the old doctrine that absence of filth was sufficient bulwark against contagion was challenged as scientists identified microscopic organisms with specific disease entities. During the next decade the development of chemical and mechanical methods for the purification of water, which required a high degree of technical proficiency in order to be efficiently utilized, and the dramatic success of specialized bacteriological techniques in reducing mortality from diphtheria contributed to shifting responsibility for health from the layman to the trained scientist. As both prevention and cure of disease were removed from the jurisdiction of enlightened common sense, new appeals for sanitary controls were phrased in terms of dependence upon qualified experts — the engineer, the chemist, and the biologist.[2]

Although the medical profession voiced proprietary rights in regard to the application of new scientific knowledge to the prevention and cure of disease, its role was not above suspicion. Despite the improved status of physicians, in part a reflection of their own efforts to improve the quality of medical education and their professional image, the right to practice medicine was still open to anyone in Massachusetts who identified himself as a "doctor"; the legislature

---

Wiebe, *The Search for Order, 1877-1920* (New York: Hill and Wang, 1967), chap. i-iii, esp. pp. 4-5, 26-31, 37-39.

2. George H. Daniels, "The Process of Professionalization in American Science: The Emergent Period, 1820-1860," *Isis*, 58:152 (Summer 1967). For a fascinating discussion of the social and scientific components of nineteenth-century water policy and its implications for policy today, see Duane D. Baumann, *The Recreational Use of Domestic Water Supply Reservoirs: Perception and Choice* (Chicago: University of Chicago Research Papers No. 121, 1969), esp. pp. 21-30, 72-75, 87-89.

refused to grant the Medical Society or any educational institution the prerogative to certify competence. Physicians who sought to establish pre-emptive rights for the care of the sick based on professional standards believed that increased interest in sanitary improvements by the state and national governments would, in time, better the position of orthodox medicine.[3]

At the same time that reformers characterized narrow political interests as inimicable to the broader picture of public well-being, Dr. Henry Pickering Walcott, president of the American Public Health Association and chairman of the Massachusetts State Board of Health, noted that the time had come when "the statesman and the sanitarian must work in harmony."[4] The physician and the layman concerned with extending social and scientific controls over the environmental and bacteriological sources of disease associated with those advocates of "good government" who were caught in the contradictory position of asking for political power and being repelled by its implications. Civil service reformers, for instance, were obliged to identify the opposition as immoral and corrupt politicians, while they saw themselves making public policy by transposing the qualities of individual virtue to the government. Public health reformers, on the other hand, were able to describe the enemy, at least partially, in the impersonal terms of science, thereby ascribing to themselves the nonpartisan interests of the total community.[5] By the end of the nineteenth century there was a recognized field of public health, designated by a body of law and

3. A letter to the editor of the Boston *Daily Globe*, June 8, 1885, summarized opposition expressed at a legislative hearing on licensing: "Our State, we are proud to say, has steadily been opposed to all medical legislation, although it has been proposed year after year by our doctors. It is class legislation of the most odious nature, that our citizens have such a horror of. The people have never asked for it; it is only the doctor's opening wedge to fetter and destroy the individual liberty of our citizens." N.S. Davis, "The Present and Future Tendencies of the Medical Profession," *JAMA*, 1:40 (July 21, 1883); George Rosen, "Politics and Public Health in New York City (1838-1842)," *BHM*, 24:461 (Sept.-Oct. 1950).

4. Henry P. Walcott, "President's Address," *Papers and Reports of the American Public Health Association*, 12:3 (1886). The American Public Health Association grew from a meeting called in New York City in 1872, leading to a national meeting the next year in Cincinnati; see Stephen Smith, "A History of Public Health 1871-1921," in Mazyck P. Ravenel, ed., *A Half Century of Public Health: Jubilee Historical Volume of the American Public Health Association* (Lynn, Mass.: privately published, Nichols Press, 1921), pp. 10-11. Membership was open to anyone interested in "sanitary studies and their practical applications," in the interest of "independence of official and governmental relationships"; see Elisha Harris, "Introductory Note," *Papers and Reports of the American Public Health Association*, 1:ix-x, xii (1873).

5. Ari Hoogenboom *Outlawing the Spoils: A History of the Civil Service Reform Movement, 1865-1883* (Urbana: University of Illinois Press, 1961), pp. ix, 190-197. Hoogenboom finds that advocacy of civil service reform was highly correlated with being "out" rather than "in" public office.

acceptable medical practice, which assigned responsibility for the control of specific diseases in Massachusetts to the State Board of Health.

As the physician and the sanitary engineer assumed ultimate authority for public hygiene, they placed themselves as intermediaries between the enemies of public health, both microbial and man-made, and the people. Often the sanitarian was in the enviable position of identifying the culprit, explaining its role, and naming the weapons of combat. Professional public health workers could determine the need and evaluate the success of preventive measures on the basis of standards established in the laboratory, where scientific methods were declared immune from private or political considerations. "Science" became for the physician, the sanitary engineer, and the laboratory investigator, a goal as well as a procedure, which gave it the authority of higher law and removed it from criticism.[6]

In contrast to the period when improved health was fused to reform of individual behavior, it was no longer possible or necessary to limit public health achievement by anything less than the commitment of the most enlightened citizens. Small wonder that, in 1915, the former president of Harvard, Charles W. Eliot, believed "that this method of preventive medicine is the one which should be universally applied for the defense of society against the evils which afflict it — such for example, as alcoholism, prostitution and war. All the beneficent forces of society should combine to *prevent* these evils," he continued. "Medical research and preventive medicine are teaching the civilized world how to deal effectively with moral, as well as physical diseases."[7]

Even in the period from 1879 to 1886, when public health was subsumed under the administrative umbrella of all state charitable interests, the work of the Health Committee was relatively free from the turmoil which characterized the departments responsible for the poor and the insane. The Board of Health, Lunacy, and Charity, meanwhile, was the target of hostile criticism from all sides, particularly after 1883 when Governor Benjamin Butler thrust it into the center of controversy over the condition of the public institutions responsible for the care of the indigent.

Butler, the symbol of opportunism and corruption to men of means in both

6. For a discussion of the conflicts faced in legitimizing scientific inquiry, see George H. Daniels, "The Pure Science Ideal and Democratic Structure," *Science*, 156:1699-1705 (July 1967), and Daniels, "Professionalization," pp. 160-166.

7. Letter from Eliot quoted in William T. Sedgwick, "American Achievements and Failures in Public Health Work," *AJPH*, 5:1108 (Oct. 1915).

political parties in Massachusetts, was elected in 1882 on the Democratic ticket. The campaign took advantage of widespread disillusion with the Republicans. Despised and feared by most traditional friends of reform and supported by the Irish and other politically and socially disadvantaged voters particularly in Boston and his native Lowell, Butler ran on the slogan of economy and honesty in state administration. Once in office, he called for a broad range of measures calculated to enhance his reputation among his constituents, singling out the Tewksbury Almshouse as an example of wasteful practices and the haven of inept officeholders appointed by Republicans.[8] His sensational charges that unclaimed corpses were dissected at the Harvard Medical School and the skins of paupers tanned "for the slipper of the aristocrat" increased tension between the governor and his indignant enemies, but resulted in few changes at the Almshouse other than the appointment of a new director.

Although the Board of Health, Lunacy, and Charity was not directly implicated in many of Butler's accusations, the atmosphere created by the investigation spilled over and led to endless internal quarrels and reorganization. Butler staged the expose' in terms of a struggle between the exploited poor and the crass patrician establishment, but members of the Board saw the attack primarily as a threat to their independence from political interference. After Butler was defeated in his bid for re-election in 1883, the Board continued to be the butt of charges and countercharges stemming from reports of improper behavior by agents responsible for relief of the "Out-door Poor."[9] Attacks on the Board

8. William D. Mallam, "Butlerism in Massachusetts," *New England Quarterly*, 33:186-188, 200-203 (June 1960); Richard Harmond, "The 'Beast' in Boston: Benjamin F. Butler as Governor of Massachusetts," *Journal of American History*, 55:268-269 (Sept. 1968). Butler surprised his opponents with irreproachable decorum at his inaugural and delivered a long speech calling for the secret ballot, woman suffrage, and a ten-hour day for railroad workers; see Hans Louis Trefousse, *Ben Butler, the South Called him Beast* (New York: Twayne Publishers, 1957), p. 246. For an assessment of Butler as a genuine political radical, see John G. Sproat, *"The Best Men": Liberal Reformers in the Gilded Age* (New York: Oxford University Press, 1968), pp. 48-49, 276.

9. Harmond, "Butler as Governor," pp. 272-274. Butler refused to reappoint Charles F. Donnelly Board chairman upon the expiration of his term in June 1883, and others, including the well-known philanthropist, Francis B. Sanborn who was Inspector of Charities, resigned. Meanwhile, the Board revised its bylaws, "especially with reference to the conduct of its officers and employees, with their powers and duties, and the methods of conducting work"; see Massachusetts State Board of Health, Lunacy, and Charity, *Fifth Annual Report* (1884), pp. xxx, xxxiii-xxxiv; *Sixth Annual Report* (1885), p. viii. The *Fifth Annual Report* was signed by only six of the nine board members; the others refusing to be associated with it. For charges involving the Department of Out-Door Poor see Boston *Daily Globe*, and Boston *Journal*, May 18, 1885. The Boston *Daily Globe*, April 18, 1885, states that Donnelly was not reappointed because Butler considered him a Cleveland Democrat.

came both from those who called for retrenchment and from advocates of an independent board of health who wanted increased financial commitment and more vigorous leadership.

Dr. Henry Bowditch, who had worked hard for the election of Butler's successor, George D. Robinson, was unable to persuade Robinson to reappoint Henry P. Walcott, the man he believed best qualified to serve the Board. Bowditch was also unable to suggest a "self-respecting physician" who was willing to fill the vacancy.[10] From the point of view held by reformers, the problem of finding the right men to give leadership in the Commonwealth became increasingly difficult in the last decades of the century. In part this reflected recognition that the origins of contemporary problems were complex, often springing from economic problems which required realistic appraisal and the application of scientific analysis. The depression which followed post-Civil War prosperity hung on in the late 1870's, aggravated by the influx of immigrants who settled in Boston. Charitable response to the plight of the poor was informed by a new sophistication about their condition, which still emphasized rehabilitation of the indigent but stressed the necessity of properly organized and rationalized aid.[11]

Searching for some thread to unravel the network of new problems, reformers who in the past had assumed the organic harmony of society found this contradicted by the evidence before their eyes. They looked fondly to what now seemed the virtuous past and were confident that they were the repository of old ideals which must somehow be infused throughout a fragmented society. The social reformer of the Gilded Age maintained his deference to traditional standards. New knowledge about the structure and function of society called for more carefully conceived, perhaps even innovative, response, but it did not alter the disposition of right and wrong, of good and evil. The American Social Science Association, first organized in Boston in 1865 to deal with social prob-

10. Henry I. Bowditch to R. C. Pitman, Oct. 30, 1885, in Bowditch, *MS* Monograph VII; Bowditch, "History of the Massachusetts Board of Health," in *MS* Monograph VIII, pp. 43-45, Holmes Hall, Francis A. Countway Library, Harvard Medical School, Boston.
11. Robert H. Bremner, *From the Depths: The Discovery of Poverty in the United States* (New York: New York University Press, 1956), pp. 123-139. For a more inclusive description of the conflicting response of postbellum reformers, see Sproat, *"The Best Men,"* and Arthur Mann, *Yankee Reformers in the Urban Age: Social Reform in Boston 1880-1890* (Cambridge, Mass.: Harvard University Press, 1954). Nathan I. Huggins' careful study of voluntary philanthropy in Boston suggests that "One way of understanding the charity organization movement is in terms of organizational reiteration of traditional standards." See his "Private Charities in Boston, 1870-1910: A Social History," unpub. diss., Harvard University (1962), p. 264.

lems created by the immigrant Irish, now became the source of useful information and of a multitude of diverse campaigns to uplift the unacculturated. In Boston the Associated Charities was established in 1879, uniting most Protestant Church-sponsored philanthropic activities and stressing the need to assimilate traditional moral values within the framework of scientific social work. Similarly, the United Hebrew Benevolent Association four years later looked to maintain its pattern of aid to the struggling Jewish immigrant, while incorporating "Yankee" techniques of organization and service.[12] Dr. Bowditch, as the leading spokesman for sanitary reform, believed that the future of "state preventive medicine" also depended on the joining of old principles with new methods.

Since Bowditch saw state public health policy as a conjugation of moral and scientific law, he saw no hope of retrieving progress from the hands of unprincipled men. While Bowditch and the *Boston Medical and Surgical Journal* despaired over the corruption which excluded men of good character from positions of responsibility,[13] the work of the Health Committee of the Board of Health, Lunacy, and Charity already indicated that professional skill could be an acceptable substitute for virtue. The annual reports of the Health Committee consistently reflected an optimism entirely absent from the records of the Superintendents of the In-door and Out-door Poor. Contrasted with the alarming increase of costs for the care of the insane and the pauper, the budget of the Health Committee was modest.[14] The Committee followed the lead of the former State Board of Health, hiring experts to gather information which was incorpora-

12. Sproat, *"The Best Men,"* pp. 56-57; Huggins, "Private Charities in Boston," pp. 93-120, 141; Barbara Miller Solomon, *Pioneers in Service: The History of the Associated Jewish Philanthropies in Boston* (Boston: privately published, Court Square Press, 1956), pp. 13-15. Although scientific social work methods were introduced to Jewish charities at this time, coordination of agencies was not meaningful until the organization of the Federation of Jewish Charities in 1895; see pp. 32-34.

13. Editorial, *BMSJ*, 113:571-573 (Dec. 10, 1885), referred to the Board of Health, Lunacy, and Charity as the "conjoint polysyllabic Board" and supported the refusal of prominent men to joint the board in its emasculated form.

14. Expenses for the Health Committee were $4,358 in 1882 and rose to $5,667 in 1884. For these same years expenses for the Inspector of Charities were $7,966 and $7,935; expenses for In-Door Poor were $22,520 and $23,294; expenses for Out-Door Poor were $15,000 and $16,944, see Massachusetts State Board of Health, Lunacy, and Charity, *Third Annual Report* (1882), appendix, p. 99; *Fifth Annual Report* (1884), appendix, p. 109. Care of the insane was included in the expenses of In-Door Poor. The reclassification of insane, making them eligible for custodial rather than hospital care, continued as an attempt to reduce expenses; see Dr. Walter Channing, "A Consideration of the Causes of Insanity," *ibid.*, pp. ccxxi-ccxlix; George D. Robinson, "Inaugural Address," *Massachusetts Senate Documents 1886* (Jan. 7, 1886), p. 28; Gerald N. Grob, *The State and the Mentally Ill: A History of the Worcester State Hospital in Massachusetts 1830-1920* (Chapel Hill: University of North Carolina Press, 1966), pp. 246-247, 252-259.

ted into general advice to the public or, when necessary, formed the basis for proposals to the legislature.[15]

Assuring pure water to the cities and towns surrounding Boston continued to be a major problem, and a small appropriation was asked for a chemist specially trained in the techniques of water examination. Although previous legislation prohibited disposal of waste directly into rivers and streams from which water was pumped for domestic purposes, the accepted theory of water purification held that water cleansed itself when the sewage was diluted and the stream flowed a sufficient distance. The critical problem was to determine at what point this was accomplished. The Merrimack River was specifically exempt from state control for, as the Committee pointed out, "the sewage of Lowell is diluted with from 600 to 1,000 times its volume of water, and then flows a dozen miles to Lawrence, much of the refuse from the mills acting as a precipitant and disinfectant to it." Altogether, the first two reports from the Health Committee encouraged the belief that the control of pollution would not be difficult once the condition was properly identified.[16]

William Ripley Nichols, professor of chemistry at the Massachusetts Institute of Technology, contributed three papers to the first *Health Supplement* to demonstrate the usefulness of specialized investigations. Concluding a highly technical paper on chemical methods of examination, Nichols wrote that the more exact quantitative analyses were unnecessary "for practical purposes . . . provided the results are interpreted with a proper knowledge of the history of the water under examination."[17] In the same year Professor W. G. Farlow of Har-

15. Massachusetts Board of Health, Lunacy, and Charity, *First Annual Report* (1880), pp. xi-xviii, listed the work of the Health Committee during its first nine months, including regulation of nuisances (although there had been no public hearings), supervision of public water under provisions of 1878 and 1879, supervision of registration of vital statistics, cooperation with physicians to "regulate the practice of medicine," encouragement of local boards and publication of circulars on certain diseases, new studies on the adulteration of food and milk, health at the Women's Prison, and the hereditary effect of intoxicating liquors. Expenses for this period were $3,998, *ibid.*, p. lxxi.

16. Massachusetts State Board of Health, Lunacy, and Charity, *First Annual Report* (1880), pp. xv, vii. For a summary of water purification theory, see C. F. Chandler, "Water Supply of Cities, Report Upon the Sanitary Chemistry of Waters, and Suggestions with Regard to Selection of the Water Supply of Towns and Citiies," *Papers and Reports of the American Public Health Association*, 1:541-552 (1875). Massachusetts law permitted use of streams for any waste disposal twenty miles above stream from its public use. Use of water in Boston increased far more rapidly than the population, due to increased plumbing facilities and changes in the standard of living; see Nelson M. Blake, *Water for the Cities: A History of the Urban Water Supply Problem in the United States* (Syracuse, N.Y.: Syracuse University Press, 1956), pp. 269-271.

17. William Ripley Nichols, "On the Examination of Mystic River Water with Remarks on Frankland's Method of Water Analysis," Massachusetts State Board of Health, Lunacy, Charity, *First Annual Report* (1880), p. 120. His other articles, also in the *Annual Report*,

vard University asserted that, although the public was increasingly conscious of the connection between germs and disease, most organisms found in water, including those which occasionally made it unpleasant to smell and taste, were in no way harmful. "Whatever truth there may be in the germ theory of disease," he wrote, "there is no doubt that designing persons impose on the credulity and fears of the public by representing as germs of disease microscopic plants which could not possibly have caused any of the diseases which have been supposed by scientific men to be produced by germs of a vegetable nature . . . The public should receive with very great caution any statements about the dangerous effect of bacteria in our waters, and, instead of worrying over the subject, had better leave the matter entirely in the hands of scientific people, who, at the present day, are the only persons who can be expected to follow the complicated and obscure relations of this difficult question."[18]

Attempts to translate this principle into effective policy led the Health Committee to contest local arrangements for sewage disposal made between manufacturers and town councils. The practice of dumping waste into the nearest available source of flowing water had been sanctioned by custom and local ruling. The law passed in 1878 to prevent pollution stated that this practice should not be construed to negate prior agreements "or to destroy or impair prescriptive rights of drainage or discharge to the extent to which they lawfully existed."[19] Under these circumstances the difficulty of interpreting the law increased every year.

After the Health Committee tried to act as arbiter of a dispute between the Boston Water Board and several suburban tanneries in 1882, it concluded that "there is . . . no permanent relief from this constant pollution but in some system of sewerage extensive enough to carry these matters to deep sea currents. Such a system is beyond the resources of any single city or town."[20] Two years later, there was effective opposition to a legislative proposal authorizing the city of Boston to purchase land surrounding the ponds and streams which sup-

---

were "Pollution of Brooks by Sulfuric Acid," pp. 19-21, and "Observations of Fresh Pond, Cambridge," pp. 97-107.

18. W. G. Farlow, "On Some Impurities in Drinking Water Caused by Vegetable Growths," *ibid.*, pp. 131, 150-151.

19. *Acts and Resolves 1878, Chapter 183*, Section 3, p. 133.

20. Massachusetts State Board of Health, Lunacy, and Charity, *Third Annual Report* (1882), pp. xli-xlv, 147-149. The 1878 law was amended in 1884 to give the courts rather than the Board the power of enforcement; see "An Act to Prevent the Pollution of Sources of Water Supply," *Acts and Resolves 1884, Chapter 154*, pp. 128-129; Samuel W. Abbott, "Water Pollution in Massachusetts," *Papers and Reports of the American Public Health Association*, 13:260-261 (1887).

plied the public reservoir, Lake Cochituate. Local manufacturers responded that if they were denied the right of drainage they would be forced to close down their businesses. "Compensation to the mill owners," they testified, "would not compensate villages which depend upon the mills for their prosperity." With good reason, the manufacturers believed that any alternative method of waste disposal would be prohibitively expensive. While the need for a general intercepting sewer to serve the communities surrounding the Mystic and Charles rivers had been recognized for close to a decade, the financial commitment such a project involved had not encouraged action. In addition, although irrigation schemes were recommended for areas where sewers to the sea were not practical, these required at least three hundred acres of well-drained land for each million gallons of sewage.[21] In the year when Butler's slogan of retrenchment had carried the day, those who sought a major state investment for public sanitation could not expect much assistance from the State House.

In this situation the advocates of state protection for public water supplies identified pure water with pure politics. They saw the selfish interests of manufacturers abetted by corrupt politicians unconcerned with the physical and social evils that would accompany pollution of the Commonwealth's natural resources. "It needs no elaborate argument from us to prove that the public health is not sufficiently attended," commented the *Boston Medical and Surgical Journal*, "where only the rich can have pure water to drink and where temptation to the poor to drink bad rum is increased. Nor shall we endeavor to show that public morality is low where important public trusts such as the management of public water supplies are made sub-servient to politics."[22] However, the position that only the expert could master information too complex for the layman put the Health Committee in an advantageous position in this debate. By turning to the professional scientist and engineer as the supervening

21. Boston *Daily Globe*, March 21, 1885; *BMSJ*, 85:418-422 (Oct. 29, 1871); *ibid.*, 91:498-499 (Nov. 19, 1874); Chandler, "Water Supply," p. 563; *Hearing Before the Joint Standing Committee on Public Health in the Matter of Restraining the City of Worcester from Polluting the Blackstone River* (Feb. and March 1882), p. 175.

22. "Bad Drinking Water and Bad Politics," *BMSJ*, 107:117 (Aug. 3, 1882). Mechanical methods of filtration were used early in the nineteenth century in Scotland, England, and Philadelphia and New York in this country; see Blake, *Water for the Cities*, pp. 258-261. The accusation that selfish private interests were responsible for inequities of regulatory legislation extended to other areas of public health. The sale of adulterated food and drink was prohibited under "An Act Relating to the Adulteration of Food," *Acts and Resolves 1882, Chapter 263* (May 28, 1884), pp. 268-269, and three-fifths of the annual appropriation must be used to prevent adulteration of milk. This verse, "The Milkman's Lament," Boston *Daily Globe*, April 18, 1885, speaks for itself:

authority, it was able to persuade the legislature of the need for further control of water pollution despite the political and financial difficulties involved.

The second report of the Health Committee included a lengthy study of sewage systems utilized by other American and European cities and concluded that no one method was adaptable to all communities. Rather these were "questions to be determined only by a competent engineer in full possession of all the facts in regard to the district to be sewered."[23] Shortly thereafter the legislature approved a special commission to propose a drainage plan for the Mystic River Valley. This commission included Ellis S. Chesbrough, a civil engineer responsible for a major sanitary engineering project on the Illinois River in Chicago, and two physicians associated with sanitary reform. The first was Dr. Charles F. Folsom, a leading member of the State Board of Health from 1874 to 1879, and of the new Board until 1881; the second was his successor on the Board of Health, Lunacy, and Charity, Dr. Henry P. Walcott, who was also a member of the Cambridge Board of Health.[24] In its report the commission suggested the establishment of a Metropolitan District Commission which would develop a general system of drainage into the Boston harbor, while interfering as little as possible with local arrangements. Although the report was favorably received, no enabling legislation followed it. Another commission, organized at the same time, was made up entirely from the Board of Health, Lunacy, and Charity. Their report of pollution in the Blackstone River recommended purchase of land close to Worcester for sewage irrigation and filtration, but again led to no action. Although the Health Committee continued to report increased pollution of water throughout the state, these statistics were "of little value," in the opinion of a contemporary physician and sanitarian, "except as furnishing material for the public printer, together with certain useful information for contractors, pump manufacturers, and others."[25]

They deal in oleomargarine,
The law don't touch 'em at all.
They adulterate coffee and paris green,
They sand their sugar and kerosene
It's sold for the best when it's awful mean;
They give a short weight, but let us try
To water the milk, there's a hue and cry,
A dreadful hubbub, you'd think by the squall,
The very heavens were about to fall.

23. Massachusetts State Board of Health, Lunacy, and Charity, *Second Annual Supplementary Report on Public Health* (1881), p. xi; Eliot C. Clarke, "The Separate System of Sewerage," in *ibid.*, pp. 25-43.

24. Chesbrough and Folsom had been members of a commission which proposed the first comprehensive sewer lines for Boston in 1875.

25. Abbott, "Water Pollution," p. 261.

The attacks upon the Board of Health, Lunacy, and Charity between 1883 and 1886 were, no doubt, in part responsible for the fact that further regulation of pollution was never assigned to the Health Committee. When the accumulated reports of uncontrolled negligence resulted in the formation of a Massachusetts Drainage Commission by the legislature in 1884, no member of the Board was asked to serve on it. However, the principle evolved in the preceding decade, when the first scientific investigations of water emphasized the technical and specialized character of this work, continued to guide public policy. Governor Robinson acknowledged the nature of past conflict over state control when he appointed men known to be spokesmen for civic reform to serve on the Commission. These five businessmen and lawyers led by John Quincy Adams in turn appointed three civil engineers headed by Eliot C. Clarke, chief engineer of the Boston sewer system, to conduct the investigation.[26] When the report was ready for presentation two years later, the Commission asked Dr. Henry P. Walcott to prepare a summary of its position. This request of Walcott confirmed the political reform stance of the Commission since Walcott had been the center of controversy in 1885 when Robinson failed to reappoint him to the Board of Health, Lunacy, and Charity. At that time Walcott had been characterized as the champion "of decency over indecency; of purity against impurity; of honor against bestial dishonor." Cognizant of the obstacles which had separated the tenet of control from the reality of negligence, Walcott asked that a special board be appointed "to guard the public interest and the public health . . . with the ultimate hope, which must never be abandoned, that, sooner or later, ways may be found to redeem and preserve all the waters of the state."[27]

The Act to protect the purity of inland waters was passed in June 1886, essentially following the recommendations of the Commission. Three months earlier an independent State Board of Health had been re-established. Now, with an engineering department responsible for the supervision of all water supplies,

26. "Resolve for the Appointment of a Commission to Consider a General System of Drainage for the Valleys of the Mystic, Blackstone and Charles Rivers, and certain other portions of the Commonwealth," *Acts and Resolves 1884, Chapter 63* (May 28, 1884), p. 388. The governor was authorized to appoint five members, not more than two from one municipality, who in turn were authorized to hire engineers. The members might be compensated, but the total appropriation was not to exceed $20,000. Besides Quincy, commission members were Solomon B. Stebbins, Edmund W. Converse, Edward D. Hayden, and Leverett S. Tuckerman.

27. Boston *Daily Globe*, June 8, 1885; *Report of a Commission Appointed to Consider a General Drainage System for the Valleys of the Mystic, Blackstone and Charles Rivers* (Boston, 1886), pp. lxi-lxii. This report was published as a separate document. See George C. Whipple, *State Sanitation: A Review of the Work of the Massachusetts State Board of Health*, 2 vols. (Cambridge, Mass.: Harvard University Press, 1917), II, 58.

sanitary reformers had reason to hope that scientific management would guard the public wealth from private abuse.[28]

Governor Robinson had found it financially inexpedient to recommend an independent board of health in 1885. A year later, prodded by the threat of cholera and smallpox and by political Independents who continued to desert the Republican party and to accuse it of failure to curb the power of patronage, Robinson asked for a new board of health. Responding also to pressure from the medical profession, he argued that "such a board can work with entire harmony within itself . . . relieved of the consideration of subjects foreign to the underlying principle of its organization. Medical and scientific men, sanitarians and specialists take a lively interest in the question, and from them a state board of health would receive most abundant aid, the benefits of which could not fail to reach the people."[29] The joint Board had failed to function effectively, and the proposal to separate responsibility for health from the administration of welfare encountered no opposition in the legislature.

The Governor moved swiftly to nominate a Board of Health which met with approval from his former critics. The choice of three doctors, including Walcott, was singled out as particularly appropriate by the Medical Society and the Boston Society for Medical Improvement.[30] The appointment of a manufacturer from Springfield and another from Williamstown tacitly acknowledged that sanitary problems accompanied the expansion of industry to the western part of the state. Hiram F. Mills, chief engineer of the Essex Company in Lawrence and a consultant to industry and municipal governments throughout the United States and Mexico, became chairman of the committee on water control and sewage, a position he would hold with distinction for the next twenty-eight years.

The Board was authorized to hire additional full-time personnel to assume specific responsibilities. A physician was to be engaged as the medical officer

28. "An Act to Protect the Purity of Inland Waters," *Acts and Resolves 1886, Chapter 274* (June 9, 1886), pp. 230-231. "An Act to Establish a State Board of Health," *Acts and Resolves 1886, Chapter 101* (March 24, 1886), pp. 82-85.

29. George D. Robinson, "Annual Address," *Massachusetts Senate Documents 1886, No. 1* (Jan. 7, 1886), p. 59. In addition, Robinson expressed opposition to pharmacists who wished to take over inspection of the purity of drugs stating that it was "unwise . . . to assign the work . . . to boards or officers who are not qualified by education or experience for such analysis and inquiry" (*ibid.*, p. 58). Sensitive to earlier criticism, he stated that separating the functions of the Board in no way implied a rebuke to the joint Board.

30. *BMSJ*, 114:499 (May 27, 1886). The other physicians were Frank W. Draper of Boston and Elijah U. Jones of Taunton.

and secretary to the Board; three engineers were to supervise the annual reports on water and sewage which towns and cities throughout the Commonwealth were required to submit.[31]   Broader powers "of a more decidedly executive character" were given to the Board, and a letter was sent to all local governments warning that the laws regarding health would be rigorously enforced to "prevent their infringement by individuals, corporations or municipalities, either from ignorance, carelessness or selfishness." The Board spoke with new authority, in part a reflection of statutory rights but even more an indication that new knowledge on the cause and nature of infectious disease required respect and cooperation beyond any other consideration.[32]

This Board was clearly destined to open a new era in public health. The application of the principle of scientific expertise to supplement and, when necessary, to replace the beneficence of individual conscience was an attempt to resolve the conflict between personal and social responsibility. On the one hand, the powers of the Board had steadily increased since 1869. On the other hand, between 1879 and 1886 opposition to control had been better defined and was less amenable to extralegal appeals which sanitary reformers had traditionally relied on; exhortations by the Board for cooperation from local boards of health and requests that manufacturers refrain from polluting water were frequently ignored or contested. In the first seventeen years of state public health the Board had conformed to its advisory function. If its advice went unheeded, the Board had but one response — more advice; if directly challenged, the Board had no power of its own and could only turn to the courts. Although the new Board was clothed with additional legal powers, in the next twenty-eight years it was rarely involved in a contest where the courts played a decisive role.[33]   Advice which had previously been hortatory assumed the power of law in its own right, complementing statutory requirements. No attempts to deal

31. The other members of the Board were Julius H. Appleton, Springfield; Thornton K. Lothrop, Beverly; and James White, Williamstown. Dr. Samuel W. Abbott was named health officer and secretary, and the engineers were Frederic P. Stearns, Joseph P. Davis, and X. H. Goodnough; see Massachusetts State Board of Health, *Eighteenth Annual Report* (1887), pp. 1, xx. The length of service of these men contrasts with the lack of permanent professional personnel in earlier years; Abbott, who had been health officer of the joint Board, served until his death in 1904; Stearns, until 1914; Goodnough, until 1930.

32. Massachusetts State Board of Health, *Eighteenth Annual Report* (1887), pp. x-xi. The Board was responsible for enforcement of laws in relation to nuisances, water and ice supplies, sewage, food, milk, and drugs, However, the Board began and ended its list of responsibilities with the need to determine and control the cause of infectious disease.

33. Robert H. Whitten, *Public Administration in Massachusetts: The Relation of Central to Local Activity* (New York, 1898), pp. 14-18, 71-74. For a discussion of changing values which led to acceptance of controls, see Wiebe, *Search for Order*, pp. 148-151, 161-163.

with these "golden years" can avoid the conclusion that part of this authority rested with the prestige that the Board acquired from the social commitment and professional competence of the men who became identified with the control of disease.

As chairman of the Massachusetts State Board of Health from 1886 to 1914, Henry Pickering Walcott became the prototype of the physician-statesman. His years in office encompassed the shift from a policy directed to the restraint of disease through sanitary engineering to a program designed to identify, control, and eradicate disease through medical means. Walcott's part in this decisive reshaping of public health practice was characteristically cautious and tactful. In his first year as chairman of the Massachusetts Board of Health he was also president of the American Public Health Association. Addressing the convention in conservative tones, Walcott suggested a middle course between the enemies of public health who opposed all efforts to regulate potential sources of disease and "the excessive zeal of the advocates of state control in medicine, who advance claims not fully justified by the present position of sanitary science." Taking as his model the skillful horticulturalist who protects his crop from physical harm but depends on nature to restore health, Walcott conceived of his role as that of a watchful citizen, protecting an innocent and ignorant public from the injuries inflicted by the urban and industrial environment, rather than as a medical scientist conquering disease.[34] The important advances in medical knowledge and the firm institutionalization of public health science which took place while he was chairman of the Board tended to obscure Walcott's involvement in the conflicts inherent to reform in this period of Massachusetts history.

Central to these conflicts was the sentiment that measures for public welfare must be removed from the arena of political conflict. This principle permitted liberal reformers at the end of the century to pronounce themselves above partisanship and to counsel moderation and adaptation rather than drastic change. Alarmed by the signs of violence in the United States exemplified by President Garfield's assassination in 1881, fearful of labor unrest epitomized by the Homestead strike of 1892, responsible citizens were reminded that laws and institutions could not of themselves change the ways of evil men. Caught between the need to maintain order in an increasingly alien world and their commitment to

34. Walcott, presidential address in *Public Health Papers and Reports*, 12:2-3. He continued later, "We may watch nature, and discover what she does, and by what organs she does it, and that is all," p. 10. Walcott was a lifelong member of the Massachusetts Horticultural Society and its president from 1886 to 1889.

an almost mystical belief in the inherent lawfulness of economic and social change, those who traditionally assumed that virtue was the primary qualification for public leadership sought for kindred spirits to fill the vacuum created partly by their antipathy to the mores of business and industry.[35]

Businessmen, with their excessive interest in making money and their lack of social and cultural refinement, must prove themselves worthy of public trust. In this setting Charles R. Codman, president of Boston's Provident Association and member of the State Board of Lunacy and Charity, wrote a candidate desiring membership on the Board that "to establish a claim you ought to be able to show not only good character & reputation but also special fitness for the position in question — some experience in dealing with charitable institutions as well as experience in dealing with matters of general business — and you ought to be able to show that you can give the time requisite & necessary for proper performance of its duties."[36] Clearly the ranks from which qualified men could be drawn was thinning; desire to serve and blameless reputation must be reinforced with both experience and leisure.

Walcott fit most of these requirements, and, although his private practice left little spare time, he had already demonstrated a willingness to endure the unpleasant notoriety which more and more often accompanied public service. The dismissal of a "subordinate" in the Lowell office of the Department of Out-door Poor who was charged with immoral behavior brought Walcott into publicized conflict with Charles F. Donnelly, chairman of the State Board of Health, Lunacy, and Charity. Although Walcott's term on the Board had expired in June 1885, when the whole matter came to public attention, he insisted on entering the controversy since the conduct of the Board as a whole was at stake. Walcott accused Mr. Donnelly and Mr. Wheelwright, Superintendent of the Out-door Poor, with making the Lowell agent a scapegoat and attempting "to conceal the real points at issue by cunning misstatements." These were, according to Walcott, the improvident spending of funds and, even more, the use of public office to hide a nest of corruption and protect guilty persons at all levels by revealing

35. This is not to dismiss the reformer's fear of immigrants or workers and the general disenchantment well documented by Sproat in "*The Best Men,*" by Mann in *Yankee Reformers in an Urban Age,* and by Barbara Miller Solomon in *Ancestors and Immigrants: A Changing New England Tradition* (Cambridge, Mass.: Harvard University Press, 1956). However, with rare exceptions, "the dangerous classes" in Massachusetts represented no real threat to public office, either elected or voluntary, until the next century.

36. Codman to F A. Bradford, March 2, 1891, quoted in Huggins, "Private Charities in Boston," p. 145.

one scandalous situation in the hope that this would divert attention from more serious crimes.

The Boston papers published the charges and countercharges at a time when Walcott's reappointment was before Governor Robinson. The *Globe* took up Walcott's case and stated that he was in disfavor because he had carried out his obligations honestly and refused to curry to special interests represented by the state's pharmacists, dairymen, members of the Board, and state officials. Walcott, for his part, maintained that his record was his best defense against the charge of inefficiency brought by his enemies. He implied that certain members of the Board, and Mr. Donnelly in particular, sought public office to improve their private interests and therefore failed to support certain regulatory measures in return for special favors granted by private business and high government officials. Walcott's friends said that he had earned the enmity of the state's drug manufacturers by insisting that they submit to impartial supervision, and that these manufacturers had been responsible for scurrilous attacks upon his professional reputation.

Although Governor Robinson failed to reappoint Walcott at this time, the fight continued in the press. The *Advertiser* accused the *Globe* of using Walcott's appointment to further its partisan attack on Republicans; the *Globe*, which traditionally supported Democratic candidates, maintained that the Republicans, who high-handedly insinuated that Democrats were the friends of corrupt political practices, were guilty of just such behavior themselves. It was the Republican Robinson rather than the Democrat Butler who abetted such impropriety, they stated, by making appointments of "non-professional men who will go along to fill vacancies."[37]

37. Walcott's charges and Donnelly's defense must be pieced together from the press since they never received official acknowledgment in the board's published reports. See Walcott's letter in the Boston *Daily Advertiser*, June 12, 1885; also Boston *Daily Globe*, April 18, 1885; Boston *Herald*, and Boston *Advertiser*, June 8, 1885; *BMSJ*, 112:611-612 (June 18, 1885). It is difficult to make sense out of Robinson's refusal to reappoint Walcott; both his political supporters and opponents urged it. One is forced to conclude that for some reason not apparent in published letters and public statements, Robinson was unwilling to join in the attack on Donnelly's honesty and disgression, which Walcott had certainly made the focal point of his criticism. Donnelly, a successful lawyer and reformer in his own right, may well have been the victim of anti-Catholic feeling. Some Democrats accused him of being a crypto-Republican, who had deserted his social class and party. Donnelly succeeded Howe on the Board of State Charities in 1875 and was appointed to the joint Board in 1879. Butler failed to reappoint him, but Robinson did so later, lending some substance to the charge that Donnelly's sympathies were with the Republicans. Donnelly continued on the Board of Lunacy and Charity until 1907. He was best known for his efforts to prevent state interference with Catholic education; see Katherine E. Conway and Mabel Ward Cameron, *Charles Francis Donnelly* (New York: James T. White and Co., 1909), pp. 18-47, 243-244.

Dr. Walcott, having made his case in a number of letters to the press and the *Boston Medical and Surgical Journal*, retired gracefully from the dispute. He not only had won support from Robinson's enemies and from the medical profession, but, in his four years as chairman of the Health Committee, he had initiated important work for the control of water pollution and the adulteration of food. What was more, undeterred by partisan concerns, Walcott had been able to work with Robinson's predecessor, Butler, as had few others of his social class and political persuasion.[38] When the State Board of Health was reorganized in 1886, Walcott and his supporters felt that their principled position was properly recognized when Robinson named Walcott chairman. Already forty-eight years old at this time, he was neither of the older generation which welcomed the Civil War as the culmination of a struggle between good and evil, nor at home with the young men who sought to reawaken enthusiasm for reform through endorsement of Cleveland's candidacy. Walcott had begun his career of public service in the "brown years" which the younger Mugwumps denounced, and for him there were no sharp breaks in the tradition which gave social and political responsibility to the educated and affluent elite.[39]

Born in Hopkinton and educated in Salem at the Fiske Latin School, Walcott had shown no evidence of strong interests beyond what was expected of him as a good scholar. Upon graduation from Harvard in 1858, he wrote his commencement disquisition on "The Women of the *Iliad* and *Odyssey*," but he was still unsettled about his future. "I may study law or I may study medicine," he wrote in the *Class Book*; "My highest ambition in life is to prove myself not unworthy of my father's name." Although he had not been drawn to any professional or business commitment, his academic record was superior, and he was elected to Phi Beta Kappa along with his classmate, Henry Adams. Adams delivered the Class Day Oration that year, chastising his fellow students for their complacency and lack of ambition for anything more than "wealth and the position which wealth gives," and for looking forward to "lives devoted neither to the welfare or the harm of others, but to simply going through the world as comfortably as may be."[40] Although Walcott may have been challenged by

38. G.H.B. [Bigelow], "Henry P. Walcott," *NEJM*, 207:1001-1002 (Dec. 1, 1932).

39. Blodgett, *Gentle Reformers*, pp. 20, 30. The difference between the energy of the younger reformers, as described by Blodgett, and Walcott's less ambitious approach, is partially a change in style between two generations.

40. "1858 Harvard Classbook," Harvard Archives, Widener Library; *Class of 1858, First Trienniel Report, July 1, 1861* (Cambridge, Mass., 1861), p. 19; *Report of the Class of 1858 of Harvard College* (Boston, 1898), pp. 139, 145; Henry P. Walcott, "Some Cambridge Physicians," *Cambridge Historical Society Publications*, 16:114 (1931); Milton J. Rosenau, "Henry Pickering Walcott (1838-1932)," *Proceedings of the American Academy of Arts and Sciences*, 68:688 (1932-1933).

these words, there is no evidence to show what caused him to turn to the study of medicine. He took the usual course, attending lectures at the Harvard Medical School and working under the distinguished Cambridge physician, Morrill Wyman. In 1861 he transferred from Harvard to Bowdoin, presumably in order to graduate sooner and serve in the Civil War. However, in June he left the United States for travel and study in Paris and Vienna; when he returned in November 1862 Walcott began the practice of medicine in Cambridge. His Civil War service consisted of four months during the summer of 1864, spent in Provincetown, Massachusetts, attached to a unit of the Massachusetts Voluntary Militia. By the end of the Civil War he had married and settled on Waterhouse Street in Cambridge where he would spend the rest of his life. When his wife died in 1879, he was left with two small sons, a busy private practice, and the companionship of the Cambridge community.

For the next fifty-two years Walcott's life revolved around his service to the Commonwealth of Massachusetts and Harvard University. By temperament, training, and habit, he was prepared to associate with those Cambridge gentlemen who devoted themselves to the ideal of making government responsive to the educated.[41] Public documents, a few speeches, and interviews with the press are almost the only records of this man whose few leisure hours were occupied with cultivating his garden and the friendship of like-minded friends who shared his comfortable world and agreed that "Character, not money or social position, but above all things character — is the most important element in success."[42]

Elected to the Harvard Board of Overseers in 1887, Walcott became a Fellow of the Corporation in 1890; from then until his resignation from Harvard's governing body in the spring of 1927, much of his time and loyalty were intimately engaged by the affairs of the university. In addition to these responsibilities and his services to the state, in both cases positions without salary, Walcott continued to care for his patients and to give advice on the wide range of ailments

41. Philip Putnam Chase describes "The Cambridge Idea" in "Some Cambridge Reformers of the Eighties: Cambridge Contributions to Cleveland Democracy in Massachusetts," *Cambridge Historical Society Proceedings*, 20:31-32 (1934): "diagnosis of political ills and the patient study and experiment in a coldly scientific spirit of the ways and means of public administration, and the persistent effort to secure the acceptance by politicians of policies based on sound principles of political science, and finally practicing of these principles when burdened with the responsibility of office." For Walcott's contribution, see Ephraim Emerton, "Recollections of Sixty Years of Cambridge," in *ibid.*, p. 58.
42. From an interview with Walcott on his resignation as chairman of the board of Massachusetts General Hospital, Boston *Sunday Post*, Feb. 17, 1929.

brought to his attention as a family doctor. In medical therapy he was a traditionalist, relying on tried and accepted treatments and eschewing innovative or radical ideas.[43]

The few months that Walcott studied abroad appear to have had little effect on his scientific interests. While other physicians were stimulated by their experiences in European universities to turn away from private practice and instead to pursue studies in pathology and bacteriology, Walcott was never drawn to laboratory investigation.[44] The optimism of scientists during the 1880's and 1890's when multiple discoveries identified specific microbic organisms responsible for a whole host of diseases did not fundamentally alter Walcott's position. He believed that contemporary obstacles to sanitary reform were no different in substance than those of the earlier period; the critical determinant was responsible leadership in all areas, including public education, public parks, and morality in public office.[45] He argued that the ability to provide these services depended on social and moral rather than technical considerations, and spoke of defending the general welfare against "the selfish interests . . . represented too efficiently for the public good by trained advocates."[46]

43. Walcott was consulted by his neighbors and friends about their own illnesses and those of their servants and acquaintances. See letters from Elizabeth C. Agassiz, April 30 and Dec. 26 (no year); from Congressman William Everett, July 16, 1894, questioning whether he had been overcharged by a Washington physician; from Arthur Gilman, April 15, 1893, asking Walcott to be health adviser to the Society for the Collegiate Instruction of Women; and from Charles P. Bowditch, July 7, 1893, for information on how to disinfect some antique furniture from France against cholera, all in the Walcott Letter Collection at the Clendening Medical Library, Kansas City, Kansas.

44. For a discussion of two leading public health physicians whose work began in the laboratory, see Charles-Edward Amory Winslow, *The Life of Herman M. Biggs, Physician and Statesman of the Public Health* (Philadelphia: Lea and Febiger, 1929), and Donald Fleming, *William Welch and the Rise of Modern Medicine* (Boston: Little, Brown, 1954). The latter book, much more than a biography, is in part a study of the knotty problem of the relation between scientific and social reform.

45. Walcott also served on the State Civil Service Commission and the Cambridge School Committee and was an adviser to various citizens groups concerned with public parks; see Charles Francis Adams to Walcott, Feb. 16, 1893, Oct. 26, Nov. 13, 1894; Henry Pickering Bowditch to Walcott, Feb. 7, 1893; F. E. Abbott to Walcott, April 2, 1893; Edward Atkinson to Walcott, June 6, 1894, in Walcott Letter Collection.

46. Henry P. Walcott, "State and Preventive Medicine in Massachusetts," *Medical Communications of the Massachusetts Medical Society*, 16:330 (1889). The extent to which lawyers were linked to "self-interest" in this period is in interesting contrast to their previous high repute: Daniel H. Calhoun, *Professional Lives in America: Structure and Aspirations 1750-1850* (Cambridge, Mass.: Harvard University Press, 1967), p. 193, sees this coming from an interaction of the content of the professions with their changing social function. For the adaptation of earlier reform attitudes to the crises of the late nineteenth century, including the transference of antiforeign sentiment from temperence advocates to those concerned with public education, see Wiebe, *Search for Order*, chap. iii, esp. pp. 57-58, 62-66.

As chairman of the American Public Health Association in 1886 he had affirmed a basic optimism in the successful outcome of a public health program based on restraint and education. Twenty-six years later his view had somewhat sharpened, and he reminded the International Congress on Hygiene and Demography that "affluence pays with what it can easily afford, but poverty pays with its life."[47] Although he claimed a special role of skill and responsibility for the physician in public health, it was as an educated citizen rather than as a trained physician that he chaired the Board of Health. In his public office he represented the conscientious layman who called on the trained specialist for advice and aid when the need arose.

For Walcott the distinction of public health practice in Massachusetts was the tradition of informed public support which gave the local board of health unique responsibility. Like public health reformers a half-century before, Walcott believed that the ultimate guarantee of health must rest with the individual person, for "[T]he Statutes of the Commonwealth have imposed on the layman the duty of practising the requirements of sanitary science, and the development of that science as distinct from the art of medicine has removed, to a certain extent, the veil that has hidden the mysteries of the caste."[48] But there were two important differences between Walcott and his predecessors. First, by Walcott's time science had become a more forceful arbiter of correct strategy; second, disease which resulted from failure to obey the rules was believed to be less an indication of individual moral culpability than of the immorality and irresponsibility of society as a whole. When Walcott spoke of the particular obligation of the state to the weak and the poor, he drew his lesson again from agriculture where the parasitic disease strikes the "tender growth . . . and when the surface of the plant is wounded."[49] The analogy recalled a romantic view of the healthy agrarian society invaded by the pathology of disruption and disorder, and Walcott beckoned the state to defend the powerless against the invading parasites of the urban-industrial complex.

Contrary to Henry Adams' Class Day prediction, Henry Walcott in his adult life never questioned the distinct responsibility he bore for the welfare of others. Although there were times when Walcott watched over the interests of the Commonwealth and Harvard simultaneously, placing him in the position of running

---

47. Walcott, "Public Health in America," *Transactions of the Fifteenth International Congress of Hygiene and Demography*, 1:70 (Washington, D.C., 1912).
48. Walcott lecture notes, from papers collected by his granddaughter, Mrs. Henry M. Keyes.
49. Walcott, "State and Preventive Medicine," p. 369.

the store from both sides of the counter, he saw no ambiguity in his role. He derived his authority for both tasks from his competence as an educated and willing servant of the institutions to which he looked for progress. Public hygiene was but one facet of the total need to shore up a distended society; sanitary reform must draw on every science, including statecraft, so that legislation might modify dangerous conditions "with the least disturbance or injury to the rights of others."[50]

It was statecraft, rather than medicine or science, which Walcott depended upon to win the struggles for improved public health in Massachusetts. Very seldom did he identify his opponents beyond the statement that they were "private" and "selfish" and "would not be tolerated in any civilized community outside of America." If Walcott did not call the enemies of progress by name, however, there is no question where he looked for its friends. Men like Charles W. Eliot, president of Harvard, could be depended upon. Beneath the formal exterior of the fifty-year correspondence between Walcott and Eliot, their mutual understanding and admiration required no explicit acknowledgment. When Eliot died, Walcott paid him the tribute they both valued most: "this life . . . was a life of service from beginning to end."

At the beginning of the twentieth century Walcott continued to affirm that the solution to conflict between the legitimate needs of the weak and the selfishness of the powerful was in the leadership of the conscientious, responsible, educated, and affluent class. Medical science had made its contribution, but Walcott's hope for the future rested with the avowal that "there has never been a period in history when wealth has been so sensible of its duties."[51] The refrain of moral commitment required a consensus of values; social responsibility required acceptance of these values as a standard. Between the years 1886 and 1914 the value of life as measured by longevity increased, and the standard of health became defined by the achievement of science. The concept of duty took on a new dimension, framed by the possibility of preventing disease rather than charitable concern for the susceptible. It was myopic attachment to an earlier tradition as well as far-sighted optimism in the ultimate balance of duty

50. Walcott, *The Physician, the College and the Commonwealth* (New Haven, Conn.: 1893), p. 8, address at the Yale Medical School graduation. In addition to serving on the Harvard Board of Overseers, as advisor on physical education, medical education for the University, and women's health for the "Harvard Annex," Walcott was acting president of Harvard during Eliot's extended absences between 1901-1905. The concept of a "distended society" is from Wiebe, *Search for Order*.

51. Walcott lecture notes, Mrs. Keyes' collection; eulogy of Charles W. Eliot, *Proceedings of the Massachusetts Historical Society*, 60:10 (1927); "Public Health in America," p. 70.

and needs that permitted Walcott to bridge the divide between moral and scientific authority. During the years that he was chairman of the Board of Health, Walcott presided over the decline of private conscience as the viable determinant of sanitary reform and the institutionalization of scientific hygiene as the incontrovertible source of preventive policy and practice.

Sanitary reform was peculiarly susceptible to the social pressures of postbellum years. If the anticipated regeneration of moral behavior proved something less than satisfactory, the emergence of more formalized therapeutic and preventive practices allowed hope for the future. Faith in science permitted a new role for humanitarian reform.

During the Civil War the Sanitary Commission had shown that the undisciplined benevolence of the volunteer could be effectively replaced by professional organization. In the last decades of the century, scientific philanthropy as well as scientific hygiene offered the chance to replace chaos with order. The social obligation of responsible citizens was increased rather than diminished by contrasts between affluence and poverty, by evidence that good will was an inadequate stimulus for reform. Scientific and social laws converged, and, when properly understood and utilized, could compensate for the frailty of errant individuals. Public health reformers were more confident than ever before that the influence of good men could be translated into statutes and institutions, that the State Board of Health could transform advice into regulation.

4 Science Defines the Methods and Goals of Public Health, 1888–1914

While sanitary engineers and laboratory scientists asserted that their knowledge of new methods to control contagious disease should determine the scope of sanitary policy, Walcott as chairman of the Board of Health retained a view that might well have limited their authority. He repeatedly hesitated to endorse the reformulation of public health goals derived from what he considered experimental work. The potential effectiveness of a preventive measure depended on statistical rather than laboratory verification, and Walcott was slow to ask legislative endorsement for procedures that strayed from the customary restraint of proven "nuisances." However, by the last decade of the century Walcott, like most middle-class Americans, came to believe that the public was best protected by the professional. It was not so much because of their knowledge as because of their superior character that "the supervision of these public interests must of necessity rest in the hands of medical men."[1] The highly trained and skilled scientists whom Walcott brought to the service of the State Board shared this view of their role and saw an analogy between their exposition of parasitism in nature and parasitism in political and social life.[2] They were a remarkable

1. Henry P. Walcott, "State and Preventive Medicine in Massachusetts," *Medical Communications of the Massachusetts Medical Society*, 16:323 (1889), and *The Physician, the College and the Commonwealth* (New Haven, Conn., 1893), p. 9. In contrast to his attitude toward physicians, Walcott appears to have had a low opinion of the competence of engineers; he specifically exempted Mills and a few others. See Walcott to C. W. Eliot, April 26, 1891 and Feb. 17, 1892, Eliot Correspondence, Harvard Archives, Widener Library, Cambridge, Mass.
2. Theobald Smith, in a speech to the American Social Hygiene Association (1905) quoted in Earl Baldwin McKinley, "Theobald Smith," *Science*, 82:575 (Dec. 20, 1935). This is not to suggest that the complex relationship between host and parasite could be simplistically applied to society, but rather that these scientists saw disease and its pre-

group of men, trained in the science of biology. Their focus on the bacteriological etiology of preventable disease placed responsibility for negligence firmly in the hands of the powerful rather than the weak. In the process of establishing the vigor and competence of the biological sciences in preventive hygiene, they challenged the identity of filth and disease and refined both the ideology and program of public health reform.

Among the professional scientists drawn to the work of the Massachusetts Board of Health, William Thompson Sedgwick and Theobald Smith were exceptional for their insight into the broader implications of their research. While both men centered their work in the laboratory, they were profoundly aware of the import of their findings for scientific methodology and of public attitudes toward the control of disease. They were unusual in their ability to question theoretic assumptions which had assumed the status of axioms and to pursue with disciplined imagination problems which less skilled and resourceful men would have put aside. They saw themselves as seekers after truth and as teachers, and in both these fields they were enormously successful. Both of them came to Massachusetts as mature men, trained entirely in American universities. In very different ways they both attracted others to emulate their careers and style of work. Sedgwick was warm, generous, solicitous, and fondly referred to by his younger colleagues as "The Chief." Smith was reserved, methodical, and demanding; his reputation for frugality was often re-established. Sedgwick worked primarily to extend the scope and accuracy of environmental controls over milk-and water-borne disease through bacteriologic techniques, while Smith's grasp of immunology led him to see the laboratory as the source of diagnostic and preventive intervention. These approaches eventually led public health officials to pay attention to the infected individual as the focus of contagion; inevitably this brought the state, as represented by the Board of Health, into a new relationship with the individual. Together with the identification of specific organisms as the causative agents of disease came the discovery of hu-

---

vention in a new way as a result of their understanding of the process of infection and resistance; see Theobald Smith, *Parasitism and Disease* (Princeton, N.J.: Princeton University Press, 1934), pp. 168-171, 192. Simon Henry Gage, Smith's teacher and friend, recounted that, when Gage was preparing an address for the American Association for the Advancement of Science in 1899, Smith suggested in jest that Gage should "Take a nice general subject such as parasitism vs. Tammany, or protective inoculation vs. political venality, and trace the relationship between leucocytosis and hoboism as illustration of the biological and sociological ills." See Gage, "Theobald Smith, 1859-1934," *Cornell Veterinarian*, 25:226 (July 1935).

man carriers of infection whom the state must control through appropriate diagnosis, prophylaxis, and treatment.[3] Both Sedgwick and Smith believed that the social effects of disease must be alleviated by first controlling the biological sources of infection.

Although Sedgwick's work as biologist to the State Board was done under the umbrella of environmental sanitation, his most significant contributions were made through the initiation of epidemiologic investigations of a specific disease, typhoid. The correlation of statistical data on the incidence of diarrheal diseases with information on the pollution of water was the foundation of Sedgwick's work. From this beginning, which had been the approved method of controlling disease since Lemuel Shattuck's sanitary surveys, Sedgwick elaborated techniques in which prevention was allied to the elimination and cure of infection. His pioneering epidemiological studies combined the methods of the biologist, the sanitary engineer, and the statistician to deal "scientifically" with pollution and skirt some of the opposition on which proposals calling for "responsible self-restraint" had foundered. When Sedgwick was asked to investigate local typhoid epidemics in the early 1890's, the work of the Lawrence Experiment Station had already made the mechanical filtration of contaminated water a reasonable alternative to the elaborate and costly sewage irrigation proposed fifteen years earlier for inland centers of population.

Legislative endorsement of a comprehensive and ultimately regulatory state water policy in 1886 had given the Board of Health the role of determining the limits of pollution which could be tolerated. As a result, the new Board moved to establish an engineering laboratory under the guidance of Hiram Mills. Two considerations were cited in requesting an additional $2,500 for the scientific study of sewage-polluted water. In the first place, a central experiment station would be more economical than investigations conducted by local water boards. Even more important, the laboratory could assure uniformity of scientific standards, particularly as new microscopic methods supplemented traditional chemical tests of potability. Beginning in 1887, the Lawrence Experiment Station conducted systematic tests to differentiate between the effectiveness of natural oxidation and that provided by stone and sand filters. At the same time the

3. E. O. Jordan, G. C. Whipple, and C.-E. A. Winslow, *A Pioneer of Public Health: William Thompson Sedgwick* (New Haven, Conn.: Yale University Press, 1924), pp. 64-65. E. O. Jordan, "The Sphere of Bacteriology," *Science*, n.s., 20:657-666 (Nov. 18, 1904). There are innumerable instances of the debates which this shift engendered; for a pertinent example, see Charles V. Chapin, "Sanitary Inspection" and the discussion following, *Journal of the Massachusetts Association of Boards of Health*, 12:170-189 (Jan. 1903).

Board opened separate microscopy, bacteriology, and chemistry laboratories for further supervision of local water supplies.[4]

These laboratoratories and the installation at Lawrence offered unmatched opportunities for scientists studying water-borne bacteria in a period when private and institutional support for research was practically nonexistent. The absence of university resources for experimental work reflected the indeterminate position of "theoretical" studies when even academic institutions needed to justify scientific scholarship by assuring its connection with the useful professions. While university scientists in all fields were considered primarily teachers, biologists held a particularly anomalous position; their discipline seldom rated the dignity of an academic appointment, let alone a laboratory. It was, instead, lumped under the catchall of "natural science."[5]

When Francis Amasa Walker brought Sedgwick to the Massachusetts Institute of Technology as assistant professor of biology in 1883, Sedgwick's first responsibility was to broaden undergraduate premedical interest in the life sciences. His experience and training made him a fine candidate for this assignment. After completing undergraduate studies at the Sheffield Scientific School of Yale in 1877, Sedgwick entered medical school. Dissatisfied with the rigid curriculum, which left no room for questioning medical theory, he transferred to the new Johns Hopkins University in Baltimore to study biology and physiology under Henry Newell Martin. At Hopkins he found a congenial and stimulating intellectual community where the student was urged to ask questions and seek answers in the laboratory rather than to memorize legends of dubious validity. After receiving his doctorate in 1881, Sedgwick stayed on for two more

4. Massachusetts State Board of Health, *Eighteenth Annual Report* (1887), pp. xxxviii-xxxix, and *Nineteenth Annual Report* (1888), pp. 25-43. Professor T. M. Drown and Mrs. Ellen H. Richards did the chemical tests at M.I.T.; microscopic studies of vegetable organisms were done by a biologist, George H. Parker, and Sedgwick reorganized the bacteriological work. See *Twentieth Annual Report* (1889), pp. xi-xii. For a description of methods, see *ibid.*, pp. 30-31. For a summary of the early work at the Lawrence Experiment Station, see Hiram F. Mills, "The Filter Supply of the City of Lawrence and its Results," in *Twenty-fifth Annual Report* (1894), pp. 545-547. The rapid increase of work can be judged by the fact that, in 1887, $600 was spent for work at M.I.T. and $727 at the Lawrence Station. The next year $1,200 was spent at M.I.T. and $7,792 at the Lawrence Station, plus an additional $16,000 for salaries. There was also a special appropriation of $25,000 spent in 1888 to investigate sewage disposal for the Mystic and Charles river valleys; see *Nineteenth Annual Report* (1888), pp. lv-lvi, and *Twentieth Annual Report* (1889), pp. xii-xiii, lxxv.

5. George H. Daniels, "The Pure Science Ideal and Democratic Structure," *Science*, 156:1702-1703 (July 1967); Charles Weiner, "Science in Higher Education," in Michael C. Hall and David Van Tassel, eds., *Science and Society in the United States* (Homewood, Ill.: Dorsey Press, 1966), pp. 176-183.

exciting years as Martin's assistant. His appointment to the Massachusetts Institute of Technology offered him a chance to communicate his enthusiasm for biology to a new generation of students, but practically nothing in the way of facilities for encouraging laboratory research. With the establishment of the Lawrence Station in 1887, Sedgwick and his students found the opportunities which the meager finances of the school could not provide.[6]

There was no reason for Sedgwick to look elsewhere for laboratory resources. Since its inception the Board of Health had relied on experts from the community to sanction its authority on controversial issues. In the first year that Sedgwick was in Cambridge he had been asked to join a colleague, William Ripley Nichols, "consultant" chemist to the Board for a number of years, in a study of the relative merits of coal and water gas.[7] As the Board became the source of state policy on water and sewage, it naturally turned to Sedgwick for help. His appointment as biologist to the Board in 1888 formalized a relationship which already existed.

In the next two years Sedgwick and his students developed and applied techniques for the identification and quantitative analysis of the microorganisms in water and sewage, inaugurating procedures for the routine water examinations conducted by the Engineering Department of the State Board of Health. These studies set the standard methods of determining the purity of water which were accepted by the Board in November 1890 and became the classic exposition of scientific methodology in this field. In the years that followed, sanitarians from other states and countries frequently consulted the Lawrence Station for aid in their own work. The impossibility of entirely preventing contamination

6. Jordan and others, *Pioneer of Public Health*, pp. 17, 28, 31, 37-38, 40, 177-178; Barnett Cohen, "Comments on the Relation of Dr. Welch to the Rise of Microbiology in the United States," *BHM*, 24:320-322 (July-Aug. 1950); Donald Fleming, *William Welch and the Rise of Modern Medicine* (Boston: Little, Brown, 1954), pp. 32, 104.

7. "A Study of the Relative Poisonous Effects of Coal Gas and Water Gas," Massachusetts Board of Health, Lunacy, and Charity, *Sixth Annual Report* (1885), pp. 275-313. This study concluded that there was a higher poisonous content in water gas; however, the conclusions were based primarily upon statistics showing a large number of accidental deaths among users of water gas in Boston and Baltimore. This investigation was part of an attempt by the coal gas manufacturers to get "scientific" support for continued monopoly of this utility, used for both heat and light. A similar situation occurred in 1886 when paper manufacturers, who were large importers of rags from European cities, attempted to get a "scientific" statement on whether smallpox and cholera could be imported through these rags and to have specific disinfecting procedures established. The case has additional interest since Louis D. Brandeis was counsel for the paper manufacturers. See Charles F. Withington, "An Inquiry into the Transmission of Infectious Diseases through the Medium of Rags," Massachusetts State Board of Health, *Eighteenth Annual Report* (1887), pp. 1-69.

of water in densely populated communities became accepted, and the investigations at Lawrence concentrated on methods for removing bacteria and inorganic matter. Innumerable experiments were conducted to determine the filtering properties of different soils, and these trials were annually repeated and reported to the Board of Health. By 1892 the Experiment Station found that it was possible to construct a system that would economically filter two million gallons of water daily and at the same time remove over 99 percent of all bacteria.[8]

While this work went on at Lawrence, the Board's Committee on Water and Sewage continued to try to restrict pollution and differentiate between benign and harmful contaminants. All but seven towns in Massachusetts with a population of 4,000 or more had public water supplies by 1891, and the three special laboratories responsible for assaying the purity of water handled over 4,000 requests for examinations as contrasted with 2,000 two years before.[9] There was a marked rise in disease rates for Lowell, Lawrence, Chicopee, and Holyoke, cities where sewage continued to pollute the water supplies. The population in other Massachusetts cities, however, enjoyed improved health, and the difference

8. *Examinations by the State Board of Health of the Water Supplies and Inland Waters of Massachusetts, 1887-1890*, Pt. II (Boston, 1890), describes the chemical and biological principles of water filtration by precipitation, mechanical filtration, and combined systems. Although sewage filtration had been practiced by some inland towns since 1876, this was essentially straining to remove silt. The Board pointed out that the water supplies in these towns were frequently "merely filtered sewage, and not so well filtered, nor as pure, as the effluent from some of the sewage filters at the Lawrence experimental station, where the supply, entirely from a city sewer, is filtered through a depth of five feet of sand," Massachusetts State Board of Health, *Twenty-first Annual Report* (1890), p. 69. See also Gary N. Calkins, "The Microscopical Examination of Water," in *Twenty-third Annual Report* (1892), pp. 397-492; George W. Fuller, "Experiments at the Lawrence Experiment Station Upon the Purification of Water by Sand Filtration," in *Twenty-fourth Annual Report* (1893), pp. 449-450. After 1881 the application of Robert Koch's (1843-1910) methods for the growth of bacterial organisms on solid media brought new precision to investigations in the bacteriological laboratory. As the work increased in all departments, the Lawrence Station became more independent of the Water and Sewage Committee, see the *Thirtieth Annual Report* (1899), p. 590.

9. Massachusetts State Board of Health, *Twenty-first Annual Report* (1890), p. lxvii; *Twenty-third Annual Report* (1892), pp. xxiii, xxxvi, 340. In 1898 there were 75 applications for advice, making a total of 583 since 1886, *Thirtieth Annual Report* (1899), p. xxx. By the end of 1902 all of the Commonwealth's 33 cities and 135 of 320 towns had public water supplies, with only 10 towns of more than 5,000 population supplied by wells. As control of public water supplies became increasingly routine, the Board was consulted by institutions and manufacturing establishments using private wells, which were generally found in poor condition; see *Thirty-fourth Annual Report* (1903), pp. 305, 18-19, 46-48, 167-168. Eleven years later all towns of more than 5,000 had public water, and 95 percent of the state population was supplied, *Forty-fifth Annual Report* (1914), pp. 245-246.

was ascribed to the successful control of the physical environment and most particularly to the extended protection of public water.[10]

The pertinence of bacteriologic research which, in the ten years preceding 1890, identified a host of specific pathogenic organisms, was not immediately apparent, so the Board focused on the general elimination of pollution as the proven method of preventing disease.[11] The benefits gained from providing the cities with pure water were a matter of record; annual reports for 1889 and 1890 cited a decrease in the proportion of urban to rural deaths and a comparable reduction in the proportion of deaths from "zymotic" as compared to other causes.[12] Although six years later laboratory diagnosis and immunologic techniques would dominate the activities of the Board of Health, the report for the year ending December 1889 suggested only further application of sanitary primciples based upon the assumption that sickness always accompanied uncleanliness.

Between 1889 and 1893 the emphasis of preventive sanitary practice in Massachusetts shifted. Policy in the preceding decade had concentrated on control of gross pollution, identification of bacterial and industrial contaminants, and filtration of sewage. There had been important modifications of earlier absolute identification of filth with disease, as the acceptance of a general "germ theory" made it possible to consider dirt the concomitant of disease rather than its causative agent. The gap between modified theory and habitual practice remained, however, while typhoid rates in Lawrence and Lowell soared.[13] In December

10. A special investigation of diphtheria in Lawrence typically accounted for the generally poor health in that city by indicating lack of precautionary measures in disposal of household wastes (Massachusetts State Board of Health, *Twenty-third Annual Report* [1892], pp. 387-415).

11. Some of the more important pathogenic organisms which were identified, largely in German laboratories in this decade were: typhoid and malaria, 1880; tuberculosis and glanders, 1882; cholera and streptococus, 1883; diphtheria and tetanus, 1884; E. coli, the organism responsible for much enteric disease, 1885; and pneumococcus, 1886. See George Rosen, *A History of Public Health* (New York: M.D. Publications, 1958), p. 314.

12. Massachusetts State Board of Health, *Twenty-first Annual Report* (1890), pp. xxx-xxxi. A slight increase in the death rate was accounted for by unusual epidemics, inaccurate birth statistics, and increased deaths from "local," i.e., constitutional causes. Increased deaths among children under five was a major concern. The death rate in 1890 was the lowest since 1879, with a corresponding decrease in deaths from "dangerous diseases"; see *Twenty-second Annual Report* (1891), pp. xliv-xlvii. The old categories "zymotic" and "constitutional" continued for another six years, although there were signs that physicians associated with the State Board considered them outdated, see *Journal of the Massachusetts Association of Boards of Health*, 2:24-28 (April 1892); see below, n. 33.

13. Supervision of water systems restricted gross pollution in most other cities, and, in a report on the geographic distribution of certain diseases, Dr. Abbott concluded that this control was responsible for a marked reduction in deaths from typhoid fever; see

1889 the Board of Health published a circular stating that "typhoid fever is an infectious disease . . . undoubtedly communicable, though not positively infectious in the restricted sense of personal contact." Although the typhoid bacillus had been identified in 1880 by Karl Joseph Eberth, a German bacteriologist, the medical profession in Massachusetts was divided on whether the organism caused or merely accompanied the disease. Bacteriologic technique made it possible to culture the bacillus from the feces of typhoid patients, but the *specific* etiology was not considered of critical importance for either diagnosis or control, and the Board was satisfied with a statement that "the poison of typhoid fever is conveyed . . . through the medium of fecal discharges."

The work of the Board of Health laboratories between 1890 and 1893 was very largely devoted to determining the means by which typhoid fever was transmitted.[14] In December 1890 Sedgwick was asked by the Lowell Water Board to investigate a typhoid epidemic in that city. Although the trained personnel at the laboratories were convinced that typhoid fever did not exist without the typhoid bacillus, as far as the city officials of Lowell were concerned effective proof awaited the painstaking epidemiologic report which Sedgwick delivered in April 1891.[15] With this investigation Sedgwick for the first time directly applied the methods of the laboratory to the practical work of a field study. Accompanied by his assistant, George McLaughlin, he personally visited every typhoid patient to determine the exact date of the onset of symptoms. At the same time he presented the explicit hypothesis that typhoid was primarily a water- or milk-borne disease, and stated the conditions that must be met to ful-

---

Massachusetts State Board of Health, *Twenty-third Annual Report* (1892), pp. 825-830. Lowell and Lawrence were permitted to continue using the Merrimack for drinking water, although sewage was emptied into it within twenty miles. Lawrence had a typhoid rate five times higher than Boston, and Lowell reported mortality from typhoid increased 340 percent between 1889-1890 and 1890-1891; see the *Twenty-fourth Annual Report* (1893), pp. 16-29, and William T. Sedgwick, "An Epidemic of Tyhpoid in Lowell, Mass.," *BMSJ*, 124:397-402, 426-430 (April 23, 30, 1891).

14. Massachusetts State Board of Health, *Twenty-first Annual Report* (1890), p. lvii; Hiram F. Mills, "Typhoid in its Relation to Water Supplies," in the *Twenty-second Annual Report* (1891), p. 525; "Tyhpoid fever is one of the diseases now generally attributed to one of the bacteria known as the typhoid bacillus." Next year, George W. Fuller, a biologist at the Lawrence Experiment Station, reported on methods for differentiating typhoid from other bacteria in contaminated water; see the *Twenty-third Annual Report* (1892), pp. 638-641. The culturing methods were an adaptation of procedures reported by Dr. Theobald Smith in a German journal of bacteriology.

15. Sedgwick's articles cited above were expanded in a number of later reports; see, especially, "On Recent Epidemics of Typhoid Fever in the Cities of Lowell and Lawrence Due to Infected Water Supply; With Observations on Typhoid Fever in Other Cities and Towns of the Merrimack Valley, Especially Newburyport," Massachusetts State Board of Health *Twenty-fourth Annual Report* (1893), pp. 667-704.

fill this theory. Sedgwick found that Lowell had five water systems, three of which were drawn more or less directly from the Merrimack River. As this had been true since 1876, his problem was to demonstrate a palpable reason for a typhoid epidemic in this year as distinguished from the past. In the course of his work Sedgwick reported that he was unable to isolate the typhoid bacillus from any of the Lowell water supplies.

He stated, however, that, far from proving the absence of this organism, this fact only pointed to the inadequacy of bacteriologic or any other method when used alone, and it substantiated the need for a flexible association of all scientific sanitary knowledge. Fecal bacteria were abundant in the water supplies, and for these, unlike vegetable organisms, the river was not a grave but a home. With utmost care Sedgwick traced the source of infection to an outbreak of typhoid in Lowell's neighboring village of North Chelmsford and then proceeded to describe the course of the organism from privies on the banks of the Merrimack to the Lowell water supply. Systematically eliminating all other possibilities and vigorously denying claims that the mill people were particularly susceptible to typhoid because of their habits and constitutional weaknesses, he concluded that "we shall look in vain for any adequate explanation of the constant excess of typhoid fever in Lowell and still more in Lawrence except to the fact that both these cities have constantly distributed to their citizens water, unpurified, drawn from a stream originally pure but now grossly polluted with the crude sewage of several large cities and towns.[16]

The investigation at Lowell was followed in the next several years by similar studies of other epidemics. With the relish of a good storyteller, Sedgwick would unravel a plot in which the villain was a bacterial organism; the victim, the unwitting public; the hero, sanitary hygiene brought to life through the application of scientific methods. Where earlier investigations were primarily concerned with the symptoms of disease as manifested in the individual and society, Sedgwick centered his study on the causative agency and a determination of its pathogenicity.

Sedgwick believed, however, that comprehending the nature of microscopic life implied more than discovery of the specific etiology of disease. Scientific inquiry into the origin, structure, and function of bacterial organisms could re-

---

16. Sedgwick, "Typhoid Fever in Lowell," p. 400, describes the fallacy of the self-purification theory; see also his "Epidemics of Typhoid," p. 699. He added that the age of the mill hands corresponded to the years of highest susceptibility and that this, compounded with the poor working and living conditions, contributed to the severity of the epidemic.

veal the mechanism which determined all life processes. He was critical of medical education which concentrated on anatomy and descriptions of disease in terms of pathological symptoms, and believed that biology could rescue scientific training from the sterile study of morphology which characterized British and American curricula. Sedgwick, no less than Lemuel Shattuck, was interested in determining the order of nature's law which could be delineated by investigating the life cycle of microbic and more complex organisms. For Sedgwick, explorations in biology had a larger purpose than the pleasure of discovery or the acquisition of knowledge about the prevention and cure of disease; they taught the "most important lesson for the conduct of life . . . that the human body has a material basis and is a *mechanism*, a *machine*." The historical study of origins, which had been given new impetus by Darwin, could now move to a more advanced stage. Sedgwick believed that the method of biological investigation was more important than its findings, for the systematic study of the origins and processes of life brought order to disparate facts and made it possible to understand both the natural and the man-made worlds.

He concluded that the history of science and the investigation of a specific typhoid epidemic were both valid sources of information about human behavior. The usefulness of science was manifold to Sedgwick; it could serve as a guide to personal health, a framework for sanitary reform, or the philosophical underpinning for a rational cosmology.[17] The relationship between research and its application was direct and inescapable, so that Sedgwick found a symbiotic relationship between the scientist teaching in the university and the scientist working for the State Board of Health; he took for granted the common interest of the academic community and the Commonwealth. The scientific method and scientists themselves were uniquely equipped to assume leadership in society, he concluded, since society was inevitably moving toward a bureaucracy based on scientific law, the law of reason. Far more explicitly than Walcott, Sedgwick

17. Quote from Sedgwick and Theodore Hough, "What Training in Physiology and Hygiene May We Reasonable Expect from the Public Schools?" *Science*, n.s., 18:356 (Sept. 18, 1903); Sedgwick, "The Origin, Scope, and Significance of Bacteriology," *Science*, n.s., 13:125-126 (Jan. 25, 1901); Sedgwick, "The Expansion of Physiology," *Science*, n.s., 25:336 (March 1, 1907). Sedgwick's integration of his scientific specialty within a broader framework had many expressions both in writing and activity: he introduced a course in the history of science for the first time in an American university; he was curator of the Lowell Institute Lectures from 1897 to 1921. For a summary of his affiliations and major publications, see Jordan and others, *Pioneer of Public Health*, pp. 116-123. See also Sedgwick, "The Outlook for Preventive Medicine," reprinted in *ibid.*, pp. 85-86.

claimed that scientists should have principal responsibility for direct hygienic intervention to promote the public health.[18]

The differences between Walcott's and Sedgwick's assumptions were not clearly defined at this time; nor did either man express the thought that conflict might eventually develop. There was no confrontation of priorities but, instead, an attempt to incorporate the concept of bacterial specificity within the older framework. Walcott's postulate, that those well endowed would exercise a special responsibility for the public health, was sufficiently flexible to include the scientist. Sedgwick, in turn, saw the acceptance of scientific law as the necessary basis for responsible social organization. During the last two decades of the nineteenth century the successful application of new scientific knowledge for the control of disease created a surge of optimism. This achievement postponed the conflict between a view that disease is primarily the social manifestation of individual ignorance and the view that disease is primarily a physiologic manifestation of the intrusion of a bacterial organism. Even the minor skirmishes that an occasional issue produced were hidden by the gradual accretion of practical accomplishment.

The policies of the State Board of Health for the protection of public water from human and industrial defilement successfully merged the concept of individual self-restraint with final judgment and disposition by the expert. The obligation of the state to prevent willful or negligent contamination of water was not likely to be contested after 1890. Since the heaviest centers of population had access to the ocean for sewage disposal, the sanitary program for the eastern seaboard concentrated on prevention of pollution rather than the treatment of polluted supplies. With the construction of a filter bed for the city of Lawrence in 1893, the work of the Experiment Station was applied for the first time on a local level, demonstrating an important advance in protective sanitary policy.[19]

18. Sedgwick, "Attitude of the State Toward Scientific Investigation," *Science*, n.s., 13:93-94 (Jan. 13, 1901). When Sedgwick wrote about "academic science" he referred to theoretical work since he saw the university as the proper setting for research. In a talk on "Scientists and Technicians in the Public Service" (1911) he said that "scientists and technicians alike, — must be employed and paid by the people, to rule over them as well as to guide them, to constitute a kind of official class, a kind of bureaucracy constituted for themselves by the people themselves," quoted in Jordan and others, *Pioneer of Public Health*, p. 134. See also *Journal of the Massachusetts Association of Boards of Health*, 2:31 (April 1892).

19. Massachusetts State Board of Health, *Twenty-fourth Annual Report* (1893), p. 559.

With the principle and methods for control of water-borne disease no longer a matter for debate, Sedgwick took the lead in pointing to the protection of milk as the next critical area for the promotion of public health. His first approach was simply to transpose successful methods of ensuring purity through the restriction of contamination. Water and milk played identical roles as vehicles for the transmission of typhoid, but in following the logic of his argument Sedgwick temporarily ignored the contradiction in his analogy. Where water could be protected from defilement, could be untouched by human hands, cow's milk, even in the simplest society, required man's interposition. The possibility of contamination was greatest in large cities where milk was touched by many hands and mouths before it reached the public. As early as 1890 Sedgwick had sent his students to count the bacteria in Boston milk. At first he believed that a system of local inspection and licensing of dealers combined with supervision of dairies could identify and eliminate contaminated milk. By the fall of 1897, after further bacteriologic studies, he concluded that pasteurization was the only sure protection from milk-borne disease.[20]

Opposition to pasteurization came from many sides and reflected not so much the absence of state authority to protect the purity of milk as uncertainty about the locus and nature of the infecting agency. Within the Board of Health there was no unanimity on appropriate policy. Physicians considered that sterilized milk was indigestible and harmful to the delicate digestive tracts of infants. Dairymen, particularly farmers from small western Massachusetts communities, already suffered from the low price of milk and saw pasteurization as an unnecessary and burdensome expense. Sedgwick and Dr. Charles V. Chapin, health officer of the Providence, Rhode Island, Board of Health, were the lone spokesmen for pasteurization at an 1897 gathering of the Massachusetts Association of Boards of Health.[21]

20. The routine procedure for discovering soured milk was to have a taster go from can to can, often using the same ladle; see Sedgwick, "On the Protection of Milk Supplies from Pollution," *Journal of the Massachusetts Association of Boards of Health*, 7:4, 11, 31 (March 1897); Sedgwick, "Bacteria and Acidity of the Milk Supply of Boston," in *ibid.*, 7:75-85 (Sept. 1897).

21. Theobald Smith joined the support for pasteurization at the fall meeting. The Massachusetts Association of Boards of Health was organized in January 1890 as a result of a call from Lemuel F. Woodward of the Worcester Board. Walcott was president of the group until 1913, and the membership came from local boards and others concerned with health issues; the large dairies regularly sent representatives. The meetings were unusually fruitful, partly due to participation of Sedgwick, Smith, and Chapin. The annual July meeting was the high point. Hosted by the Boston Board, the group would go by launch to the Quarantine Station on Gallop's Island for a shore dinner and meeting. After 1932 divisions representing professional specialties were established, and in 1936

At the meeting Sedgwick argued that although it was indeed necessary to produce milk under the cleanest possible conditions, "milk ought to be Pasteurized at the very latest very soon after it is drawn from the cow." Robert Burns, representing the large Boston Dairy Company, presented the dilemma most clearly. "I myself am afraid to drink milk without knowing the source from which it comes," he said, "and, when I go among my poor families, I hardly know how to tell them to Pasteurize their milk . . . [in order to] get the best results. We want to get the source pure, and as fresh as we can, and get it as soon as we can from the supply into the hands of the consumer; but it seems to me, while restrictive laws are very necessary, and I thoroughly agree with the suggestions of the committee, that something might be done tentatively in the way of education, certain measures that they could take without great expense, which I think, would help the matter."[22] The "restrictive laws" prescribed by the Board of Health involved standards of cleanliness which required individual vigilance at every point from the farmer to the consumer.

The Board continued to endorse the motto "Be Clean" as the core of its policy. Conforming to this principle ten years later, Walcott rejected a proposal from Nathan Straus to replicate a New York experiment and distribute "sterilized" milk to the poor of Boston as part of an effort to reduce infant deaths from summer diarrhea. In 1907 Walcott believed that the best way to guarantee clean milk for the consumer, even in the urban slums, was to prevent contamination. He responded to Straus's philanthropic offer by reiterating Massachusetts' superiority of control over supply and transportation of dairy products. "The additional handling which pasteurization requires," he wrote, "would with us constitute a serious addition to the danger always imminent from unclean or infected hands — which has always appeared to me as the principal source of mischief."[23] If the Board had accepted the proposition that pasteurization was

the group was reorganized as the Massachusetts Public Health Association. The *Journal of the Massachusetts Association of Boards of Health* began publication somewhat irregularly as a quarterly beginning in January 1891, when the group had ninety-five members. See Francis P. Denny, Roy F. Feemster, and Samuel C. Prescott, "Fifty Years of Public Health in Massachusetts: A Brief History of the Massachusetts Association of Boards of Health, 1890-1936, and its Successor the Massachusetts Public Health Association, 1936-1940," pamphlet of the MPHA, n.p., n.d.: pp. 5-8, 17, 21.

22. Sedgwick, "Milk Supply of Boston," p. 84; *Journal of the Massachusetts Association of Boards of Health*, 7:100 (Sept. 1897).

23. Walcott to Jerome D. Greene, Feb. 20, 1907, Eliot Correspondence, Harvard Archives: "State and Preventive Medicine," p. 325. Discussion of pasteurization continued to draw the same advocates and opponents; see *American Journal of Public Hygiene and Journal of the Massachusetts Association of Boards of Public Health*, 14:38-57 (1904-1905). A report from the State Board of Health in 1906 stated unequivocally that pasteu-

a necessity, it would have implied that its supervisory and educational programs were insufficient to protect the purity of milk. Reliance on pasteurization would, in Walcott's view, terminate the ultimate responsibility of the individual to preserve conscientious cleanliness. For Walcott, whose concept of prevention rested on enlightened restraint of the human rather than the bacterial organism, the price was too high to pay.

Underlying the changes that did take place in the program of the Board in the last decade of the nineteenth century were hesitant shifts in the attitude toward disease itself. In 1884 the legislature passed a law requiring the family and physician of any person sick with "small-pox, diphtheria, scarlet fever or *any other disease dangerous to the public health*" to give notice to the selectmen or local board of health.[24] The purpose of this notification was avowedly to prevent further contagion through contact with the infected person or members of his family. Since in many instances the selectmen doubled as the board of health or if a board did exist it functioned only upon call, compliance with the statute depended upon the cooperation of individuals directly involved with the sick person. From 1886 to 1892 the State Board in its annual summary of reports from local boards noted that, for the most part, measures for the protection of health were limited to garbage and sewage disposal. Attention to specific disease was almost entirely restricted to the larger cities where there was a demand for separate infectious disease hospitals to care for the poor.

The concept of contagion remained sufficiently vague to support a demographic study as the necessary basis for a "thorough knowledge of the natural history of infectious diseases." Although with increased municipal organization the reporting of infectious disease continuously improved, the Board requested more stringent legislation "for the purpose of tracing the course and origin of epidemics."[25] By implication the purpose of registration was not primarily to

---

rization had a deleterious effect and "too much reliance should not be placed upon municipal milk stations and philanthropic distribution." The remedy for milk-borne disease was clean milk and breast feeding of infants; see *Monthly Bulletin* of the State Board of Health, 1:134 (Dec. 1906); 2:46 (Feb. 1907); 2:185-186 (Aug. 1907). Beginning in 1929, all milk sold in Boston was pasteurized or certified, and other cities followed.

24. "An Act Concerning Contagious Diseases," *Acts and Resolves 1884, Chapter 98* (March 21, 1884), pp. 77-78; a fine was levied against the individual for noncompliance, and notification of the school committee in each town was mandatory. "An Act to Prevent the Spread of Contagious Diseases Through the Public Schools," *Acts and Resolves 1884, Chapter 64* (March 7, 1884), p. 50; any member of a family in which smallpox, diphtheria, or scarlet fever was present could not attend school until two weeks after the patient recovered or died.

25. Abbott, "On the Geographical Distribution of Certain Causes of Death in Massachusetts," Massachusetts State Board of Health, *Twenty-third Annual Report* (1892),

identify the sick individual and restrict his activity but, rather, to provide additional data and enhance the usefulness of vital statistics. By 1893, however, attention had turned to the actively infected individual, and the legislature required local boards of health to notify the State Board of all dangerous diseases at the time of diagnosis.[26]

Larger cities and towns complied with the new provisions, but more than half the towns with a population of 5,000 or less failed to do so. Lack of response from these smaller towns was partly the result of failure to assign official responsibility; it also reflected disagreement over what precautionary steps were necessary to prevent disease. In 1893 disease was still considered as primarily coincident with the overcrowding of an urban environment. Even when the specific disease was acknowledged to be contagious, susceptibility was accepted as an inevitable concomitant of bad living conditions.[27] This conclusion led the State Board back to the position that its effective responsibility was limited to establishing an environment that would allow the individual to seek good health stimulated, they hoped, by the best educational experience.

Five years later the annual reports from the cities and towns showed a marked increase in the reporting of some contagious diseases, particularly diphtheria and typhoid, and by 1907 the Board had persuaded the legislature of the need for a more extended medical framework in the registration of morbidity. An act passed that year gave the State Board the entire responsibility for naming the diseases henceforth to be classified as dangerous, leaving "no discretion to individuals and local authorities in defining the terms." In August a list of sixteen

---

p. 760, 877-888, and "Isolation Hospitals for Infectious Diseases," in the *Twenty-fifth Annual Report* (1894), pp. 691-716. Diseases continued to be classified as "zymotic" or "constitutional" despite Abbott's efforts to abandon such distinctions "since the modern discoveries of bacteriologists have shown the true character of diseases of this class," *Journal of the Massachusetts Association of Boards of Health*, 5:88 (Dec. 1895); 6:10-17 (March 1896).

26. "An Act Relative to Notices from Local Boards of Health in Cases of Diseases Dangerous to the Public Health," *Acts and Resolves 1893, Chapter 302* (May 3, 1893), pp. 938-939.

27. Massachusetts State Board of Health, *Twenty-fifth Annual Report* (1894), pp. 446-448. See also report from Boston Board in *Twenty-third Annual Report* (1892), p. 884: "One of the evils which this Board is called upon to combat is the practise [sic] of overcrowding which prevails in the tenement-houses in certain sections of the city . . . The two principal causes of overcrowding are, first, the inclination to live in a densely inhabited neighborhood; and, second, to economize. The people who are addicted to this habit are, with some rare exceptions, uncleanly in their habits and not accustomed to good sanitary surroundings, and evince little desire to improve them. That they are aware that they are violating some law or sanitary regulation is clearly shown by their uniform habit of concealing the truth as to the number of occupants in their habitations."

reportable diseases was issued, including meningitis, tuberculosis, measles, whooping cough, and scarlet fever. The steps that finally brought each case of contagious disease into the domain of public surveillance entailed a tentative recognition that the distinction between personal hygiene and public sanitary measures was not absolute.[28] It accompanied a shift in the attention of the Board of Health from the environment to the laboratory.

   Laboratory techniques for the diagnosis of disease were a distinct adjunct to preventive methods available up to 1894. Clinical identification of individual cases of disease was independent of whatever aid the state laboratories might offer, and the environment remained the focus of control. It was the attempt to restrict the spread of diphtheria among urban school children that first led to reliance on laboratory diagnosis of specific etiology and the differentiation between causes and conditions of contagion. As with the typhoid bacillus, laboratory identification of the Klebs-Loeffler bacillus did not automatically establish its causative role in diphtheria for Massachusetts physicians. An epidemic of diphtheria in Worcester during the winter of 1892 stimulated discussion of the relation of the organism to infection. Dr. Samuel W. Abbott, speaking as secretary of the State Board, maintained that confusion arose from a failure to distinguish between the source of the disease and the situation which nurtured it. "We are apt to say that overcrowding and damp cellars are causes of diphtheria," he said. "I do not think so," he continued. "[T]hey are merely conditions . . . These conditions are no more causes than is the soil in which a tree grows the cause of a tree. The real cause of the tree is the seed. If you furnish the seed with light, air, heat and moisture it will grow and become a tree. The same is true of the germs of diphtheria, if you furnish them with the proper conditions they will flourish." The very next year the Boston Board of Health specified that, in mild or convalescent cases of diphtheria, medical inspection by a

28. Quote from Massachusetts State Board of Health, *Thirty-ninth Annual Report* (1907), p. 5. For reports from towns, see *Twenty-seventh Annual Report* (1896), pp. 766, 772-775, 777-778; *Twenty-eighth Annual Report* (1897), pp. 870-872, 878, 884-885, 888-894; and *Thirty-fourth Annual Report* (1903), pp. 576-590. For legislation see "An Act to Authorize the State Board of Health to Define What Diseases are to be Dangerous to the Public Health," *Acts and Resolves 1907, Chapter 183* (March 8, 1907), p. 139; "An Act to Provide for the Compulsory Notification of Tuberculosis and Other Diseases Dangerous to the Public Health," *Acts and Resolves 1907, Chapter 480* (June 6, 1907), pp. 436-438. The specific diseases mentioned were smallpox, diphtheria, and scarlet fever, or eye irritation in a less than two-week-old infant. Failure to notify could result in a fine of up to one hundred dollars. Studies of infantile paralysis were begun by the State Board in this same year. See also E. O. Jordan, "The Problems of Sanitation," *JAMA*, 50:494 (Feb. 15, 1908).

physician could not rule out a continued infectious condition; the only dependable criterion for "the actual disappearance of the specific germs of disease" was by means of bacteriological investigation.[29]

Although the official reports of the State Board for 1893 did not single out the control of diphtheria for any special consideration other than isolation and disinfection, by the next year the local boards in Worcester, Waltham, Lowell, and Boston took steps to establish bacteriology laboratories for the free examination of throat cultures submitted by local physicians. In addition these boards began the free distribution of diphtheria "anti-toxine," which reports from France and Germany had shown to be effective in reducing diphtheria mortality and conferring a short-term immunity from the disease.[30]

At this time the State Board had no laboratory facilities or personnel available for the diagnosis of diphtheria, but it undertook to make antitoxin available. The Board announced, in October 1894, the appointment of Dr. J. L. Goodale who would set up the laboratory and have access to horses and other animals needed for the production of antitoxin. Initial arrangements were makeshift to say the least; the horses used for the inoculation that would produce immune blood serum were stabled at Harvard's Bussey Institution at Forest Hills, and the processing of antitoxin was to be done by Dr. Goodale in a small laboratory at the State House. Although there was no suggestion that the state should provide smallpox vaccine at this time, the Board apparently foresaw this possibility and prefaced its description of the advantages of immunization from diphtheria with a review of the benefits conferred by vaccination.

Although there was no information on when or how the antitoxin would be made available, the Board took this opportunity to redefine the limits of state responsibility for the prevention of disease: "Public hygiene is a life saving department of work," said the announcement, "and the operations of a board of health which pertain to the management and control of infectious diseases should constitute one of the most important functions not only of general but also of local health organizations. The saving of human lives, both individually and col-

29. *Journal of the Massachusetts Association of Boards of Health*, 2:24 (April 1892); Massachusetts State Board of Health, *Twenty-fifth Annual Report* (1895), p. 752. Boston began medical examinations of school children with the appointment of fifty physicians in 1894, *Twenty-sixth Annual Report* (1895), p. 821.

30. Massachusetts State Board of Health, *Twenty-sixth Annual Report*, pp. 820-821, 840, 856-857, 860. Worcester was the first city to set up a bacteriology laboratory; the others called in physicians to do the diagnostic work. Boston established a plant to produce antitoxin on Gallop's Island under the direction of Dr. Harold C. Ernst of Harvard Medical School; other cities purchased antitoxin from Germany or the New York City Board of Health.

lectively, adds to the wealth and efficiency of the population, and such work deserves the highest praise and encouragement."[31] The intervening accommodation which gave substance to this sentiment and permitted the State Board to produce and distribute antitoxin between 1895 and 1904 was the close relationship of Walcott, President Eliot, and Harvard University.

Despite these initial steps to provide preventive therapy, Dr. Walcott's reluctance to initiate the production and distribution of antitoxin is a matter of record. He hesitated to seek state support for a venture which he viewed as experimental, and it was not until 1903 that Walcott requested that the legislature appropriate money to build its own vaccine and antitoxin plant. A few years before he had privately expressed his doubts as to the propriety of the state manufacture of antitoxin "as a public enterprise – from the ease with which the agent can be obtained and the purity of it." In a letter to President Eliot he acknowledged the certainty that many lives had been saved through the free distribution of this product, but pointed out that this would be true for a number of other remedial agents. "This is the only instance of which I have knowledge," he continued "where a health authority adopts measures for the care of disease, measures which are not preventive."

Although Walcott continued to believe the only preventive measures available to the state were education or environmental control, he noted that the legislature did not share his hesitation. Speaking at a meeting of the Massachusetts Association of Boards of Health in 1902, Walcott described his cautious departure from traditional public hygiene. The Board of Health had been compelled to produce antitoxin, he explained, because a commercial product of "untrustworthy character" had appeared for sale. No enabling legislation was requested at that time since "we never have asked the permission of the legislature of Massachusetts to save human life." Consequently, the work was carried on for nine years under the regular appropriation without additional expense to the state.[32]

The initial therapeutic management of infectious disease under state auspices had been accomplished with minimal commitment. During these years the state rented housing for the laboratories and stables from Harvard and shared equipment and personnel whose services and salaries were divided between the university and the State Board of Health. The right of the state to manufacture and distribute an item available on the market was not assured, but meanwhile

31. *Journal of the Massachusetts Association of Boards of Health*, 5:24 (April 1895); Massachusetts State Board of Health, *Twenty-sixth Annual Report* (1895), pp. cvii-cviii.
32. Walcott to C. W. Eliot, March 1901, Eliot Correspondence, Harvard Archives; *Journal of the Massachusetts Association of Boards of Health*, 12:127-128 (Oct. 1902).

the antitoxin laboratory was given an acceptable institutional setting in which to mature. Shortly after the first announcement that the state would produce the serum and make it available without charge, all facilities for this work were transferred from the State House to Forest Hills. The move coincided with the appointment of Dr. Theobald Smith, assistant professor of applied zoology at the Harvard Medical School, as part-time pathologist to the Board of Health. His duties included supervision of antitoxin production and direction of a newly organized State Board of Health Bacteriological Department which was to carry on "experimental and executive work in the investigation of infectious diseases."[33]

Theobald Smith was a thirty-six-year-old experimental scientist when he accepted an appointment at Harvard in 1895. He had already made significant contributions to understanding the transmission of infection and the nature of disease. As an undergraduate at Cornell, his extraordinary intellectual abilities in the study of language and mathematics as well as the biological sciences had indicated the likelihood of scholarly success in a number of disciplines. After graduating in 1881, he went on for a degree at the Albany Medical College. Both his own inclination and his teachers' advice moved him toward a career in research. In 1884 he was recommended by Cornell to Dr. Daniel Elmer Salmon, chief of the United States Bureau of Animal Industry in the Department of Agriculture, who was looking for an assistant to study the diseases destroying large numbers of cattle and hogs. Smith's work during the next eleven years as

33. Massachusetts State Board of Health, *Twenty-seventh Annual Report* (1896), p. viii. Clearly Walcott was responsible for bringing Smith to Harvard and for the arrangements which facilitated sharing laboratory equipment and space with the Board of Health; see Walcott to C. W. Eliot, Aug. 20 and Sept. 1, 1895; July 16 and Sept. 7, 1896. As the volume of work increased, Smith took over; see Smith to Eliot April 27, May 30, and July 17, 1896, all in Eliot Correspondence, Harvard Archives. The Bussey Institution at Forest Hills, Jamaica Plain, was Harvard's school of agriculture and horticulture. A large tract of land was donated by Benjamin Bussey's will in 1835, but the accompanying endowment was insufficient to support the full-scale program inaugurated in 1872. Francis Parkman, the historian, taught horticulture briefly, and the faculty often donated their services when income from the estate was depleted following burning of the Bussey stores in 1872. The State Board laboratory crowded the already limited space until 1904 when the state constructed its own building on Harvard land; see Walcott's description of the arrangement in *Journal of the Massachusetts Association of Boards of Health*, 12:131 (Oct. 1904). Harvard's program was reorganized in 1907 as a graduate School of Applied Biology. For the Bussey Institution, see Governor John A. Andrew, *Massachusetts Senate Documents 1863, No. 1* (Jan. 9, 1863), pp. 46-58; William Morton Wheeler, "The Bussey Institution," in Samuel Eliot Morison, *Development of Harvard University, 1869-1929* (Cambridge, Mass.: Harvard University Press, 1930), pp. 508-513.

director of the pathology laboratory of the Bureau earned him an international reputation. His identification of the etiology of hog cholera and swine plague, along with the development of the technique to produce artificial immunity from these diseases, and his brilliant investigation of Texas cattle fever, which revealed that the tick was the insect vector responsible for the spread of the disease, were of far-reaching practical and theoretical importance.[34]

These studies initiated Smith's lifelong work on the cause and communication of disease. He ultimately concluded that prevention could not be realistically achieved through the elimination of pathogenic parasites as such, but only through an evaluation of the correspondence between the host and the invading organism, which could lead to appropriate control. "Too often it has been assumed that parasitism was abnormal and that it needed only a slight force to reestablish what was believed to be a normal equilibrium without parasitism," he wrote in 1934, the last year of his life. "On the contrary," he continued, "biology teaches us that parasitism is a normal phenomenon and if we accept this view we shall be more ready to pay the price of freedom as a permanent and ever recurring levy of nature for immunity from a condition to which all life is subject." His first work on hog diseases introduced the theoretical and practical application of a revolutionary approach to protection from disease through artificially induced immunity; his paper, published with Dr. Salmon in 1881, "On a New Method of Producing Immunity from Contagious Diseases," opened the way for the eventual use of biological products to protect human life.[35]

Smith's work had started with animal diseases, and he returned constantly to comparative studies as the most testable source of useful generalization. At the same time he differentiated between this older method and the newer experimental techniques in which the same phenomena were consciously controlled in order to observe, measure, and record some specific aspect of the biological

34. Simon Henry Gage, "Theobald Smith 1859-1934," *Cornell Veterinarian*, 25:208-213, 218 (July 1935). Claude E. Dolman, "Texas Cattle Fever: A Commemorative Tribute to Theobald Smith," *Clio Medica* (London), 4:1-31 (1969), indicates that a series of personal and professional circumstances made Smith eager to leave the Bureau of Animal Industry by the fall of 1894. Dolman quotes a letter from Smith to Simon Henry Gage, his teacher and close personal friend, relating that Smith had been invited to Massachusetts by Walcott in January 1895. The letter, dated Feb. 17, 1895, says that Smith had accepted the position as director of the serum laboratory for the Massachusetts State Board of Health. There is nothing in the letter as quoted by Dolman to indicate that Smith anticipated a Harvard appointment at this time, although when he arrived in Boston on May 6 he moved directly into a house on the Bussey property belonging to the university.

35. Smith, *Parasitism and Disease*, p. 4; Daniel Elmer Salmon and Theobald Smith, "On a New Method of Producing Immunity from Contagious Diseases," *Proceedings of the Biological Society of Washington*, 3:29-33 (1884-1886).

process. All of Smith's investigations were marked by the consciousness that the choice of method implied the limit of realizable goals. Recognition of this boundary was not only significant for his research; it also set him apart from those who looked to the laboratory as the final answer to preventing disease. Smith acknowledged that control of disease was indeed inhibited both by inadequate powers for the sanitarian and by the selfishness of private citizens who interferred with measures destined to benefit the general welfare. However, the problems faced by the scientist in the laboratory were even more complex than those social obstacles which impeded practical application of scientific knowledge; permanent and fixed solutions were contrary to the nature of life. The principle which guided Smith obviated any simple utilization of laboratory findings, no matter how expertly derived or hypothetically beneficial, since "the character of infectious disease is due to the host as well as the parasite . . . and . . . the interaction of the two organizations causes modifications in both."[36]

When Smith was invited to come to Harvard in 1895 by President Eliot, it was with the hope that Smith's work in comparative pathology would strengthen the Veterinary School, which had been founded in 1882. The school never flourished, and Smith was appointed to the faculty of the Harvard Medical School; he moved with his family into a small house on the Bussey estate in Forest Hills and began work in a laboratory especially equipped for him in a nearby building. With the removal of the state laboratory for processing serum to the Bussey Institution in the fall of 1895, Smith took over supervision of this new phase of work for the Board.[37]

Although Smith had achieved eminence as an independent scientific investiga-

36. Smith, *Parasitism and Disease*, pp. ix-x; Theobald Smith, "Public Health Laboratories," *BMSJ* 143:492 (Nov. 15, 1900). In this same article Smith acknowledged "the frequently discouraging encroachments of politics upon the functions and functionaries of the laboratory." But he focused on internal problems where "[t]he difficulty lies less in the perversity of the experimenter than the perversity of his environment," meaning the biological environment.

37. Harvard's efforts to establish a veterinary school began in 1882 and ended unsuccessfully in 1901; see Frederick C. Shattuck and J. Lewis Bremer, "The Medical School 1869-1929," in Morison, *Development of Harvard University*, pp. 568-569. Both Eliot and Smith felt Smith's appointment could aid the State Cattle Commission, especially in the control of bovine tuberculosis. A "scientific institution not directly interested in the practical execution of the work . . . " could lay "the groundwork for any legislation . . . " and "would be in a position to supply the State with tuberculin, mallein and reliable vaccines and exercise a control over the products on sale"; see Theobald Smith to C. W. Eliot, "Proposed Scope of Work in Comparative Pathology," Eliot Correspondence, Harvard Archives. For a description of the "coextensive" functioning of the State Board of Health laboratories and Harvard's facilities, see Smith, "The New Antitoxin and Vaccine Laboratory, A Ten Years Retrospect of the Production and Distribution of Diphtheria Antitoxin," in Massachusetts State Board of Health, *Thirty-seventh Annual Report* (1906), p. 529.

tor and would have preferred to continue his research free from the responsibilities of managing the antitoxin plant, the opportunity for work was limited by the resources available. Smith's career, like Sedgwick's, reflected the status of the medical and paramedical professions at the end of the nineteenth century. While chemists and physicists had already asserted their independence from the justification of utility and set their professional goals from within the structure of their own disciplines, Smith pointed out that the biologists' work was circumscribed because "material and resources were extremely scant and this meagerness determined the direction and scope of all research."[38] When George F. Fabyan gave a substantial gift to Harvard in the spring of 1896 for the study of comparative pathology, Theobald Smith was immediately named to fill the endowed chair. From September 1896 until the summer of 1914 when he left his laboratories at Bussey to go to the Rockefeller Institute for Medical Research, Smith divided his time between Harvard Medical School and the State Board of Health.[39]

Fortunately Smith's responsibility for elaborating the production of diphtheria antitoxin made it possible for him to continue research in the broad field of immunology. The problems which arose from the first clinical use of antitoxin stimulated Smith to further laboratory exploration on the variability of organisms, the nature of selective susceptibility, and the process of acquired immunity from infection. It would be incorrect to say that Smith was uninterested in the practical outcome of his work. His scrupulous concern for accuracy made him insist that physicians receiving antitoxin from the state submit throat swabs for laboratory diagnosis and report the course of all diphtheria cases whether treated with serum or not.[40] At the same time, what engaged Smith's attention

38. Letter from Theobald Smith in *Journal of Bacteriology*, 27:20 (Jan. 1934); Smith, address to Sixth Annual Meeting of Harvard Medical School Alumni, June 23, 1896, *Bulletin of the Harvard Medical School Alumni Association*, No. 9, 1896, pp. 51, 53-55.

39. C. W. Eliot to George F. Fabyan, April 3, 5, and 8, 1896. Smith was first invited to the Rockefeller Institute in 1902; he declined, stating, among other reasons, that his work at the Bussey was just beginning to show results. See Smith to W. H. Welch, Feb. 11, 1902. By 1908 the press of state work was so great that Smith suggested the appointment of a resident director, but added "I should be very sorry to completely sever my connection with it, for it offers a certain material basis for research not to be duplicated here," Smith to Eliot, July 26, 1908; all the above are in Eliot Correspondence. For further material on Smith's understanding of the relationship between Harvard and the state, see his speech at a dinner given in his honor in June 1914 in a collection from this occasion in Holmes Hall, Countway Library. See also *The Harvard Medical School, 1782-1906* (n.p.:n.d.), pp. 157-161, a volume authorized and written by the faculty to record the history of each department.

40. First state circular on diphtheria antitoxin reprinted in Massachusetts State Board of Health, *Twenty-seventh Annual Report* (1896), p. 690; the annual reports divided data according to whether or not bacteriological diagnosis had confirmed clinical judgment.

was not the usefulness of his research for, as he frankly stated, his "interest in a problem usually lagged when certain results could be clearly formulated or practically applied." The setting did provide the necessary materials, but he felt that "discovery should come as an adventure rather than as a logical process of thought . . . The joy of research must be found in the doing."[41] It was not a matter of choice but a matter of reality for Smith; scientific investigation could not be harnessed to social justification. Nevertheless, he was deeply concerned with the relationship between theory and practice and aware that the state laboratories had a triple function.

First, production of the antitoxin required not only strict attention to the purity and strength of the product but vigilance as to its use and constant study of the possibility of extending similar techniques to other diseases. Within the next twenty years, the state introduced biologics for the control of smallpox, typhoid, meningitis and ophthalmia neonatorum.[42] Second, control of contagious disease depended in part upon identification of the human sources of infection through accurate bacteriological methods. The laboratory established at the State House in 1894 continued this work under Smith's direction, and within five years routine tests were performed for malaria, tuberculosis, and typhoid, as well as diphtheria. Third, acceptance of laboratory diagnosis by an increasing number of physicians caused local communities to establish independent laboratories of their own. As a result, in 1903 Dr. Walcott indicated that any city of fifty thousand should expect to make such facilities available.[43] While these

41. Letter from Theobald Smith in *Journal of Bacteriology*, pp. 19-20.

42. The laboratory also produced tetanus antitoxin in 1888-1889, but stopped because conditions were not adequate to assure freedom from contamination; see Smith, "The New Antitoxin and Vaccine Laboratory," p. 539. "An Act Relative to the Production and Distribution of Antitoxin and Vaccine Lymph," *Acts and Resolves 1903, Chapter 480* (June 26, 1903), p. 526; "An Act Relative to the Prevention of Ophthalmia Neonatorum," *Acts and Resolves 1910, Chapter 458* (April 27, 1910), p. 403; "An Act Relative to Specific Material for Anti-typhoid Inoculation to be Furnished by the State Board of Health," *Acts and Resolves 1912, Chapter 104* (Feb. 16, 1912), p. 78; Massachusetts State Board of Health, *Forty-fifth Annual Report* (1914), pp. 2-3, a circular stating that the Board was prepared to furnish a curative serum for cerebrospinal meningitis.

43. Massachusetts State Board of Health, *Twenty-eighth Annual Report* (1897), p. 709, announcement that the laboratory would make diagnostic tests for tuberculosis; *ibid.*, pp. 701-702, announcement that blood smears will be examined for malarial parasites; *Thirty-second Annual Report* (1901), pp. 727-729, announcement that Widal test will be performed on blood serum for diagnosis of typhoid. Physicians in the wealthier communities surrounding Boston were most easily persuaded to use antitoxin; see reports from Newton as contrasted with Holyoke, Chicopee, Lowell, and Marlboro in the *Twenty-seventh Annual Report* (1896), pp. 766. 772-775, 777-778. A year later the small towns showed greater interest, *Twenty-eighth Annual Report* (1897), pp. 870-872, 878-879, 884-885, 888-889, 892-894; by 1897 most physicians used antitoxin, *Twenty-ninth Annual Report* (1898), p. 597. On the need for municipal laboratories, see Walcott in *Journal of the Massachusetts Association of Boards of Health*, 12:126 (Jan. 1904).

laboratories were the foundation of a radically new concept — that the prime function of a board of health was to reduce the incidence and destructiveness of disease by medical means — Theobald Smith continued to stress that scientific prevention was dependent on knowledge of the *process* as well as the *etiology* of disease. He suggested that the laboratory also opened the way to disentangling "the interwoven lines of force which enter into the making of disease" and was the best place to evaluate the suitability of new methods. From the point of view of the victims of disease, the process of prevention had moved from the reformers' lectern to the bedside; it was no longer necessary to understand the laws of nature in order to obey the mandates of science. But Smith believed that the scientist must also take responsibility for determining not only how scientific sanitary hygiene should be implemented but what was to be its focus.[44]

As early as 1888 Smith had viewed the contest against disease as a complicated interrelationship expressed as "Grimm's law of disease"[45]:

$$\text{disease} = \frac{\text{virulence}}{\text{resistance}}$$

A scientific and technical understanding of the implications of this relationship was the prerequisite for the formulation of public health policy. Perhaps the most fruitful outcome of this phase of his work was his differentiation between the tuberculosis organism which infects cows and that responsible for human disease. Measures for the control of tuberculosis were linked in Massachusetts, as elsewhere, to the determination of its etiology. However, recognition that tuberculosis was a contagious rather than a hereditary or a constitutional disease did not preclude disagreement over the best means of control since the manner of contagion and the outcome of infection remained unclear.[46] While the state

44. Smith, "Public Health Laboratories," p. 492. There was much discussion at the quarterly meetings of the Association of Boards of Health over the source and implementation of public authority; see *Journal of the Massachusetts Association of Boards of Health*, 12:170-189 (Jan. 1903); 14:83-84, 101-105 (May 1904). The Association took issue with the American Medical Association for presuming to set standards of public hygiene. For a recent comment, see Geoffrey Edsall, "Public Health and the Laboratory," *AJPH*, 40:1368–1371 (Nov. 1950).

45. From a letter to Gage quoted in Gage, "Theobald Smith," p. 215. It is an interesting comment on Smith's breadth of knowledge that he used an analogy pertaining to the development of language.

46. Smith's work influenced other scientists at first more decisively than public opinion and legislation. In 1908 Koch indicated Smith's contribution on this question. Smith's first important publication on tuberculosis was "A Comparative Study of Bovine Tubercule Bacilli, and of Human Bacilli from Sputum," *Journal of Experimental Medicine*, 3:451-511 (July and Sept. 1898). A preliminary article appeared two years earlier: "Two Varieties of Tubercule Bacillus from Mammals," *Transactions of the Association of American*

offered laboratory tests for the diagnosis of pulmonary tuberculosis beginning in March 1896, another decade passed before this procedure was widely used.[47] It was another case where the identification of the causative organism did not at first affect treatment or prevention, in this case complicated by the many forms in which the disease was manifested.

Smith was among the very few who maintained, at the beginning of the century, that infection from bovine tuberculosis through the consumption of milk and meat was of minor importance. While he advocated tuberculin testing of cattle and the removal of infected cows from the herd, he vociferously attacked reliance on these measures as antiscientific, uneconomical, and mistakenly carried on in the name of public health. He believed that limited knowledge on the process of the disease made it necessary to focus on the major source of contagion, pulmonary tuberculosis, and to resist popular pressure for measures that were not useful. In an article published in 1908 reviewing the history of social and scientific prevention of tuberculosis, Smith intimated that the number of controls for a disease was inversely related to knowledge about the disease. Once again, he urged that public health measures be restricted to specific scientific and medical methods. Prevention of tuberculosis could be accomplished in three ways: suppression of contagion, increasing resistance to infection, and destruction of the bacillus after infection. Of these three methods, only a combination of the first two was available. Since the spread of disease was greatest from advanced cases, Smith advocated that the state inaugurate a program for the hospitalization and treatment of advanced cases, thereby removing them as a source of infection.[48] When the nation's first state hospital for the treatment

---

Physicians, 11:75-95 (1896). For discussion on the nature of tuberculosis, see *Journal of the Massachusetts Association of Boards of Health*, 4:2-21 (Sept. 1894). T. M. Prudden wrote in *Harper's Magazine* (1894): "Tuberculosis has in this country been officially almost entirely ignored in those practical measures which health boards universally recognize as efficient in the suppression of this [infectious] class of diseases," quoted in Richard H. Shryock, *National Tuberculosis Association 1904-1954: A Study of the Volunteer Health Movement in the United States* (New York: for the National Tuberculosis Association, n.p., 1957), p. 51.

47. See Massachusetts State Board of Health, *Twenty-sixth Annual Report* (1895), pp. lviii, lxxv, for first concern with bovine tuberculosis and suggestion that tuberculosis should be listed as contagious; *Twenty-seventh Annual Report* (1896), pp. xv-xix, tuberculosis was officially designated as contagious; *Thirty-first Annual Report* (1900), p. 674, recorded 360 specimens received during the first two years of diagnostic testing.

48. *Journal of the Massachusetts Association of Boards of Health*, 8:30-31 (March 1898). Smith, "A Comparative Study of Bovine and Human Bacilli," pp. 506-507; *Bulletin of the Harvard Medical School Alumni Association*, No. 9, 1896, pp. 61-63. Theobald Smith, "Certain Aspects of Natural and Acquired Resistance to Tuberculosis and their Bearing on Preventive Measures," second Mellon Lecture delivered at the University of

of tuberculous patients was opened in October 1898, Massachusetts launched a pioneer program.

While the State Board of Health had no specific responsibility for hospital care of tuberculous patients until 1920, the state rapidly expanded its effective role. Although the Massachusetts Hospital for Consumptive and Tubercular Patients at Rutland attempted to restrict its early admissions to patients with a favorable prognosis, popular and medical support of this combined therapeutic and preventive approach led to the construction of four more institutions. State Hospitals in North Reading, Lakeville, and Westfield had opened by 1910, and the city of Boston had established a hospital in Mattapan.[49] The State Board of Health continued to stress the infectious nature of tuberculosis, the need for early diagnosis, and the broad range of hygienic preventive measures. While deaths from tuberculosis continued to decline, the number of diagnostic tests performed annually increased eight-fold between 1896 and 1912, and elaborate programs for the dissemination of information on tuberculosis were pursued by both state and voluntary organizations.[50] The complicated problems which con-

---

Pittsburgh, 1916, pp. 26, 34-39. Smith's views were summarized in an article in the *AJPH*, 2:518 (Feb. 1908): "Now it is possible that we may be threatened again by legislative schemes to pay off the public treasury money to defray the immunization of young cattle according to von Behring's scheme. What the State can justly do is pay for suitable experiments to study this method and to prepare the vaccine, but nothing more. If the State has money to spare, it should be reserved for the care and housing of human consumptives."

49. Until 1910 each hospital was under a separate board of trustees; the first was established for Rutland in 1895. The North Reading Hospital opened in 1907, the other two in 1910. In February 1910 hospital boards of trustees were replaced by the "Trustees for the Massachusetts Hospitals for Consumptives," and in 1920 the legislature placed all tuberculosis work under the Department of Public Health; see Paul Dufault, MS "The Story of the Rutland State Sanatorium," pp. 1, 17, 22-23, in files of Division of Health Education, Massachusetts Department of Public Health. "An Act Relative to the Maintenance of Tuberculosis Dispensaries in Cities and Towns of Ten Thousand Inhabitants or Over," *Acts and Resolves 1911, Chapter 576* (June 22, 1911), pp. 600-601, imposed a fine of up to five hundred dollars for towns failing to provide care of indigent tuberculous patients; "An Act Relative to the Maintenance of Isolation Hospitals by Cities and Towns," *Acts and Resolves 1911, Chapter 613* (June 30, 1911), pp. 635-636; see also William C. Hanson, "The Maintenance of Isolation Hospitals by Cities and Towns in Massachusetts for the Reception of Persons Ill with Diseases Dangerous to the Public Health," *Monthly Bulletin* 7:60-64 (Feb. 1912).

50. Although deaths from tuberculosis declined steadily long before the identification of the tubercle bacillus, at the beginning of the twentieth century agreement about the contagious nature of the disease increased attention to diagnosis and prevention. Until 1904, however, lack of care for patients with advanced disease remained the rule; see Shyrock, *National Tuberculosis Association*, pp. 68-69. Massachusetts showed a greater rate of decreased mortality than other states where records were kept; see Hiram F. Mills, "The Supression of Tuberculosis," Massachusetts State Board of Health, *Forty-sixth Annual Report* (1914), p. 701. After August 1901 all forms of tuberculosis were declared

trol of tuberculosis continued to present caused Smith to emphasize again both the special area in which state preventive medicine should function and the absolute authority it should exercise within its proper scope.[51]

Smith's forceful guidance played an important part in setting the tone and conditions under which the laboratories of the State Board would extend their influence. The success of the antitoxin program in reducing mortality from diphtheria and the expectation that further application of immunologic techniques would fundamentally alter the contest between man and disease gave the scientist pre-emptive rights which the sanitarian had never enjoyed before. In addition, the new stature of the laboratory accompanied changes in the assumptions underlying policies of the Board of Health. By reducing the importance of the environment as the critical factor in the prevention of disease, it permitted the Board to relegate gradually to other agencies supervision which it had previously exercised, or even to view certain measures as superflous. The work of the laboratory led the Board to define the existence and character of an increasing number of the most dangerous diseases and to provide medical means for their control. Since mortality rates for these diseases were highest among children and the poor, these gave scientific justification to a program which had previously relied on a tradition of moral and social concern. Finally, because the laboratory scientist and the physician possessed specialized information and skill, these tended to place their judgment above contest. The right to sanction what steps were needed to protect the public health became the province of the specially trained and authorized.

These reassessments of the purpose and scope of the legitimate functions of the State Board of Health were in many respects an analogue of what Robert Wiebe has referred to as "the search for order" which characterized American political and social thought at the turn of the century. In the area of public health the smallpox epidemic of 1900-1902 again demonstrated the ineffective-

---

"dangerous to the public health" and therefore reportable (*ibid.*, p. 690). An exhibit on tuberculosis organized by the State Board at Horticultural Hall in Boston from Dec. 28, 1905, to Jan. 7, 1906, was attended by 25,953; see *Thirty-eighth Annual Report* (1906), pp. 2-20, and Boston *Herald*, Dec. 24, 1905; the population of greater Boston was 595,380 at this time. For a summary of activities on tuberculosis see Edwin A. Locke, ed., *Tuberculosis in Massachusetts* (Boston: Wright and Potter, 1908), a report prepared for the International Congress on Tuberculosis, Washington, D.C., 1908; "Control of Tuberculosis," *Monthly Bulletin* of the Massachusetts State Board of Health, 7:180-199 (May 1912). For the growth of voluntary organizations to combat tuberculosis, see Shryock, *National Tuberculosis Association*, esp. pp. 55-112. The National Tuberculosis Association was founded in 1904.

51. Theobald Smith, "Animal Diseases Transmissable to Man," *Monthly Bulletin* of the Massachusetts State Board of Health, 4:275-276 (Dec. 1909).

ness of isolation "in the struggle of a dense population against such a pervasive virus" and the State Board argued that protection could only be guaranteed if the state supervised the preparation of vaccine lymph and if qualified physicians performed the vaccination. While druggists maintained that state manufacture of vaccine would be an unnecessary infringement of their prerogative, Dr. Smith, as director of the state laboratories, avowed that the perishable nature of vaccine and the extreme care which must be exercised to insure its potency required Massachusetts to support compulsory vaccination by insuring proper supplies.[52] Smith also stressed the importance of accuracy in the preparation of diphtheria antitoxin and the necessity of guaranteeing adequate dosage. Acceptance of antitoxin by physicians had increased distribution by the state from 1,700 doses in 1895 to 33,000 in 1899, and an epidemic in 1900-1901 had entirely depleted available stock.[53] By the beginning of the twentieth century the State Board assumed that its responsibility to advise included the obligation to provide private citizens the means of protection. In 1903 the Board asked the legislature for an appropriation to build its own plant for the production of diphtheria antitoxin and smallpox vaccine.[54]

The state finally faced the question of whether or not the Board should be authorized to manufacture these items, already available through commercial establishments. During March of 1903, the legislative Committee on Public Health held hearings at which the representative of the Massachusetts State Pharmaceutical Association testified concerning his inspection of the laboratory

52. *Journal of the Massachusetts Association of Boards of Health*, 12:130-137 (Oct. 1902); Massachusetts State Board of Health, *Thirty-fourth Annual Report* (1903), pp. xv-xvii; Smith, "The New Laboratory," in *Thirty-seventh Annual Report* (1906), p. 540; Smith, "The New Laboratory of the Massachusetts State Board of Health for the Preparation of Diphtheria Antitoxin and Vaccine," in *Journal of the Massachusetts Association of Boards of Health*, 14:231-232, 236 (May 1904).

53. Massachusetts State Board of Health, *Twenty-eighth Annual Report* (1897), p. 655. During the twelve months preceding April 1904, 117 towns and cities received antitoxin, an increase of 23 over the previous year; almost 28,000 individuals received treatment, bringing the total number receiving antitoxin since 1895 to just under 13,000; the death rate from diphtheria in the epidemic year was a little over 5 per 10,000 but it was estimated that without antitoxin it would have been over 14 per 10,000; see *Thirty-fifth Annual Report* (1904), pp. 530-532, 535, 541.

54. "An Act Relative to the Production and Distribution of Antitoxin and Vaccine Lymph," *Acts and Resolves 1903, Chapter 480* (June 26, 1903), p. 526; there was no specific appropriation for this work until the following year. See *Acts and Resolves 1904, Chapter 95* (Feb. 18, 1904), p. 66, which contained an appropriation of $8,000; Massachusetts State Board of Health, *Thirty-fourth Annual Report* (1903), pp. xxxviii-xli. For support of this measure, see Frank L. Morse, "The Recent Epidemic of Smallpox in Massachusetts," *Journal of the Massachusetts Association of Boards of Health*, 13:60-63 (July 1903).

at the Bussey Institute. Mr. Bartlett, representing the commercial manufacturers, addressed himself to one question: whether or not the state laboratory afforded the proper scientific conditions to protect the purity of antitoxin. In contrast to "reputable plants like Parke, Davis and Company and H. K. Mulford," he found at the state laboratories that "the whole impression of the plant is one of crudeness and filth, far, far behind the times . . . As I passed through the gate and down the street," he said, "I cast one look behind, and when I contemplated that this great museum of comparative Biology and Bacteriology that we have heard so much about at the hearings, really consisted of two unsanitary and filthy stables, I could sympathize with the present inhabitants of Greece as they reflect on their former greatness and their shattered idols. I must say as a son of Old Massachusetts I turned and went away with sadness at the spectacle, saying, 'O tempora! O mores!' Only one conclusion can be drawn from these facts and that is that Massachusetts in this respect is crude, primitive and far, far behind the methods of the time in the manufacture of these products and should stick to inspecting and not attempt to manufacture them."[55]

The response of the State Board showed the authority which science had conferred on its public representative. The duty of the state extended beyond protection of the purity of biologic products and included responsibility for the application of preventive therapy. While agreeing that conditions at the state laboratories were far from perfect, Dr. F. L. Morse, director of the bacteriology laboratory for the Somerville Board of Health, assured the public that every provision had been taken to insure the safety of antitoxin provided by the state. "It is standard in everything but price," he said at the public hearing. "The State produces this at a cost of less than twenty-five cents a bottle. The druggists charge something like two dollars a bottle for what they sell."[56]

Theobald Smith protested the serious implications that Bartlett's accusations had for public policy in general, claiming that the manufacturer's testimony encouraged the uninformed to make judgments they were not competent to make and brought on political manipulation of matters that should be left free of such intrusion. "The fact is that antitoxin is prepared inside of the horse," he wrote, "but next to the horse, the most important steps are those carried on in the laboratory." Further, he specified that the difference between a public and a private laboratory is that the first finds its chief incentive in the service of science, while the second is of necessity primarily concerned with making money. Citing

55. Typescript of Barlett testimony with Theobald Smith folder, Harvard Archives, Widener Library.
56. Boston *Daily Advertiser*, March 12, 1903.

the need to combine manufacture, research, and controlled application of scientific remedies, he stated that, as far as commercial manufacturers were concerned, "they have thus far not contributed anything of value to the problem of serum therapy and vaccines . . . Progress will come only through laboratories aided by the universities, by special funds and by public institutions authorized to prepare such biological products."[57]

The legislature, after some debate, authorized the State Board to build a new laboratory for the production of vaccine and antitoxin. The move from the old plant was accomplished in the summer of 1904 without interrupting production. The new building was next door to the old one and again on Harvard property, but in many ways the slight change in location was the least significant aspect of the move. The immunity conferred by smallpox vaccine and diphtheria antitoxin was accompanied by at least a partial immunity for the State Board from what had been considered unwarranted interference from political interests. Since 1886 when Henry Walcott had been appointed chairman of the Massachusetts State Board of Health, partisan interests in various guises had been seen as threatening the responsible exercise of care for the public health. What had started with an attempt to isolate and protect the Board from "dirty politics," ended with the assignment to the Board of areas of responsibility identified as specifically exempt from political interference. If the focus of responsibility had narrowed, the prestige and power of the Board had increased. The position of the fifteen District Health Officers first appointed in 1907 to carry out the work of the State Board was an indication of this change. Assigned to different districts throughout the state, their early reports had concentrated on establishing local boards of health and inspection of unsafe factory conditions.[58] By 1910 their reports were filed by reference to prevalent diseases rather than geographic districts, and their work was more strictly medical. When factory inspec-

---

57. Letter from Theodore [*sic*] Smith, *BMSJ*, 148:431-433 (April 30, 1903).

58. "An Act to Provide for the Establishment of Health Districts and the Appointment of Inspectors of Health," *Acts and Resolves 1907, Chapter 537* (June 19, 1907), pp. 518-521. The Health Officers were to be practical and discrete persons, learned in the science of medicine and hygiene." They were to inform themselves on the sanitary conditions of their districts, and on all contagious diseases; also, they were to watch over the health of all minors employed in factories. They were to inspect factories for ventilation and cleanliness and to give advice on structural improvements although they had no right to enforce any code of safety. For a description of the districts, see Massachusetts State Board of Health, *Thirty-ninth Annual Report* (1908), pp. 3-5. Walcott stated that public concern over bovine tuberculosis and the health of minors in factories was the greatest stimulant for this legislation; see *AJPH*, 3:272 (Aug. 1907). He saw this as the culmination of the struggle against political interference; see Walcott to C. W. Eliot, July 26, 1907, Eliot Correspondence, Harvard Archives.

tion was taken over by the State Board of Labor and Industries in 1912, the Board of Health stated that its officers could now limit themselves to the "all-important field of investigation of the occurrence of diseases dangerous to the public health and to co-operating with local health agencies in the control of such diseases."[59]

Walcott, who saw disease in the individual and in society as an expression of disorder, had looked to the established sources of restraint as the best guarantee of an effective State Board. Yet he was in many ways the beneficiary of the new view that the real business of public health was to dispel acceptance of the filth theory of disease and replace it with scientifically authorized medical intervention. The new breed of sanitarian described prevention in specific terms and protected the power of the Board by assigning responsibility to a clearly identified authority. When Walcott retired as chairman of the Board of Health in 1914, a letter from 2,200 of his fellow physicians paid tribute to his service and hailed the enviable reputation the Board had achieved under his leadership.[60] A significant component of this new stature came from a commitment to science which Walcott had helped to bring into being without fully understanding or sharing its assumptions. When the Board of Health was reorganized later that year as the Department of Health, the new divisions of responsibility signaled that the search for overarching laws of health was outmoded. More and more, health could be most successfully defined as freedom from an increasingly long list of specific diseases.

59. Massachusetts State Board of Health, *Forty-fourth Annual Report* (1913), p. 589.
60. *BMSJ*, 170:819-820 (May 21, 1914); see Boston *Evening Transcript*, May 19, 1914, for editorial comment.

5 The New Politics and the New Public Health, 1914–1936

The reorganization of Massachusetts public health work in 1914 did not result from official dissatisfaction with policy or program. On the contrary, administrative changes reflected the optimism with which the Board of Health viewed the future. Confidence that the identification of contagious disease, the isolation of infected persons, application of immunologic techniques, and the conscientious protection of the environment could be successfully amplified — all supported the assumption that mortality and morbidity rates would continue to decline. Consequently, the new Department of Health was organized into six divisions which indicated no important departure from accepted preventive practice, and the competence of the Water and Biologics Laboratories encouraged new services along established lines.[1] Although there was much talk about "The New Public Health," there was little evidence before 1920 that this involved anything more than efficient administration of measures that had been well established during the previous quarter-century.

1. The principle of full-time professional direction for each area of responsibility was recognized with the appointment of salaried specialists to direct four of the divisions. However, Dr. Rosenau continued the practice of Dr. Smith, dividing his time between the State Laboratories and the Harvard Medical School; Professor Selskar M. Gunn continued full-time responsibilities at the Massachusetts Institute of Technology while directing the Division of Hygiene (Massachusetts Dept. of Health, *First Annual Report* [1916], pp. 6, 22, 26–27). A distinction should be made between the professionally oriented public health worker who emphasized increasing efficiency within a scientifically defined area of responsibility and the more grandiose vision of public health propounded in reformist journals. See Charles V. Chapin, *Sources and Modes of Infection* (New York: Wiley, 1910), or Milton J. Rosenau, *Preventive Medicine and Hygiene* (New York: D. Appleton, 1913), as contrasted with a series of articles by Alice Hamilton and Gertrude Singer on "The New Public Health," *Survey*, 37:166-169 (Nov. 18, 1916); 37:456-459 (Jan. 20, 1917); 38:59-62 (April 21, 1917).

Among enlightened public health officials, there was considerable agreement that only two obstacles impeded further progress: first, the danger that public health would become enmeshed in politics; second, the possibility that the continued exercise of restraints that were either outmoded or could more properly come under the jurisdiction of the police would negate the affect of scientifically authorized measures. The cult of efficiency, which influenced public health as much as business, education, and the conservation movement, suggested that conflict could be resolved and that the discrepancy between the ideal and the actual could be mediated through the rational application of scientific knowledge.[2]

The optimistic tranquillity which resulted from accepting the premise that there would be no radical innovation in the years ahead produced a large measure of consensus in public policy and support for the Department of Health. Because of the successes registered by the State Board of Health, it had been for many years capable of absorbing contradictory attitudes within the rubric of preventive medicine and remaining aloof from outside interference. Proclaiming that the promotion of health depended upon the efficient implementation of clearly defined scientific principles of hygiene did not, however, obviate the underlying assumption that these rules required a commitment on the part of the citizen to adjust personal behavior.

While it was true that the application of bacteriologic techniques to control contagious disease required no new social reforms, by the beginning of the new century sources of infection were shown to be more often people than things, and it became difficult to determine at what point public health encroached upon the duties of physicians or the rights of their patients. Even agreement that the Health Department should limit itself to stringently scientific and medical measures of proven value suggested a corollary of debatable merit: that the practice of medicine was to some degree a function of the state. Furthermore, although the demise of the filth theory had established the authority of the laboratory, mortality and morbidity surveys now indicated that diseases of uncertain etiology claimed more victims than contagion.

Only one "degenerative" disease was listed among the first five causes of death in 1910, but twenty years later the situation was reversed, and pneumonia, which

2. Samuel Haber, *Efficiency and Uplift: Scientific Management in the Progressive Era, 1890-1920* (Chicago: University of Chicago Press, 1964); Raymond E. Callahan, *Education and the Cult of Efficiency: A Study of Social Forces That Have Shaped the Administration of the Public Schools* (Chicago: University of Chicago Press, 1962); Samuel P. Hays, *Conservation and the Gospel of Efficiency: The Progressive Conservation Movement 1890-1920* (Cambridge, Mass.: Harvard University Press, 1959).

was not amenable to prevention through immunization, remained the sole contagious disease in this category. Quite obviously different scientific methods were necessary to prevent, or at least to mitigate, suffering from noncontagious disease. Perhaps this implied different behavior on the part of the cooperative individual as well. Addressing the Massachusetts Medical Society in his first year as Commissioner of the new Department of Health, Dr. Allan J. McLaughlin warned that significant reduction in the incidence of these noncontagious diseases could only be affected "by spread of the gospel of right living and personal hygiene through the medium of popular education."[3] Even when the laboratory had offered protection to the ignorant as well as to the knowledgeable, it was not unusual for public health workers to question the value of legislation and ordinance alone. In the words of one spokesman, the "non-intelligent masses rebel against rules they do not understand, and evade all they find safe to ignore."

Enthusiasm over decreased typhoid, diphtheria, smallpox, and even tuberculosis mortality rates only accelerated concern over how to influence those individuals who seemed impervious to education. Such an approach had implications beyond the boundaries of public health practice. As early as 1903, at a meeting of the Massachusetts Association of Boards of Health, Mrs. Ellen H. Richards had warned against the dangers inherent in "our custom to give vote and bath first and educate up to privilege afterwards." "In other words," she continued, "the law can be carried out only when the constituency is sufficiently enlightened as to its value affecting themselves."

Mrs. Richards and her contemporaries believed in the power of education. The physician, or even better the public health nurse or sanitary inspector, could give friendly instruction and, "instead of leaving irritation and animosity behind him, be welcomed as a friend and helper."[4] In the next twenty years it was less

---

3. George Hoyt Bigelow and Angelina Hamblen, "Changing Causes of Death," *NEJM*, 202:216 (Jan. 30, 1930); *BMSJ*, 173:152 (July 29, 1915).

4. Ellen H. Richards, "Educational Sanitary Inspection," *Journal of the Massachusetts Association of Boards of Health*, 13:33-34 (July 1903). Ellen (Swallow) Richards was the first woman to play a significant role in Massachusetts public health. She grew up in New Ipswich, New Hampshire, the childhood home of Lemuel Shattuck, where both of her parents were schoolteachers. Graduated from Vassar College in 1870, she was the first woman to enter M.I.T., where she received her B.S. in Chemistry in 1873. Her long career as a teacher in this institution began with assisting William R. Nichols in his studies of water pollution for the State Board of Health in 1871. She was in charge of the Board of Health Laboratory until it moved to the State House in 1897. Her interests led to the scientific study of nutrition and home economics, and she coined the word "euthenics" to describe the scientific control of the environment. As a teacher and lecturer she was identified with numerous movements for scientific social reform, both in the university and the home. See Caroline L. Hunt, *The Life of Ellen H. Richards* (Boston: Whitcomb & Barrows, 1912).

clear what the friendly sanitary inspector might have to say and even less certain that he would be welcomed into the homes of the ignorant. Efforts to improve the health of the very young and the aged, who made up a disproportionately large share of the annual mortality statistics, uncovered contradictory attitudes toward disease and the diseased. These attitudes were only temporarily breached by the exhortation to educate and inform. By the 1920's, differences over the most efficient *means* of disseminating information to mothers in an effort to reduce maternal and infant deaths revealed profound fissures in what had previously seemed near unanimity on the *purpose* of public health policy.

Dr. Charles V. Chapin, one of the earliest spokesmen for "The New Public Health," had argued in 1911 for a vigorous program confined to strictly scientific preventive measures. There was little more reason for health departments to assume responsibility for street cleaning and control of nuisances, he said, than "that they should work for free transfers, cheaper commutation tickets, lower prices for coal, less shoddy in clothing or more rubber in rubbers, — all good things in their way and tending towards comfort and health."[5] Yet if conditions which led to poor health and premature death were not amenable to quarantine, immunization, and sanitary engineering, did this absolve the state of responsibility to prevent their occurrence or diminish the burden of ill health? Without directly addressing himself to this query, and frequently not of his own volition, the professionally trained public health worker gradually assumed more inclusive responsibility for the prevention of sickness. Although it is certain that in the decade before the Great Depression the Massachusetts Department of Public Health initiated new programs which implied that disease was a social as well as a biological phenomenon, it is far less clear how the Department arrived at the stage where it felt competent to exercise newfound authority. Furthermore, these modifications were accompanied by far-reaching changes in the way that the professional and the public defined health and the nature of state responsibility.

One symptom of this change in attitude was the frequent substitution of the phrase "public hygiene" for what had previously been called "public health." Health had come to mean freedom from specific disease. Hygiene, however, which had once referred primarily to general cleanliness, now appeared as a hyphenate — "social-hygiene," "mental-hygiene," or "dental-hygiene" — and sometimes in an even more ambiguous context.[6] Although public health offi-

---

5. Chapin, *Sources and Modes of Infection*, p. 28. See also Edwin O. Jordan, "Profitable and Fruitless Lines of Endeavor in Public Health Work," *Science*, 33:834-835 (June 2, 1911).

6. Sensitivity to this ambiguity was not exclusively the result of historical hindsight;

cials were not naïvely innocent of the relationship between health and behavior, they were far from unanimous in their endorsement of measures which further diffused their responsibilities.

The pressure upon health officials to assume new powers did not originate exclusively from concern with the social concomitants of disease or from a more comprehensive description of pathology. The Department's regard for more efficient utilization of its resources was matched by the rhetoric of a new breed of elected state officials who challenged the separation between politics and reform. In the early part of the twentieth century advocacy of social reform in Massachusetts ceased to be synonomous with political nonpartisanship. In the two decades preceding social security legislation, the struggle to win the votes of the immigrant and laborer beset Massachusetts Republicans and Democrats alike with intraparty conflicts which threatened to displace the traditional upholders of political morality from office. If in the past, "Politics" with a capital "P" was viewed as inimical to the integrity of charitable interest in relief of misfortune and the improvement of social conditions, "politics" with a small "p" now was viewed by some successful officeholders as a necessary stimulus to further progress.[7]

With regard to public health reform, respect for the scientist and the physician tended at first to channel this sentiment into the traditional relationship between the state government and the Department and to shelter public health from the fray of politics. Even while the insurgents sought adherents from elements in the population, such as the Irish who had more often been the object of social reform rather than its originators, improved public health remained an acceptable objective.

However, by the third decade of the century, public health became everybody's business in quite a different sense than originally proposed by the Department. Scientific prevention required the identification of the cause of disease, but as the cause of noncontagious disease became a matter of dispute, the function of the Department of Public Health was also opened to contro-

---

see the caustic comments of Dr. George H. Bigelow, Massachusetts Commissioner of Public Health (1925-1933) in *Commonhealth*, 13:49 (July-Aug.-Sept. 1926), and 16:101 (Oct.-Nov.-Dec. 1929).

7. There are special studies of Massachusetts politics which are crucial in evaluating the reform movement of this period; for a contemporary work, see Solomon Bulkley Griffin, *People and Politics Observed By a Massachusetts Editor* (Boston: Little, Brown, 1923). Two more recent books are particularly helpful: Richard M. Abrams, *Conservatism in a Progressive Era: A Study in Political Theory* (Cambridge, Mass.: Harvard University Press, 1964); J. Joseph Huthmacher, *Massachusetts People and Politics, 1919-1923* (Cambridge, Mass.: Harvard University Press, 1959).

versy. Just as public health lost its isolation from the external currents of political pressure, the era of good feeling was further threatened by divergent claims to authoritative diagnoses of society's ills and the proliferation of more inclusive preventive measures. In the search for optimal methods to promote health, it became almost mandatory that the physician, the sanitary engineer, and the laboratory scientist be joined by the politician and a host of professionally trained workers in the paramedical and social sciences.

There was very little in the *Annual Report of the Massachusetts State Board of Health* for 1913 to suggest the need for administrative reorganization on the state level. The various departments noted a steady increase in the volume of work during the past year: the Antitoxin and Vaccine Laboratory provided 21,014 ampules of antityphoid vaccine and made antimeningitis serum available for the first time; three special investigations of poliomyelitis, originally initiated as a result of the 1910 epidemic, were completed; inspection of milk supplies increased markedly with the cooperation of the largest dairies. Another example of the way that public support stimulated the Board's work was the acceptance of preliminary steps to control venereal disease, leading to the recommendation of a special laboratory for the diagnosis of syphilis and gonorrhea. However, these reports or suggestions for future activity did not entail any departure from established lines of work. All that was required was a modest increase in appropriations to extend existing facilities. Even the usual urgent request for laboratory space received little prominence in the 1913 *Report*, perhaps because of recent legislation authorizing the maintenance of county bacteriologic laboratories when properly supervised by the State Board of Health.[8]

The State Board, in one way or another, affected every citizen of the Commonwealth by 1914. All of the cities and towns with a population of more than five thousand had public water supplies. In addition to the general supervision of public water and sewage facilities, the Board investigated complaints brought against private water companies serving some of the smaller towns. The Board

8. Massachusetts State Board of Health, *Forty-fifth Annual Report* (1914), pp. 2-5, 7-8, 477, 535-557. The need for laboratory accommodations became urgent again in 1917, when Harvard asked the state to vacate the Forest Hills plant as soon as possible; see *Third Annual Report* (1918), p. 13. The issue lay quiet again until the 1920's; see correspondence between Benjamin White, first full-time director of the Laboratories, and Commissioner Eugene R. Kelley, Oct. 8, 1920, April 14, 17, 1922; President A. Lawrence Lowell of Harvard to White, Sept. 30, 1920; Kelley to Lowell, April 14, 1922, all in files of Massachusetts Department of Public Health, Institute of Laboratories, Jamaica Plains. Mark W. Richardson, "The State Board of Health and Its Relation to the Milk Problem in Massachusetts," *Monthly Bulletin*, 6:20-22 (Jan. 1911).

was also charged with ensuring the purity of many foods sold across the counter, including items kept in cold storage. Another responsibility of the Board was to determine the strength of proprietary drugs and to make certain that alcoholic liquors met standard requirements. The Board was even charged with the examining and licensing of plumbers. Pamphlets on health and dangerous diseases were likewise distributed to local boards of health, to physicians, and to the general public.[9]

All these labors were accomplished with a working force of ninety-one persons. This number included not only trained scientists who took charge of the laboratories at the State House, at Forest Hills and at the Lawrence Experiment Station, but clerks and stable hands as well. Many of these employees, including the twelve district health inspectors, were hired only on a part-time basis. By comparison with other state health departments, the Massachusetts Board of Health spent little money. The total appropriation for 1913 was $189,000, which included a balance of $2,000 left over from the previous year. This efficient utilization of personnel and low rate of expenditures contributed to the good reputation of the Board within the state and on the national level. In a letter to Governor Foss, written in 1911, Dr. Charles V. Chapin had pointed to the "absolute freedom from every form of favoritism" as the distinguishing component of public health service in the Bay State.[10]

The freedom from political strife which the Board of Health had enjoyed since 1886 was only partly due to its reputation for competence. Year after year an almost unbroken line of Republican governors and legislators had acceded to the requests of Dr. Walcott, chairman of the Board. Apparently the role of the Board as a regulatory agency was entirely consistent with the expectations of the state's political leadership. The Board's power to give advice was liberally interpreted, and the district health inspectors, food inspectors, and sanitary engineers reported no significant opposition to their suggestions. If manufacturers

9. Massachusetts State Board of Health, *Forty-fourth Annual Report* (1913), pp. 20-22, 55-56, and *Forty-fifth Annual Report* (1914), pp. 6-8, 11, 17, 40-42. Under "An Act to Provide for the Supervision of Water Companies by the State Board of Health," *Acts and Resolves 1909, Chapter 319* (April 26, 1909), pp. 263-264, the Board had the power to advise private companies, but complaints about rates or services had to go first to the local town authorities.

10. Charles V. Chapin, *A Report on State Public Health Work Based on a Survey of State Boards of Health* (Chicago: American Medical Association, 1915), pp. 191-192; Massachusetts State Board of Health, *Forty-fifth Annual Report* (1914), pp. 45-51. The total budget reported here is slightly larger than that given by Chapin because special appropriations were included. Letter from Chapin to Eugene N. Foss, accompanied by evaluation of the Massachusetts State Board of Health (1911), typescript with Charles V. Chapin Papers, Rhode Island Historical Society, Providence, Rhode Island.

found the Board's restriction of industrial waste disposal, or the recommendations to safeguard health which followed visits of factory inspectors, unwelcome, their complaints went unheeded.

Public utilities, railroads, and corporate businesses in Massachusetts had long been subjected to regulatory "advice" from state commissions. Civic responsibility to protect "the public interest" from ignorance, irresponsibility, or selfishness — whatever its source — had long been assumed by successive generations of enlightened Republicans whose candidates for public office were drawn from the old stock of native Americans. This conservative political establishment had never yielded its substantial power to immigrant groups or their children, although such new citizens made up more than half the state's population by 1900. Yet Massachusetts workers were protected from the evils of long hours and unsanitary factory conditions to a degree unknown in other industrialized states. As Richard M. Abrams has shown, in the first years of the twentieth century what was new, progressive legislation in less forward-looking states, appeared in Massachusetts as amendments to already existing statutes.[11]

These real accomplishments had taken place in quite a different atmosphere, however, from that which prevailed in the Bay State by 1910. At the turn of the century the annual state and municipal elections had failed to reflect the preponderance of urban and immigrant voters, but by the end of the next decade Yankee-Republican hegemony in the Commonwealth was no longer assured. Governor Eugene Noble Foss was the first Democrat since the Civil War to be elected to three successive terms. The first Irish-American to win state-wide office, David Ignatius Walsh, followed him in 1914. Although these elections were indicative of important changes within the state, it is significant that in regard to public health the insurgents adopted the rhetoric of their predecessors. The tradition that politics and public health reform were inimical was still viable. Successful politicians from both parties agreed with public health officials that sanitary policy would be effective only to the degree that it continued to be free from political interference.

Although the attitude toward the Board of Health remained unchanged, important differences in the language of reform politics raised alarm among those able and conservative men who had traditionally led the state's numerous commissions and boards. Governor Foss was a Yankee businessman whose political life had begun as a dissident Republican, but his first inaugural address in January 1911 was a call to give the government back to the people. What proved to be the longest legislative session in the state's history opened with the charge

11. Abrams, *Conservatism in a Progressive Era*, pp. 5-14, 131-133.

that a crisis existed which would require extensive changes in administration and legislation in order to protect the rights of labor, women, and children. "Representatives of monopolistic interests have usurped the prerogatives of the people," said Foss, causing the Boston *Advertiser* and the *Herald* to predict ruin for the state in the hands of an unscrupulous and ambitious reformer.

A more sympathetic journalist writing in the conservative *Harper's Weekly* was less impressed with the governor's radicalism than with his pledge to bring order and economy to public administration. After an interview with the newly elected governor, Charles Johnston reported enthusiastically that Foss was the "unique example of a business man of wide experience and demonstrated ability called upon to conduct the business of a great State on business lines, given unusual freedom to investigate the entire field of the State's business matters, and point the way to put them on a business basis."[12]

Although Foss directed a sharp eye to the affairs of the various commissions, which he did not favor "as a means of transmitting business . . . for . . . their tendency is not in accord with popular or representative government," his investigation of the Board of Health revealed no evidence of abuse of authority or patronage. On the contrary, the report submitted by Dr. Chapin indicated that the Board had attracted young men of exceptional ability who served the state well at nominal salaries. Dr. Chapin's only criticism was that pride in the reputation for conservatism and economy had led the Board of Health to proceed too slowly, and it is "possible," he admonished, "that this commendable purpose be carried too far."[13] Apparently there was no need to alter the composition of the Board or to modify its powers.

The only important change in responsibility for public health during the Foss administration was the shift of factory inspection from the district health inspectors to the Board of Labor and Industries. The Board of Health, in turn, made few requests, but did note that the work of the health inspectors had increased so much that even when relieved of factory inspection their duties required the full-time attention of professionally trained personnel.[14]

12. For a summary of legislation passed under Foss, see Richard B. Sherman, "Foss of Massachusetts: Demagogue or Progressive?" *Mid-America*, 43:88-89 (April 1961). Sherman sees 1910-1913 as the height of Progressivism in Massachusetts. Foss, "Inaugural Address," *Massachusetts Senate Documents 1911, No. 1*, Jan. 5, 1911, p. 4. For press reactions, see Sherman, "Foss of Massachusetts," p. 87. Charles Johnston, "A Talk With Governor Foss," *Harper's Weekly*, 55:7 (Sept. 2, 1911).

13. Foss, "Inaugural Address," 1911; typescript of Chapin evaluation which accompanied letter to Foss (1911).

14. "An Act to Provide a State Board of Labor and Industries," *Acts and Resolves 1912, Chapter 726,* Section 5 (June 10, 1912), p. 836. Massachusetts State Board of Health, *Forty-fifth Annual Report* (1914), pp. 5-6.

Recognition that the work of the health inspector was central to the efficient execution of public health policy suggested that prevention of disease required specialized training and exclusive responsibility. At the same time, while the Board continued to exercise certain "police powers," Dr. Walcott looked forward to the day when these powers would be transferred to a more appropriate agency. However, Dr. Walcott saw no particular need to reorganize the Board at the state level. He reiterated the principle that the main prerequisite for public health service remained, in 1914 as it had been in 1886, "to keep politics absolutely out of the health question."[15]

When Foss was succeeded by David I. Walsh, Dr. Walcott felt the need to reaffirm this principle. Shortly before Walsh's inaugural, in January 1914, Walcott had a frank talk with the newly elected Governor. Dr. Walcott was satisfied that, although no specific proposals had emerged from the conversation, Governor Walsh shared his concern for maintaining the Board's independent role.[16] Although the meeting was entirely cordial, there was little real basis for understanding between Walcott and Walsh. Walcott believed in the politics of restraint, and Walsh had already demonstrated in his election campaign that he was committed to the politics of pressure. Walcott looked forward to the continuation of a Board of Health composed of laymen and physicians dedicated to civic responsibility who would voluntarily lend their prestige to carefully conceived, scientifically authorized measures to prevent disease. Walsh, on the other hand, planned for a Department of Health led by professionally trained public health experts who would execute the affirmative responsibility of the state for the social welfare of its citizens.

David Ignatius Walsh was a politician of consummate skill whose oratorical talent brought new voters to the Democratic party.[17] Born in 1872, the ninth of ten children, Walsh's election to the state's highest office came only fifteen years after his first serious venture in politics. Everything about Walsh was unusual, even his parents' response to the overwhelming odds they faced as Irish

15. Walcott to Dr. George C. Shattuck, Jan. 3, 1914, George C. Shattuck Papers, Holmes Hall, Francis A. Countway Library of Medicine, Harvard Medical School, Boston, Mass.

16. *Ibid.*; for Walsh's preliminary proposals, see files of speeches prepared for 1913 campaign, David I. Walsh papers, Dinand Library, College of the Holy Cross, Worcester, Mass.

17. Biographical material on Walsh from William Joseph Grattan, "David I. Walsh and His Associates: A Study in Political Theory," unpub. diss., Harvard University (1957); Dorothy G. Wayman, *David I. Walsh: Citizen Patriot* (Milwaukee, Wisc.: Bruce, 1952); John H. Flannagan, Jr., "The Disillusionment of a Progressive: U.S. Senator David I. Walsh and the League of Nations Issue, 1918-1920," *New England Quarterly*, 41:483-504 (Dec. 1968), supports the view of Walsh as a liberal reformer in his early political career.

immigrants in the semirural factory towns of central Massachusetts. Walsh's father, Thomas, had worked in a Leominster comb factory until 1880, when unemployment forced him to move to nearby Clinton; there his in-laws, the Donnellys, found work for him in the carpet mill. Five years later Thomas died, leaving his wife, Bridget, to raise the children.

While other families in similar circumstances often neglected education in order to gain another breadwinner, the Walsh children attended the local high school. One daughter went on to normal school, and the oldest son trained for the law and opened practice, only to die in his twenties. Young David showed considerable promise at high school, but had no plans for further education; upon graduation he began work as a grocery clerk. His mother and four sisters arranged for him to go to college, however, and somehow they raised the two-hundred-dollar annual fee for Holy Cross College in nearby Worcester. With only his younger brother left at home, David entered the small Catholic college and graduated in 1893. Out of a class of twenty-eight, five went into medicine, eight into the priesthood, and eight chose the law.

David Walsh returned to Clinton, but two years later he entered law school at Boston University with the hope that this would qualify him for a serious political career. He had been involved in town affairs since his adolescence and knew the obstacles to success which faced even the most able Irish-Catholic boy. With over one-third of the Massachusetts population Roman Catholic, only a handful had ever been elected to the legislature, and none to state-wide office. In his successful campaign for election to the Massachusetts House in 1899 and 1900, Walsh made it clear that he was the spokesman for a specific constituency — the immigrant and the laborer — rather than the proponent of disinterested, neutral government.[18]

Walsh saw the opportunity to reverse the fortunes of the disadvantaged through partisan politics, specifically within the Democratic party. The issue of genteel reform versus "bossism" had split the Democrats along class and ethnic lines. Foss's victories had done little to diminish these divisions, kindled by the appearance of an effective Irish machine in Boston and fanned by Yankee distrust and clannishness.[19] Walsh was hardly an acceptable figure to old-time Democrats, but he was an effective public speaker and surprised the politically astute with his successful campaign for Lieutenant Governor in 1912. Both parties

18. The original typescript copies of Walsh's public addresses from his many campaigns for office are deposited at the Dinand Library.

19. Abrams, *Conservatism in a Progressive Era*, esp. pp. 249-294; Huthmacher, *Massachusetts People and Politics*, chap. i.

adopted a reform platform in that year, and Woodrow Wilson won the Massachusetts electoral vote, placing the state in the Democratic column for the first time. Walsh's forthright espousal of government responsibility for social welfare, however, caused considerable discomfort in both camps.

A year later, state politics was further fragmented as four candidates entered the gubernatorial contest. Walsh won a bitter battle for the Democratic nomination, only to have Foss file papers as an Independent.[20] Once again, all candidates advocated "reform" in a campaign where the epithet "progressive" ceased to be a distinction. The Democratic nominee reminded the voters that "only sixty years ago the Republican party was organized to resist the encroachment of the slave oligarchy . . . Then it began to decay. Selfish interests began to take possession of it . . . In 1896, under the leadership of Mark Hanna, its bondage to special privilege became complete . . . To put the matter squarely," Walsh concluded, "the Democratic party of today is the Republican party of fifty years ago . . . The Progressive party has no call to exist."

Elected by a plurality of fifty thousand, he announced that his victory was a mandate for affirmative government in the interest of the working man. Just a few weeks before he had told gatherings at Lawrence and Lowell that the interests of labor "must be more and more considered by all classes, as carrying with it the welfare of the rest."[21]

In his campaign Walsh often turned to the question of improved public health. Here was a dramatic issue that lent itself to his advocacy of vigorous state government. Before his election he proposed that the Board of Health be reorganized to include responsibility for charity and insanity. The population of the state had increased by 75 percent since 1886 when the joint Board of Health, Lunacy, and Charity had been dismembered; but, said Walsh, costs in these areas had increased by 69 percent. Sidestepping the cry for economy, the candidate maintained that the increased expense would be justified if services improved equivalently.

Taking advantage of the good repute of the Board of Health, Walsh accused the Republicans of "wasteful extravagance . . . from failure to give the State Board of Health due authority."[22] He maintained that the legislature had paid insufficient attention to the recommendations of the Board. For example,

20. Grattan, "Walsh," pp. 134-152; Walsh Letterbooks, Walsh papers.
21. Typescripts of speeches delivered by Walsh in 1913 campaign, and in Cambridge and Somerville, Oct. 30, 1914, Walsh papers.
22. From material on "public health" prepared for both 1912 and 1913 campaigns, and incorporated into a number of speeches used in both these years, Walsh papers.

money had been spent needlessly to establish a leper colony against the Board's advice, while the Board was not given sufficient funds to carry on other activities. Actually, there was little evidence that the Board had been denied at any time, but it was clear that Governor Walsh found public health reform a suitable vehicle to demonstrate the proper role of government.

Walsh wrote later that he would have liked to reorganize all the state's supervisory boards, but he turned his attention first to the Board of Health because it seemed "especially timely." Although he gave up the idea of a joint Board of Health, Charity, and Insanity, he announced in his inaugural address that he would sponsor legislation for "a salaried Board of Health, with a Health Commissioner appointed by the Board subject to the approval of the Governor." Four months later he took the initiative and asked for a paid commissioner as well as full-time district health officers and three new departmental divisions: infant and child hygiene, communicable disease, and education. In the intervening months, Walsh went outside the state for advice from the federal public health service and the New York City Health Commissioner, Hermann Biggs. It was Walsh, rather than any member of the Massachusetts Board of Health, who pressed for state reorganization. Moreover, it was Walsh who conducted the negotiations which resulted in the release of Dr. Allan J. McLaughlin from the United States Public Health Service to serve as the first Commissioner at a salary of $7,500.[23]

Walsh's assertion, during his 1914 campaign for re-election, that the reorganization was the result of his "persistent and determined efforts and against great odds," seems to be without foundation. Walsh initially sought support from the Massachusetts Medical Society, which offered no opposition and made only one suggestion — that the health officers should be physicians in good standing.[24] It was also true that the proposals for division heads to be exempted from Civil Service and the five-year term for the Commissioner were mildly contested in

23. Walsh, "The Ideals of a Governor," *New England Magazine*, 52:206 (March 1915); "Inaugural Address," *Massachusetts Senate Documents, No. 1* (Jan. 8, 1914), pp. 32-33; "Message Relative to the Protection of Public Health," May 8, 1914, in *Messages to the General Court, Official Addresses and Proclamations of . . . Governor David I. Walsh* (Boston, 1918), pp. 76-79. Letters from Walsh and members of his staff to Herman Biggs, Health Commissioner of New York City; to Woodrow Wilson; to Surgeon General George W. McCoy; and Dr. Victor G. Heiser, Bureau of Internal Affairs — all written from May 12 through the end of September 1914 and collected in Walsh Letterbook VII. Walsh to McLaughlin, Sept. 30, 1914, informing of his confirmation as Commissioner, in Walsh Letterbook III. All of these letters are in Dinand Library.

24. *BMSJ*, 170:819 (May 21, 1914).

the press.[25] At one point Dr. Milton Rosenau, a member of the Board who had spoken for reorganization at the first legislative hearing, withdrew his support because he felt the bill did not provide adequate provisions for enforcement and was too dependent on "moral suasion." But, on the whole, both physicians and legislators supported the principle that public health work should be guided by professionally trained men under a central authority, and the bill was passed on July 6, 1914, with hardly a ripple of opposition.[26]

Beneath the unanimity of support for administrative reorganization, the new Department of Health had been assigned a role which was hardly commensurate with Dr. Chapin's dictum limiting public health measures strictly to the scientific control of disease. It was Governor Walsh, not Dr. McLaughlin, who said that the "consensus of opinion among publicists is to the effect that one of the chief causes of poverty, discontent and restlessness is due to physical unfitness and disease." Somehow the successful campaign against disease was to serve as the model for a campaign against all social ills.

At a conference of Massachusetts public health officials in April 1915, Charles W. Eliot, president emeritus at Harvard, joined Walsh in greeting the millennium. In a speech called "The Main Points of Attack in the Campaign for Public Health," he listed tuberculosis, venereal disease, alcoholism, and prostitution as the fields for immediate attention. "It is for the boards of health, in cooperation with the medical profession and the courts, to apply to these scourges the principles of preventive medicine," he announced.[27] Small wonder that in later years Governor Walsh claimed his sponsorship of health legislation as his most significant contribution to public welfare. However, there was no more real agreement between Walsh and Eliot than there had been between Walsh and

25. Boston *Evening Transcript*, May 15, 1914. The issue of civil service requirements has remained a difficulty for the department; see "Report of the Special Commission to Study and Investigate Public Health Laws and Policies," *Massachusetts House Documents 1936, No. 1200* (Dec. 2, 1936), pp. 45-50. The Commissioner and the directors of divisions were exempted from civil service until 1942. When these positions were filled from the civil service roster, it became even more difficult to get adequately trained personnel, and a number of incumbent division directors were found to have minor physical impairments which would have originally removed them from consideration. From an interview on May 1, 1968, with Dr. Herbert L. Lombard, retired director of the Division of Cancer and other Chronic Diseases.

26. *BMSJ*, 171:119-120 (July 16, 1914); "An Act to Create a State Department of Health and to Amend the Public Health Laws," *Acts and Resolves 1914, Chapter 792* (July 7, 1914), pp. 969-972.

27. Typescript of 1914 campaign speech by Walsh, Walsh papers; speech by Eliot published in *AJPH*, 5:623 (July 1915).

Walcott. It was impossible for the public health expert to close the gap between Eliot's idea that state preventive medicine would teach the poor and the ignorant how to resist the temptations of alcohol and Walsh's idea that the paramount responsibility of the state was to serve the economically disadvantaged.

After Dr. McLaughlin came to Massachusetts he set the pace and the direction for reorganization. Assuming office in November 1914, he made it clear that the Department would be run on a businesslike basis. He predicted that a far-sighted public health program would eventually require something like $360,000 annually, or 10 cents per capita, but he scrutinized existing expenditures with an eye to reducing unnecessary waste. As a result of his economy measures, the two Boston offices for inspection of food and drugs were combined in 1915, so that several clerical and supervisory positions were abolished. One man who had formerly worked as a food inspector for $2,500 was now named a veterinary inspector at a salary reduced to $1,800. By the end of his first year Dr. McLaughlin was pleased to announce that, through careful attention to administrative details, two new division directors and an epidemiologist had been appointed without any substantial budgetary increase.[28]

Dr. McLaughlin agreed with a report published by the American Medical Association in 1915, that the central concern of state sanitary policy must remain the control of contagious disease.[29] In his first report he noted that syphilis, a contagious and preventable disease, annually accounted for more deaths in Massachusetts than diphtheria, typhoid, scarlet fever, measles, influenza, and whooping cough combined. However, the traditional reporting procedures for identifying and controlling contagious disease were inappropriate in this instance. Recognizing that physicians would object to registering the names of patients with venereal diseases with public health authorities, McLaughlin suggested a system of coded numbers. The state had already facilitated the diagnosis of syphilis through the establishment of the Wasserman Laboratory in June 1915, and he estimated that 1,800 blood specimens would be submitted in the coming year. To encourage this project, McLaughlin advocated that the state make inexpensive treatment available through the production and free distribution of Salvarsan to all dispensaries, hospitals, and physicians, Although this step would involve considerable expense, Dr. McLaughlin felt it was justified. But he cautioned, "let us be practical and consider syphilis as a public

28. Massachusetts Department of Health, *First Annual Report* (1916), pp. 7-10, 13.
29. Charles V. Chapin, *A Report on State Public Health*, p. 4.

health problem, leaving the academic discussion of its moral and social aspects to others."[30] It seemed that public health officials were not entirely prepared to accept the proffered role of public censor.

The control of other contagious diseases presented additional conflicts. In December 1914 the Department published an amended list of thirty-two reportable diseases considered to be dangerous to the public health. At the same time, the Division of Communicable Diseases reminded local boards of health that they were responsible under law for meeting the medical expenses of those families unable to afford necessary treatment "without such assistance in any sense pauperizing the recipient or the recipient's family." Within a few months, the Department of Health was faced with complaints from a number of cities. The effect of this directive was to encourage "certain classes of the population to seek public aid for diseases that either were trivial in character or were of such a chronic nature that the practical effect tended to their perpetual support at the expense of the community, when no such action would be taken by these individuals and their families if they had been obliged to accept such relief from the overseers of the poor as had hitherto been the case." Responding to the pleas of such populous cities as Lowell, Cambridge, and Worcester, the Department held a hearing in August and reduced the number of reportable diseases to eighteen.[31] It appeared that the Department of Health would have to voluntarily curtail what had previously been agreed upon as the efficient exercise of minimum responsibility.

Problems associated with this dilemma were postponed, however when America became involved in World War I. The traditional optimism which had characterized public health reform for over thirty years was hardly shaken by figures which showed that one-half of all men between twenty-one and thirty years old drafted for military service were rejected. A careful study of the unfit only emphasized the extent to which preventable disease was responsible for later damaging defects. Meanwhile, an article surveying public health in the United States

30. Massachusetts Department of Health, *First Annual Report* (1916), pp. 19-21. Salvarsan had been purchased from Germany at a cost of $3.00 to $4.50 per dose until the outbreak of World War I.

31. "An Act Relative to the Expense of Caring for Persons Infected with Diseases Dangerous to the Public Health," *Acts and Resolves 1909, Chapter 380* (May 13, 1909), pp. 348-349; Massachusetts Department of Health, *First Annual Report* (1916), pp. 548-551. It should be noted that venereal diseases were not reported to the Department at this time.

indicated that Massachusetts had already taken preliminary steps to ensure a healthier citizenry in the future.[32]

The ability of the Massachusetts Health Department to meet the crises which arose during the war seemed to justify this appraisal. As many new cases of tuberculosis were detected through physical examinations at the time of induction, the Department appeared to be buoyed by this fresh opportunity for future work. Responding to evidence that the incidence of venereal infection increased among civilians as well as soldiers under stress of wartime living conditions, the Department reversed its original position and recommended mandatory registration of all active cases of syphilis and gonorrhea. Fifteen clinics were opened for diagnosis and treatment of venereal disease. The sanitary and medical problems which arose with the opening of a camp for training thirty thousand young men at Ayer were quickly met through the appointment of civilian health officers.[33]

During the wartime emergency it seemed appropriate for the government to assume a variety of far-reaching responsibilities. For a while, at least, the Health Department was relieved of the need to arbitrarily restrict the scope of its policies. But, even in the euphoria evoked by total commitment to wartime preparedness, Dr. McLaughlin noted that the proper allocation of limited resources must be determined by the Commissioner. He reminded the legislature that although other state agencies, such as the Department of Education, might become involved in programs to protect the public health, "no State money should be expended for the prevention of disease unless under the supervision and control or by the advice of the State Department of Health."[34]

In principle the reorganized Department was in a position to meet all the requirements set by Dr. Walcott, Governor Walsh, and Commissioner McLaughlin. A man specially selected because of his training and experience in public health work presided over a distinguished, unpaid Public Health Council of physicians and concerned laymen. Six full-time health officers worked in the field to give advice and encourage law enforcement. Three new divisions supplemented the established work in sanitary engineering, food and drug inspection, and the biol-

32. C. B. Davenport and Albert G. Love, "Defects Found in Drafted Men," *Scientific Monthly*, 10:5-25 (Jan. 1920); Alice Hamilton and Gertrude Seymour, "The New Public Health," *Survey*, 38:60 (April 21, 1917), and "The Health of the Soldier and Civilian: Some Aspects of the American Health Movement in War-time," *Survey*, 40:89-94 (April 27, 1918).

33. Massachusetts Department of Health, *Third Annual Report* (1918), pp. 16-19, 21-27.

34. *Ibid.*, p. 11, and *First Annual Report* (1916), p. 21.

ogics and diagnostic laboratories. There was every reason to expect that these administrative steps would encourage a vigorous and comprehensive health policy in which expedient and farsighted programs would be initiated without political interference and could be entirely directed by sound professional judgment.

Yet within a few years it was evident that neither the goals of the Department nor the effective means of reaching these goals could be defined by the rigorous pursuit of businesslike methods, or the firm application of the principles of scientific hygiene. Efficiency could not foreclose discussion on the larger questions of the purpose of public health policy. Was there any assurance that the prevention of disease might not open the door to more malignant tendencies, such as excessive dependence on the state?

This was hardly a novel question, but it assumed greater urgency when the control of contagious disease seemed so close at hand. In the past, moral commitment to the general welfare had been a sufficient basis for weighing advantages of public health and welfare services against possible ill effects. The salaried public health official, such as Dr. McLaughlin, accepted his responsibility to make the benefits of sanitary science available to the public. Did recognition that enjoyment of these benefits required education in personal hygiene imply that the Department must judge the merit or efficacy of instruction? Did not such decisions involve ethical considerations which were as inappropriate to sanitary science as the collection of garbage or the inspection of plumbing? At the end of World War I it was clear that decisions about the purpose and effect of state preventive medicine could no longer be free of conflict. It was also clear that the participants in this struggle would be far more diverse than in the past. What remained to be resolved were the specific issues and the higher principles to be invoked.

The Massachusetts Department of Health had clearly established its authority to determine public guidelines for the control of contagious disease by the end of the second decade of the twentieth century. In the next ten years, as attention shifted to illness which was not amenable to prophylactic immunization, public health authorities redefined their responsibilities so that promotion of health rather than prevention of disease became the primary objective of public health policy.

In some respects the Department returned to the view of the first State Board of Health, which had conceived its role as both the guardian of public health and the tutor of personal behavior. This was a time — announced an article in the *American Journal of Public Health* — to reinterpret the motto of the New

York City Health Department, that "public health is purchasable — within natural limitation a community can determine its own death rate." This slogan now bore directly on the individual as much as on the public authorities. Personal hygiene must supplement and amplify the progress already achieved through identification of the sources of infection, immunization, and control of the environment. In 1915 Lee K. Frankel, vice-president of the Metropolitan Life Insurance Company and an advocate of social insurance, singled out self-indulgence as the reservoir of personal irresponsibility. "There is a moral obligation," he said, "as well as a physical one not too [sic] succumb to the temptation of overeating, over-drinking, absence of exercise, and overwork," if the promise of a longer and healthier life for coming generations was to be fulfilled.[35]

However, particularly in the years after the war, it was more usual to decry undesirable personal behavior as ignorance, and to describe reform in terms of pedagogy. Advances made in the scientific control of disease during the fifty years since the State Board of Health had been established had recast the lines of instruction in personal hygiene to emphasize persuasive guidance rather than threats of punishment. Although differences of opinion often were expressed as arguments over the best method of teaching mothers how to care for themselves and their children, or over who should determine the scope of public responsibility for patients with chronic diseases, disagreement over "how" and "who" barely covered a larger area of contention. Assurance that programs designed to reduce excessive infant mortality, for instance, were grounded in science could not alter the fact that the remedial measures proposed were calculated to cure social ills as often as specifically medical problems.

Justification for these departures from traditional procedures came slowly. Social services, maternal and child welfare programs, and hospital care for the patient with cancer were intended to alleviate misfortune rather than to prevent specific diseases, and it was reasonable to call for the investigation of a situation which bred an undesirable condition and, at the same time, to offer aid and instruction to its victims. The search for scientific prevention did not allay pressing needs, and, while public health spokesmen continued to seek the source of disease, they were sensitive to the need for intermediate solutions. What had originally been seen as a palliative, however, gradually became the core of prevention.

In Massachusetts, one impetus for innovation resulted from the Department's inability to control contagious disease. The influenza epidemic that hit the

35. Lee K. Frankel, "Science and the Public Health," *AJPH*, 5:287 (April 1915).

United States in 1918 was particularly virulent in the Bay State. Although the Division of Communicable Diseases had credited its system of reporting and the adoption of an "endemic index" with preventing separate outbreaks of seven other contagious diseases from reaching epidemic proportions, these methods were ineffectual in curtailing the spread of influenza.[36] Efforts to develop a prophylactic vaccine were abortive, and, at the height of the epidemic, the Department's effective contribution was limited to keeping records and directing additional medical assistance to stricken communities.

The epidemic accented the question of what the proper role was for those representatives of the Division of Communicable Diseases who had most frequent contact with the public, the district health officers, and their newly appointed nursing assistants. Two years before, Dr. Eugene R. Kelley, director of the Division, believed that the main task was to standardize quarantine regulations and to improve the application of epidemiological data. As a result of these successful efforts, he concluded that the control of contagious disease in Massachusetts was well in hand. District health officers, he believed, could limit their responsibilities to field surveys and advice to local boards of health.[37]

When Dr. McLaughlin was recalled to Washington in April 1918, Dr. Kelley, who was appointed Commissioner, faced a new situation. With influenza virtually uncontrolled, Kelley tentatively suggested that, although medical social service lay outside the usual province of state responsibility for public health, further study of this kind of work was in order "merely as a matter of preventive medicine."[38]

While this particular suggestion was not immediately pursued, there were a number of additional indications that the Department was moving toward a broader definition of its role. As Commissioner, Kelley chaired the Massachusetts Health Committee, a new organization which was to serve as a clearinghouse for all governmental and voluntary health activities within the state. First

36. Massachusetts State Department of Health, *Fourth Annual Report* (1919), pp. 16, 197-198. There were 145,262 cases of influenza and 11,000 deaths reported in the epidemic year.

37. Massachusetts State Department of Health, *First Annual Report* (1916), pp. 546-551, and *Third Annual Report* (1918), pp. 195, 202.

38. Massachusetts State Department of Health, *Fourth Annual Report* (1919), pp. 4, 29. Kelley pointed out that the Massachusetts General Hospital and other institutions functioning in urban areas were already providing outpatient care and social service, but in smaller communities there were no agencies for this work. Eugene R. Kelley (1882-1925) was born in Maine and received his M.D. from Johns Hopkins in 1906. After a brief private practice he went to the state of Washington, where he was Commissioner before coming to Massachusetts to head the Division of Communicable Diseases in 1915; see *BMSJ*, 193: 701-702 (Oct. 8, 1925).

convened in July 1918, the group was to guide educational campaigns "to make Uncle Sam's boys fit for fighting and to cut down on the sickness and death rate for the Commonwealth."[39] Professor Charles E. Bellatty of Boston University was hired as executive director. Although the Committee had no real independent function, it was clear from its membership, which included all the state's charitable and welfare agencies, that the promotion of health was not considered exclusively a medical problem.

A month earlier, Professor Bellatty, "a publicity engineer of high standing," was appointed editor of the Department's official journal. On his advice the monthly *Public Health Bulletin* was changed to the quarterly *Commonhealth*. Available free to any citizen, it soon adopted a popular style and carried articles on such subjects as children's health and nutrition, clearly directed to its lay readers.[40] Thus, the Department sought to enlist the interest and support of the concerned public. More willing than before to share its authority, the Department also accepted more inclusive obligations.

The newly christened journal devoted more space to articles on the health of infants and children, or "child conservation" as it was aptly called, than any other subject. No new phase of the Department's work illustrated the augmented responsibilities of public health officials better than the campaign to reduce excessive maternal and infant mortality. No issue was more likely to arouse public concern, and no problem was more intricately imbedded in a complex of medical, social, and moral components.

Before the 1914 reorganization of the Health Department, the prevention of sickness among children had not been singled out for special consideration. The health of the Massachusetts child who worked, the child who was sick with diphtheria, or the infant who was nourished with cow's milk, was incorporated into the general concerns of the State Board of Health. The movement which later identified the unique nature of children's health needs stemmed from the work of the Division of Hygiene, which was established to promote instruction in the principles of personal health. Despite the fact that Dr. McLaughlin in-

39. *Commonhealth*, 5:179-180 (July 1918). Two years later, at the behest of the Massachusetts Medical Society, the group was reorganized as the Massachusetts Central Health Council. Although state health officials continued to participate, the leadership was then drawn primarily from voluntary health organizations; see *BMSJ* 182:588 (June 1920); 183:88 (July 15, 1920).

40. *Commonhealth*, 5:223 (August 1918) has an appeal for articles from all "who appreciate the value of newspaper publicity for the furtherance of public improvements." In subsequent issues articles had such titles as "Food and the Calorie," "Food for Children from Two to Six," "Infant Feeding," and "The War Against Venereal Disease."

cluded within the scope of the Division responsibility for "infant mortality, child welfare, medical examination of school children, industrial hygiene and health instruction in general," the first director, Professor Selskar M. Gunn of the Massachusetts Institute of Technology, was only available part-time.

The proposed plan of work was both ambitious and ambiguous, possibly because it was unclear what means were available to implement the projected campaigns. Although the Commissioner stated that fully 50 percent of the Department's annual budget could well be allocated to instruction in hygiene, no less than $30,000 for child welfare alone, the original budget was a mere $15,000. At first it seemed that attention to children was primarily justified by their particular susceptibility to instruction since adults too often reacted to hygienic precepts with skepticism or apathy. Dr. McLaughlin attributed the negligent attitude of many adults toward their personal health to poor training in childhood, although he hoped that all but the incorrigible could be interested in the health of future generations.[41]

The Division of Hygiene made its initial report after barely six months' work. Professor Gunn announced that a large number of slide shows, movies, and lectures had been sponsored for educational purposes. The most important accomplishment, however, was an investigation of infant mortality. The preliminary study indicated that children born to mothers who worked in the Lowell mills were less likely to live through their first year than children born under more favorable circumstances, but it suggested no specific remedies.[42]

Without doubt this state investigation was stimulated, in part, by developments on a national level. The child welfare movement received much of its early impetus and support from social workers who, at the turn of the century, began to seek legal protection for the abused child and public recognition of the special status of children. Two presidents, Theodore Roosevelt and William Howard Taft, endorsed the proposal of a Children's Bureau. When this bureau was established in 1912, Congress charged it with the duty of investigating "all matters pertaining to the welfare of children and child life among all classes of our people."

Although the birth registration area included only fifteen states, the Bureau's first undertaking was a "democratic" survey of infant mortality; that is, the investigators gathered a broad sample of infant and maternal deaths, representative of all classes and social conditions. Julia Lathrop, the Chicago social worker

41. Massachusetts State Department of Health, *First Annual Report* (1916), pp. 22-27.
42. *Ibid.*, pp. 787-791.

appointed by President Taft as first Chief of the Bureau, concluded that, although in many instances the conditions which caused death were preventable, a baby's chance for health in the first year of life increased with the father's income.[43]

The findings of the Children's Bureau indicated that poor medical care was but one of the factors contributing to excessive infant mortality. The Bureau urged the states to improve birth registration, and itself organized conferences on child labor and the economic and social bases of child welfare standards, as well as on the health needs of children. Taking pains not to offend the medical profession, Miss Lathrop emphasized that the popular pamphlet, *Infant Care*, issued for public distribution in 1914, was not designed to replace the physician, "but rather to furnish such statements regarding hygiene and normal living every mother has a right to possess in the interest of herself and her children." After the war, however, when the American Medical Association reversed its original position of support for the Children's Bureau to one of outright opposition to any government involvement in medical care, the Bureau was the object of increasing criticism from physicians.[44]

The Massachusetts Department of Health, meanwhile, also intensified its campaign to reduce the high infant death rate. With vital statistics generally deemed the measure of effective health policy, it seemed to Dr. Kelley that education directed toward mothers was more likely to yield quick results than measures for the control of disease emanating from the Biologics Laboratory or the Division of Sanitary Engineering. As in his earlier reaction to the influenza epidemic, Dr. Kelley, in 1919, indicated some doubt about the efficacy of traditional epidemiologic and immunologic programs. Although these methods could account for the near eradication of typhoid, he could give no assurance that the Department had contributed significantly to the reduced incidence of tuberculosis. Since he believed that most infant deaths resulted from a general disregard of hygiene and failure to meet nutritional requirements, rather than from any spe-

43. For an account of the founding and early years of the Children's Bureau, see Dorothy E. Bradbury, *Five Decades of Action for Children: A Short History of the Children's Bureau* (Washington, D. C.: Government Printing Office, 1962). At its inception the federal program for child welfare reflected the interest in improved medical care for all sections of the population which, before the war, was expressed in broad support for health insurance and old-age assistance; see James G. Burrow, *AMA: Voice of American Medicine* (Baltimore: Johns Hopkins Press, 1963), pp. 132-151; Alton A. Linford, *Old Age Assistance in Massachusetts* (Chicago: University of Chicago Press, 1949).
44. Lathrop quoted in Bradbury, *Five Decades of Action for Children*, pp. 9-10; Burrow, *AMA*, pp. 139, 152-158, 160-164.

cific disease, the cure was "more intensive work on the part of the authorities for prenatal, maternity and infant care." He, therefore, supported the proposal for maternity benefits which had been introduced, for the third time, in the 1919 legislative session.[45]

Actually several bills advocated a variety of different kinds of financial and medical aid to expectant mothers, but none was reported for final consideration. Reflecting rather widespread support for some form of maternity assistance, Governor Calvin Coolidge opened the 1920 session of the legislature with the assertion that Massachusetts was "committed to the policy of aiding children by assisting the mother to care for them." In his second inaugural address, which otherwise advocated a policy of retrenchment rather than reform, Coolidge called for extending "medical aid and nursing care to needy and expectant mothers." Coolidge, who would again face this issue as President, knew the value of a time-honored platitude. "Motherhood should be honored and childhood protected," was a sentiment above political contest.[46] Coolidge was not alone in his desire for a facile solution to what still seemed a transparent problem.

Three bills, differing in whether aid should be money or services and differing in whether services should be available to all or only to the needy, were introduced to the legislature in 1920. Discussion of the proposed measures was almost entirely limited to consideration of what method would be most propitious. The Department of Public Health supported the principle that more health information and nursing care was the primary requisite of any program. Dr. Kelley blamed lack of adequate financial support for the inefficacy of measures being administered by the Division of Hygiene, but raised no question concerning the underlying purpose of continuing work. Clearly, education of the uninformed was the necessary ingredient for improved maternal and child hygiene. Since the Department stated that there was almost as much ignorance of proper hygiene among the well-to-do as among the poor, it was evident that diffusion of information was its central task. Dental hygiene and nutrition received special attention in 1920, and through all these activities it seemed that attitudes

45. Massachusetts State Department of Health, *Fifth Annual Report* (1920), pp. 6-8: furthermore, Kelley pointed out that "a sound nutritional and physical foundation in early life is necessary for combatting infection in later life," *Sixth Annual Report* (1921), pp. 5, 11. Massachusetts infant mortality rates were 15 percent higher than those for New York City at this time. For a brief history of various proposals beginning in 1916, see Merrill Champion, "Maternity Benefits," *Survey*, 45:864-865 (March 12, 1921).

46. *Massachusetts Legislative Documents, Senate, No. 1* (Jan. 8, 1920), pp. 7-8.

could be improved, enabling the Department to foster healthful habits and a receptive frame of mind.[47]

The Massachusetts Medical Society and the Massachusetts Homeopathic Medical Society supported the maternity benefits bill which required that medical and nursing services be provided by physicians through contract with the Department of Public Health, no matter what the mother's financial situation, as long as she would abide by the instructions of the Department and had resided in the Commonwealth for one year prior to delivery. Dr. Alfred Worcester, president of the Massachusetts Medical Society, was aware of differences among physicians over the desirability of the state's becoming involved in any aspect of medical care. He surveyed all doctors registered with the society, and only 22 percent of the 3,560 members responded, with slightly better than two-to-one favoring some form of aid.[48]

Influenced unduly, perhaps, by the somewhat equivocal support of the medical profession, the legislature was still unable to settle on a satisfactory plan for maternal aid. Instead, an interim commission was established to investigate the matter further. The commission was made up of Dr. Kelley; Robert W. Kelso, the Commissioner of Public Welfare; Dr. Worcester; Mr. Edward E. Whiting, a newspaperman; and Mrs. Helen A. MacDonald, representing women's organizations. Dr. Merrill Champion, Director of the Division of Hygiene, was appointed to conduct the investigation.

Dr. Champion's report was accepted by the commission and submitted to a special legislative session in December 1920. It took issue with the Children's Bureau finding that maternal and infant mortality rates were related to poverty. On the contrary, Dr. Champion reported that in Massachusetts more than half the maternal deaths "came from families where the total income was undoubtedly sufficient to pay for medical care," and where, "in the opinion of competent observers," housing conditions were fair or good. A study of one thousand

47. Massachusetts Department of Public Health, *Sixth Annual Report* (1921), pp. 4-7. For a discussion of the beneficial effects of proper hygiene, see Samuel A. Hopkins, "Some Things Everyone Should Know About the Mouth," *Commonhealth*, 7:321 (Sept.-Oct. 1920). In 1920, as part of the reorganization of state government, the name of the Department was changed to the Massachusetts Department of Public Health, although the annual reports continued to be numbered consecutively from 1915. The changes in state administration had little effect on the Department because of the earlier reorganization, but it was now given supervision of the four state tuberculosis sanatoria (Rutland, Westfield, Lakeville, and North Reading), and the Penikese Leper Hospital.
48. The legislation originally supported by the MMS and the MHMS was the Young Bill: *BMSJ*, 182:121-123 (Jan. 23, 1920); 182:789-790, 285-286 (March 11, 1920); 183:230 (Aug. 19, 1920); 183:608-609 (Nov. 18, 1920).

infant deaths showed that 50 percent had not been treated by physicians, indicating that mothers not only failed to care adequately for their newborn infants, but they also neglected to seek the medical assistance they could afford. The logical conclusion, wrote Dr. Champion, "seems to be that mothers and infants die in Massachusetts largely because of lack of hygiene. This conclusion justifies us in continuing the plan we have always followed of directing our efforts towards the education of our citizens in matters of personal hygiene. It further confirms our belief that this can most effectually be done through the extension of public health nursing service in the homes of the citizens of the Commonwealth."

Although there was considerable disagreement among doctors as to the validity of the commission's findings, especially in regard to the extent of unnecessary infant and maternal deaths, the report avoided many problems when it did not recommend any form of maternity benefits. Since education and information were the best methods of improving personal hygiene, the legislature was absolved of responsibility for passing any further legislation. Physicians could be satisfied that this outcome "would involve no interference with the present relationship between physician and patient"; of the 1,500 answers to a questionnaire sent to 6,000 practicing physicians, the overwhelming majority had opposed both cash benefits to mothers or free medical care furnished through the state. And Dr. Champion believed that a conservative estimate could project that an additional appropriation of $300,000 would bring an end to 39 percent of all maternal and infant deaths as the result of more comprehensive educational and nursing services administered by the Department of Public Health.[49]

It was entirely logical that the following year Commissioner Kelley should recommend that the Commonwealth accept funds made available by the federal government through the Sheppard-Towner Act for the extension of child welfare work. Noting that "certain groups of citizens are opposed to the fundamental principle of Federal or State 'benefits,' whether they take the form of cash payments to mothers or free medical or nursing service," Dr. Kelley believed there was no objection to "a campaign of hygienic education" which he understood to be the goal of the federal legislation.[50]

49. Boston *Herald*, June 4, 1920; Champion, "Maternity Benefits," pp. 864-865; "Report of the Special Commission to Investigate Maternity Benefits," *Massachusetts House Documents, No. 1835* (Dec. 1920).
50. Massachusetts Department of Public Health, *Seventh Annual Report* (1922), pp. 19-20. The Sheppard-Towner Act (67th Congress, 42 Stat. 224), of 1921, provided that participating states receive funding from the federal government for the purpose of "promoting the welfare and hygiene of maternity and infancy." Money was to be distributed

Supported by both candidates in the 1920 presidential campaign, the Sheppard-Towner Act was based, according to Julia Lathrop, on the precedent of matching grants-in-aid to the states for agricultural education. Although she did not say so, the precedent was equally derived from the provisions of the Chamberlain-Kahn Act, which made money available to the states during the war for the control of venereal disease. Since Massachusetts had already accepted federal money under twenty-two different provisions, including the Chamberlain-Kahn Act, Dr. Kelley had no reason to expect opposition to the Sheppard-Towner Act, which would give Massachusetts approximately $41,000 for the first year, and $36,000 for the four years following. Not only would these funds contribute substantially to the hard-pressed state budget, but Dr. Kelley found the federal support entirely consonant with the Department's educational program.

Moderate opposition to accepting Sheppard-Towner funds was expressed immediately in the editorial columns of the *Boston Medical and Surgical Journal*. Within a few months district medical societies raised further objections based, at first, on skepticism about the statistics provided by the Children's Bureau.[51] In the next months, while those who had remained proponents of state maternal benefit plans shifted their support to federal aid, the physicians who had earlier questioned the propriety of introducing any form of medical assistance into the educational programs of the Department of Health were joined by individuals and groups who opposed Sheppard-Towner as an unwarranted invasion of state and individual rights.

Leading the campaign against any extension of federal power, and focusing first on maternal aid and later on the movement to regulate child labor, was a national organization founded in Boston in 1922 — the Sentinels of the Republic. Headed by Louis Coolidge, former Assistant Secretary of the Treasury, this

---

to the states meeting certain minimum requirements involving the establishment of a special bureau to carry on investigations and educational work and appropriating matching state funds. Standards were set by a Federal Board of Maternity and Infant Hygiene, composed of the Chief of the Children's Bureau, the Surgeon-General, and the Commissioner of Education. The Children's Bureau was responsible for administration of funds, providing one of the major points of attack for the opposition. The original appropriation was for five years; after a bitter fight, it was renewed for two years with the provision that this would be terminal.

51. *BMSJ*, 185:360-361 (Sept. 22, 1921); 186:200 (Feb. 9, 1922). For discussion of national support and opposition to Sheppard-Towner, see Edward R. Schlesinger, "The Sheppard-Towner Era: A Prototype Case Study in Federal-State Relationships," *AJPH*, 57:1034-1040 (June 1967); J. Stanley Lemmons, "The Sheppard-Towner Act: Progressivism in the 1920's," *Journal of American History*, 55:776-786 (March 1969).

organization secured support from such well-known, civic-minded citizens as former governor William A. Gaston, Mrs. Barrett Wendell, and Mrs. Frank B. Sanborn. For the next ten years the Massachusetts-based Sentinels and their Washington secretary, Mary G. Kilbreth, mounted a growing and quite successful campaign against child welfare and security legislation.[52]

The Sentinels of the Republic viewed Sheppard-Towner, and the Children's Bureau in particular, as participants in a conspiracy for the federal usurpation of state's rights. With increasing virulence, the Sentinels charged that the national government was about to inaugurate compulsory prenatal examinations, restrict the personal choice of medical care, and teach birth control. When the Sentinel's third president, Alexander Lincoln, ran for Attorney General of Massachusetts in 1926, the same year that Congress was to renew the Sheppard-Towner appropriation, Miss Kilbreth wrote him that it was "absolutely essential to take some dramatic action of that kind that will arrest the attention of the public to what is going on" in Washington. She believed that Massachusetts should lead this campaign since it had already taken the initiative against federal child welfare programs.[53]

The Commonwealth, one of three states refusing to accept Sheppard-Towner funds, led a short-lived legal battle to have the law declared unconstitutional.[54] Although the Massachusetts Medical Society expressed grave doubts concerning the wisdom of accepting federal assistance for work which might intrude on the professional prerogative of physicians, it was certainly not the center of opposition. The Department of Public Health, on the other hand, clearly favored accepting the support of the federal government for the extension of educational programs. There appeared to be agreement with this position in the legislature; the speaker of the Massachusetts House of Representatives, B. Loring Young, made a strong case for Sheppard-Towner since the legislation met previous objections by specifically prohibiting the use of these funds for maternity benefits,

52. Alexander Lincoln Papers, Schlesinger Library, Radcliffe College, folder A-109-1, 3, 5, 6.

53. Kilbreth to Lincoln, April 6, 1926, Lincoln Papers, folder A-109-9. Originally the Sentinals planned to campaign for a state referendum based on the Public Opinion Law of 1920, but gave this up in favor of lobbying. When the appropriation was renewed Miss Kilbreth considered it a major victory since the terms prohibited further funds after 1929.

54. Forty states accepted Sheppard-Towner funds in the first year. By 1925 Massachusetts, Connecticut, Illinois, Vermont, Rhode Island, Kansas, and Maine still refused to participate, but by the end of 1927 only the first three remained adamant. See Lemmons, "The Sheppard-Towner Act," p. 782; *BMSJ*, 189:1080-1081 (Dec. 27, 1923); 193:1176 (Dec. 17, 1925).

indicating that "the intent of Congress is to promote health and not miscellaneous and undefined social theories."[55]

Some historians have indicated that Massachusetts' fragile reform coalition broke up as ethnic and class tensions rose in the second and third decades of the twentieth century. This analysis implies that immigrant groups, both new and older Irish, saw victory at the polls undermined by their endorsement of social welfare measures. If this were so, then one would expect to see Irish Democrats joining resistance to federal and state maternal and child welfare legislation following John F. Fitzgerald's narrow margin of defeat in the 1922 gubernatorial campaign.

Opposition to these measures in Massachusetts was not, however, voiced by ambitious Irish-Catholic politicians at this time. Although officially the Catholic Church certainly did not encourage the state or federal governments to intervene in the schooling or child-rearing practices of its members, the Church issued few calls against maternal and child welfare legislation until 1924. "Honey Fitz," James Michael Curley, and David Walsh already represented different factions among Democratic voters, but until 1924 they all maintained their stance as reformers. At the beginning of the election campaign that year, when Curley ran for Governor and Walsh for the United States Senate, both supported the child labor amendment. After Cardinal O'Connell came out in opposition, Curley shifted his position, but Walsh remained silent. The defeat of both Irish Democratic candidates in 1924 marks a turning point in their public attitudes toward welfare legislation. When Walsh successfully ran for the Senate seat vacated when Lodge died two years later, his rhetoric had shifted completely. Walsh, who between 1914 and 1924 had been the proponent of vigorous government, now saw "big government" and "big business" as equal threats. He became a leading opponent of federal child labor legislation and the "federal bureaucracy" in all its aspects. It was not until 1926 that Mary Kilbreth, secretary of the Sentinels, was able to write that "I am hopeful, though not sure, that the National Catholic Welfare Conference is being swung into opposition." Organized opposition to maternal and child welfare legislation by "old stock" Americans of conservative stamp was well under way in 1924 when Cardinal O'Connell attacked the child labor amendment as a threat to the rights

---

55. *BMSJ*, 185:735 (Dec. 15, 1921). Kelley supported Sheppard-Towner before a public hearing of the Joint Legislative Committee on Public Health and Social Welfare, adding that in general he "opposed interference by the Federal Government in matters which . . . could be left to State and local agencies" (see *ibid.*, 186:333 [March 9, 1922]).

and duties of parents.[56] With varying degrees of alacrity, Fitzgerald, Curley, and Walsh jumped on a rolling bandwagon.

It is difficult, however, to assign responsibility for the initial action against federal child welfare legislation taken by the Commonwealth in 1923. After consultation with the state's Attorney General, J. Weston Allen, the legislature decided not to accept federal money for its child and maternal health program.[57] Asserting that such funds represented an unconstitutional diversion of federal revenues collected from the taxation of income and claiming that Congress had no right to interfere in matters which belonged under the jurisdiction of the several states, Massachusetts brought action against the Treasury Department. The Commonwealth was represented by Alexander Lincoln, president of the Sentinels, who argued that since Massachusetts' citizens contributed more than 5 percent of the total income taxes collected throughout the United States and would receive back less than half of this $56,000 as its share of Sheppard-Towner funds, the state was faced with an "illegal option . . . to yield its sovereign power or to give up its share of appropriations."[58]

When the Supreme Court refused to hear the complaints, claiming that these arguments were fundamentally political and that the state did not have sufficient interest in the controversy to present the suit, the *Boston Medical and Surgical Journal* feared this would be interpreted as endorsement of a dubious trend in legislation. The editors urged Massachusetts legislators to continue their principled opposition "to a system which will be of no appreciable advantage to us and an experiment for others." Three years later, the *Journal* urged that Sheppard-Towner be allowed to terminate after its first five-year term. But at the same time, the *Journal* called the federal government to task for allocating only 10 percent of the annual budget to health needs. Physicians insisted that any program with a medical component should be directed by the United

56. Huthmacher, *Massachusetts People and Politics*, pp. 70-74, 107. Kilbreth to Lincoln, Feb. 1, 1926, Lincoln Papers, folder A-109-9. Dorothy Kirchwey Brown, *The Case for Acceptance of the Sheppard-Towner Act* (Washington, D.C.: National League of Women Voters, n.d.). Mrs. Brown, the wife of the prominent Boston attorney LaRue Brown, wrote this pamphlet as chairman of the Child Welfare Committee of the League. When they returned to Boston from Washington in 1920, where Mr. Brown had been Assistant Attorney General during the war, Mrs. Brown continued her activities in behalf of child welfare reform which began when she worked briefly in the Children's Bureau. As a leader of the League, she continued to work for civic reform and was aware of the various currents of support and opposition to this legislation. In an informative interview in the fall of 1969, Mrs. Brown confirmed the support of child welfare measures by Massachusetts Irish political leaders between 1920 and 1926.

57. *BMSJ*, 186:717-723 (May 25, 1922).

58. Lincoln Papers, folders A-109-9, 10.

States Public Health Service. At the same time, they accused the Children's Bureau of being willing to allow the program to lapse unless the funds were administered through its own agencies.[59]

Each year, as reports publicized the progress of maternal and child health programs, opposing groups came forward with contrary principles and facts. It seemed impossible to evaluate the advantages of measures undertaken on their merits since both friends and enemies agreed that they were but a shadow of things to come. When Grace Abbott, who succeeded Miss Lathrop as Chief of the Children's Bureau in 1921, announced a substantial reduction in maternal and infant mortality, the American Medical Association and the Massachusetts Medical Society cast doubts upon the accuracy of the federal statistics.[60]

Other insidious educational materials had a far more pernicious intent. Dr. M. Victor Safford, Deputy Commissioner of the Boston Health Department, claimed that as concern for the child became "a prominent occupation," the unwary would be faced with subtle campaigns to promote birth control. Moreover, he suggested that the proposed constitutional amendment "may start the operation of a corps of Federal officials to prevent boys and girls from developing industrious habits at a time of life when such habits must be developed if they are to be acquired at all." While the Sentinels of the Republic warned the country against further federal invasions of privacy and affronts to medicine, a southern physician speaking at the national convention of the American Medical Association attacked Massachusetts for its newfound and unseemly disavowal of federal aid to the states.[61]

The Massachusetts legislature, committed both to rejecting funds for maternal

59. *BMSJ*, 188:965 (June 14, 1923); 190:1142 (June 26, 1924); 194:646-647 (April 8, 1926); 195:732 (Oct. 7, 1926).

60. Grace Abbott, *Ten Years' Work for Children* (Washington, D.C., Government Printing Office, 1923), pp. 3-4, 10; *BMSJ*, 186:200 (Feb. 9, 1922).

61. *BMSJ*, 191:776 (Oct. 23, 1924); *JAMA*, 79:963 (Sept. 16, 1922). In Washington, Congressman Alben Barkley of Kentucky, noting physicians' fears of government intervention in medical matters, urged that Sheppard-Towner be under the direction of the Children's Bureau since, he believed, this would be more likely to avoid the danger of the government's practicing medicine than if the program were directed by the Surgeon-General; see *JAMA* 77:1913 (Dec. 10, 1921). Although Sheppard-Towner expired in 1929, some congressmen continued to advocate federal child welfare as part of a Children's Bureau extension program. The Sentinels of the Republic led the successful fight to defeat these proposals (Newton Bill and the Cooper-Jones Bill in 1930 and 1931). The Children's Bureau bore the brunt of the attack, and after 1931 Miss Kilbreth believed that it had been "completely exposed. It's a safe target for political attack now," she wrote; see Kilbreth to Lincoln, March 6, 1931, Lincoln Papers, folder A-109-10. David I. Walsh, then Senator from Massachusetts, played a prominent role in the campaigns against maternal and child welfare legislation.

and infant hygiene and to extending public health measures to reduce mortality rates, appropriated an additional fifteen thousand dollars to the Division of Hygiene for the balance of 1922. At the time the Division reported that although infant deaths between one month and one year of age were slowly but surely declining, there was very little change in the death rate of the newborn. Attributing the first decrease to improved state and municipal sanitary controls of water and milk and the consequent decrease in diarrheal disease, Dr. Champion reiterated that further progress was dependent on education in personal hygiene.[62] In the next few years, there were virtually no changes in the implementation of the program other than an increase in the quantity of work. Having agreed that its role was to stimulate local boards of health, voluntary nursing associations, and physicians to perform their established functions, the Division concentrated on reaching these groups.

At the same time, the Department paid more attention to and greater enthusiasm was engendered for steps taken by the Division of Communicable Diseases to prevent and control the diseases of later childhood. Distinctly medical programs were developed for the prevention and control of tuberculosis and diphtheria as the Department of Public Health energetically advocated the immunization and care of susceptible and sick children. Even though prevention of tuberculosis was founded on the promulgation of proper hygiene, rather than any specifically medical prophylaxis, these measures were justified by an elaborate scientific diagnosis which left no room for vague social theories of etiology.[63] Detection and decisions about the management of the patient were determined by physicians, and the prolonged treatment frequently required was continued under professional supervision at the state sanatoria. Under these conditions, by common consent, the Department of Public Health played host to the diseased.

While the Division of Hygiene continued its educational campaigns, the Division of Communicable Diseases organized programs for immunization against diphtheria through Schick testing and the use of toxin-antitoxin, and for the early identification and isolation of tuberculosis through X-ray, tuberculin test-

---

62. Massachusetts Department of Public Health, *Eighth Annual Report* (1923), pp. 5, 152. The legislature also agreed to a sum of $50,000 for the following year, still far short of the $300,000 suggested by Dr. Champion in 1920.

63. Massachusetts Department of Public Health, *Ninth Annual Report* (1924), pp. 4-13. The Department described three discrete types of tuberculosis, roughly corresponding to the age of patients: infantile, adolescent, and adult. Although these classifications were not considered absolutely rigid, they did suggest different preventive and therapeutic care for each category.

ing, and hospitalization, along with the establishment of a children's sanatorium at Westfield. The control of specific disease was assigned exclusively to the Division of Communicable Diseases, and the Division of Hygiene depended more and more upon its cooperation with the State Department of Education.[64] Within the Division, infants and mothers shared attention with the elderly and the chronically diseased. As the Department of Public Health took on responsibilities for reducing the fifty thousand deaths caused annually by noncontagious diseases, it became necessary to reorganize these services and to create a Division of Adult Hygiene with a special cancer section in 1928. The new Division of Child Hygiene at the same time retained its "legal responsibility to fact find in regard to causes of sickness among mothers and children." However, with the appointment of Dr. M. Luise Diez, the first woman to head any major phase of the Department's work, came the admission that "limited resources in this field can be most effectively used by educating the educators, be they teachers, parents, public health nurses, or responsible nonprofessional persons. This is accomplished by all the methods from the didactic lecture to the casual conversation and the service demonstration."

It seemed that very little had changed in public health practice since Massachusetts had first agreed that children's health required special attention. Yet death rates among children had declined, and the diseases of childhood claimed fewer victims. The questions remained: were these results derived from the work of the Department of Public Health? If so, were they the result of new habits and attitudes engendered by the policies of the Division of Hygiene? Seven years later, in 1936, a special commission reported that although Massachusetts' maternal mortality rates were not higher than those of other states, they would be further reduced "if known scientific information . . . were uniformly applied throughout the Commonwealth." The same was true of infant deaths. Prevention and cure rested with "education of the parent in the . . . rudiments of hygiene . . . avoidance of contact with infectious diseases and active immunization . . . simple basic rules for the care of illness . . . and the elimination of conditions conducive to serious accidents."[65]

In a sense, evaluation of the underlying purpose of child and maternal welfare legislation was left to its critics. Coincident with their attacks on the federal bureaucracy, they questioned whether the health needs of a particular group

64. Massachusetts Department of Public Health, *Tenth Annual Report* (1925), pp. 11, 18.

65. Massachusetts Department of Public Health, *Fourteenth Annual Report* (1929), pp. 11, 123, 130.

should receive the benefits of special legislation — whether the specific circumstances could be isolated from the conditions affecting the entire population.[66] The attempt to alleviate symptoms had permitted the Division of Hygiene to avoid the original issue: if excessive infant and maternal mortality rates were caused by failure to obey the rules, was the ultimate cure education or the enforcement of regulations? Was ignorance primarily the result of unfortunate social conditions or personal obduracy?

"The outstanding public health problem of the present day," announced Dr. Herbert L. Lombard in 1929, "is the control of the chronic diseases of middle life."[67] This was not a parochial judgment from the first director of the Division of Adult Hygiene; rather, it was the dominant view of the Department of Public Health. A marked departure from the Department's outlook in 1914 when the control and possible eradication of contagious diseases were major concerns, this new position derived both from the analyses of epidemiologists and the growing public expectation that social responsibility for health included measures to mitigate the hardships created by chronic, noncommunicable disease.

Yet, as in the case of earlier proposals to protect the health of mothers and children, it was not clear that the Department shared public sentiment. With respect to cancer, the public seemed to expect a combination of state medical and welfare services to alleviate the pain and hardship of prolonged illness. As early as 1915, resolutions had been introduced in the legislature requesting more than the statistical studies on the incidence of cancer which the Board of Health had reported beginning in 1896.[68] The Department supplemented its epidemiological work, after 1919, with a cancer diagnostic service furnished through cooperation with the Harvard Cancer Commission. But the Department

66. It is interesting to note that although this kind of question was not raised, and I would suggest *could* not have been raised at this time by the advocates of a more inclusive health policy, they were precisely the grounds for attack from conservative groups. See William C. Woodward, "Federal Domination over State Health Activities," *American Medical Association Bulletin*, 25:68-77 (March 1930).

67. Herbert L. Lombard, "The Chronic Disease Problem in Massachusetts," *Commonhealth*, 16:103 (Oct.-Nov.-Dec. 1929).

68. Herbert L. Lombard, "The Massachusetts Cancer Program," and an "autobiographical record" distributed by the Massachusetts Department of Public Health in 1959, pp. 5-6. Although medical opinion was divided as to whether there was a real increase in cancer, or whether the apparent increase was an artifact of better diagnosis, there is no doubt that the public believed cancer had become a greater threat to life; see George H. Bigelow and Lombard, *Cancer and Other Chronic Diseases in Massachusetts* (Boston: Houghton, Mifflin, 1933), pp. 100-111.

consistently failed to support various bills intending to place medical and hospital care of the cancer patient under state supervision. Even when the Department somewhat reluctantly took over responsibility for the four state tuberculosis sanatoria and the leprosy hospital in 1920, Dr. Kelley rejected the legitimacy of providing public facilities for cancer patients. Instead, he preferred the traditional role of state health agencies — that of giving advice by providing dependable diagnostic services to physicians and distributing informational pamphlets published by the American Society for the Control of Cancer to the layman.[69]

The safest path for "adult hygiene," at least one epidemiologist believed, was to follow the guideline set by work in maternal and child hygiene. If "the principle of 'keeping the well child well' works" she wrote, "We should carry the principle on into adult life . . . new interest would be created in personal and individual health . . . for the increased efficiency and greater enjoyment of life."[70] However, if the Department accepted the position that lack of proper hygienic information was responsible for the health deficits of early childhood, it was difficult to apply this view to those over fifty years of age, as death rates for the population as a whole declined from 19.2 per 1,000 in 1870 to 14.3 in 1920.

This leap in logic would have necessitated the development of a specialized hygiene for those persons in the middle and later years of life who had somehow resisted the edification of early hygienic instruction. Dr. Merrill Champion's investigation of maternal and infant hygiene in 1920 had revealed no important correlation between social and economic conditions and the fluctuation of morbidity and mortality rates.

Five years after Dr. Champion's investigation, Dr. Lombard was brought to the Department to begin a series of studies on the epidemiology of cancer. His conclusions, first reported in 1927 and continuing into the next decade, showed that the significant variables in the incidence of noncontagious disease were age, sex, economic status, density of population, and nationality. One survey in addition indicated that there were more than 500,000 Massachusetts citizens whose health was impaired by chronic disease, and that approximately one-third of these did not receive medical care. Since only one-half of the chronically ill in the lowest socioeconomic group obtained even occasional medical attention, compared with four-fifths of those who were well-off, Dr. Lombard concluded

69. Massachusetts Department of Public Health, *Fifth Annual Report* (1919), p. 26, and *Sixth Annual Report* (1920), pp. 10-12.
70. Mary R. Lakeman, "Path-Finding in Adult Hygiene," *Commonhealth*, 17:50 (Jan.-Feb.-March 1930).

that "probably the principal reason for failure to procure medical advice is poverty."[71]

This assessment added to the difficulty of determining what services the Department might appropriately provide. The coincidence of poverty and chronic disease did not establish a causal relationship, and, although untreated illness might eventually contribute to indigency and therefore to the welfare costs of the state, this did not necessarily clarify the responsibilities of the Department of Public Health.[72] There was widespread agreement in the medical community, including those physicians who worked in public health, that the scientific nature of prevention and therapy required the establishment of standardized controls to assess the effectiveness of all measures employed. It would be inefficient, uneconomical, and contrary to the precepts of medicine, to engage in meliorative programs that could not be carefully evaluated. If the acceptable criteria of a viable public health program, "the prevention of a given disease, the lessening of sickness and death from specific and related causes, and the promotion of health to a discernable degree,"[73] were to be maintained, the Department's powers would have to be confined to the prevention of disease. These primarily self-imposed strictures had placed public health administration in a favorable position to influence both legislation and public respect; the image of scientific hygiene could not be forfeited without seriously impairing the authority of the Department of Public Health.

Confounding this view was the Department's commitment to its humanitarian role: "we ought to be doing *something*," wrote Dr. Kelley, "something practical, financially feasible, scientifically sound, and phychologically acceptable to the public."[74] Even Dr. Kelley's usual caution was affected by the belief of social scientists in the 1920's that the collection and analysis of facts would

71. Herbert L. Lombard, "The Chronic Disease Problem in Massachusetts," *Commonhealth*, 16:104-105 (Oct.-Nov.-Dec. 1929), and "The Chronic Disease Problem in Massachusetts," *Proceedings of the National Conference of Social Work* (Boston, 1931), p. 149. Lombard's second article and one presented at the same meeting by George H. Bigelow ("The Massachusetts Cancer Program," pp. 152-162) report most of the investigations conducted in Massachusetts between 1927 and 1930.

72. Bigelow and Lombard, *Cancer and Other Chronic Diseases*, pp. 71-72. There was considerable disagreement as to whether the main problem was that poverty created conditions conducive to chronic disease or whether chronic disease increased dependence among those whose economic condition was already marginal. The Department of Public Health tended to stress the former, and the Department of Public Welfare, the latter.

73. Edgar Sydenstriker, "The Measurement of Public Health Work," *Annual Report of the Milbank Memorial Fund* (1926). See also W. S. Rankin, "Elimination of Politics from Public Health Work," *JAMA*, 83:1285-1289 (Oct. 25, 1924).

74. Kelley, "Cancer and the Health Administrator," *AJPH*, 14:561 (July 1924).

open the way for realistic manipulation of the social conditions depriving people of the opportunity for health. But it was necessary, Dr. Kelley believed, to maintain a distinction between what health needs were and what it was possible to accomplish. Whereas the Department should cooperate with other government agencies and with volunteer groups as well, priorities for state policy should be assigned by the Department itself.

It was hardly a criticism of Dr. Kelley that neither "needs" nor "possibilities" could be established along the hard lines which would have facilitated decisions about priorities. However, in the optimistic 1920's it was quite usual to talk as though these criteria could be established if enough data were accumulated and enough money spent. As a result, halfway measures were often considered expedient and innovation postponed awaiting the confirmation that was supposed to be right around the corner. In the meantime, perhaps the proper role of the Department of Public Health would be less open to dispute if questions of larger purpose could be postponed a while in favor of more immediate and mundane goals.[75]

This was precisely what Dr. Kelley attempted in his seven years as Commissioner. Having begun his term with the broadest vision and pride in the pioneering role of the Department he headed, he gradually narrowed his definition of a permissible role for the state in the pursuit of public health. At the outset of his work in Massachusetts he had insisted that prevention necessitated standardized quarantine and mandatory immunization for smallpox and diphtheria. Two years before his death, Kelley urged that the physician's "attitude of scientific inquiry" made his first duty "leadership in matters of social welfare." An article published posthumously warned that public health departments are constantly being pressed to perform services and functions beyond the province of the state, services and functions which "should revert to the consultation room of the general practitioner to be carried on privately on a fee basis precisely the same as curative medicine is now and always has been." During his relatively brief term, this moderate man who had gently attempted to gain support for mildly innovative policies was time after time rebuffed by both the medical profession and the legislature as no other spokesman for public health had been in over fifty years. He suffered not only the strain of administering a demanding

75. See Henry F. May, "Shifting Perspectives on the 1920's," *Mississippi Valley Historical Review*, 43:407-408 (Dec. 1956); Edgar Sydenstriker, "The Vitality of the American People," in *Recent Social Trends in the United States*, 2 vols (New York: McGraw-Hill, 1933), I, 602-660; Harry H. Moore, "Health and Medical Practices," in *ibid.*, II, 1061-1113; Bigelow and Lombard, *Cancer and Other Chronic Diseases*, preface. This last book is dedicated to Kelley, in recognition of his guidance during the "critical early formative period" of the chronic disease policy in public health.

public health program, but he was also troubled with poor health; at forty-two years of age he took his own life on September 27, 1925.[76]

The combination of pressures which resulted in the reformulation of Massachusetts public health policy in the second quarter of the twentieth century was more diverse than in any period heretofore. New measures grew in part out of defeat since contagious disease seemed to have reached the irreducible minimum possible without more complex knowledge of social factors influencing the etiology and epidemiology of specific infection. Accepting a somewhat skeptical estimation of the degree to which public health measures directly affected the reduction of contagion, a 1925 doctoral dissertation by Dr. Edward G. Huber at the Harvard School of Public Health suggested that it would be economical to divert a substantial portion of public health funds to education and other efforts to secure public cooperation.

Dr. Huber, a physician in the Army Medical Corps who retired from the army to join the Massachusetts Department of Public Health some ten years later, criticized the medical profession for its antagonistic attitude toward state-supported preventive medicine. He implied that if physicians could be persuaded to utilize medical prophylaxis, the Department of Public Health could concentrate on more general measures for the promotion of health and the encouragement of uniform health standards. Dr. Huber chided the public health officer for his exclusive focus on communicable disease. Such a policy was an error, he wrote, because the public was interested in the problems of chronic disease and would support the Department more readily if it took a broader view of its responsibilities. It would be both efficient and expedient, he concluded, for public health to be identified at this time with education rather than medicine.[77]

76. Compare Kelley, "The Modern Public Health Movement," *Commonhealth*, 8:259-267 (Nov.-Dec. 1921), "The Medical Graduate," *BMSJ*, 189:806-810 (Nov. 22, 1923), and "Remarks on Certain New Developments in Public Health," *BMSJ*, 183:1180 (Dec. 24, 1925). Obituary, *BMSJ*, 193:701-702 (Oct. 8, 1925). The Boston *Herald*, Sept. 28, 1925, reported that Kelley was despondent because the legislature rejected his pleas for higher salaries for public health personnel.

77. Edward Huber's study was supported by the Massachusetts Medical Society and published serially in nineteen installments as "The Control of Communicable Diseases Prevalent in Massachusetts, With a Study of Mortality Due to Them During the Past Seventy-Five Years," *BMSJ*, 195:87-89 (July 8, 1926) – 195:933-942 (Nov. 11, 1926). He stated that an additional reason for not relying exclusively on the traditional means of controlling contagious disease was that variables of host and infecting organism were not responsive to available scientific determinants. Edward Godfrey Huber (1882-1946), a member of the second class at Harvard School of Public Health, returned to Massachusetts as an epidemiologist in the Division of Tuberculosis of the Department of Public Health in 1935. He remained closely associated with the department in various capacities even after his main responsibilities became teaching and administration at the Harvard School of Public Health, where he was Professor of Public Health Practice and Associate Dean at the time of his death.

Dr. George H. Bigelow, who succeeded Dr. Kelley as Commissioner, seemed at first to share this point of view. His first reports stressed the need for the district health officer to be a "generalist" rather than a "specialist," and emphasized that the local physician was the indispensible element in preventive medicine and should deal directly with the patient. State-supported clinics, were they the tuberculosis and venereal disease dispensaries already in operation or the proposed cancer clinics, were stopgaps at best and should be reduced to a minimum. With an eye to their eventual dissolution, the Department issued a pamphlet, *Preventive Medicine From Your Family Physician.*[78]

Within a few years this trend was transformed. Profoundly influenced by nonprofessional demands for more comprehensive public health care, the Department of Public Health resumed its role of physician to the public, and "education" became another word for programs that fell short of success. Beginning in 1915, the legislature annually considered petitions authorizing the Department of Health to establish some form of medical care and hospital facilities for the patient with cancer. No epidemic of contagious disease in Massachusetts, and none of the Department's own recommendations for legislative action received the insistent attention demanded by the families and friends of cancer victims. Although the Department charged that routine public health services in rural communities were grossly inadequate and submitted annual requests to have the sale of unpasteurized milk prohibited, this type of advice went unheeded or was subjected to arguments which prevented favorable action.[79]

The medical profession certainly did not encourage augmented public health services at this time. No spokesman for the Massachusetts Medical Society appeared before the legislature to urge the adoption of a state cancer program. In fact, the *Boston Medical and Surgical Journal* completely disregarded all legislative motions for the investigation of cancer in the state. Instead, it remarked that the backwardness of a small number of physicians was responsible for the failure of patients to seek medical advice.[80]

Despite this lack of support from the Department and the medical profession, the legislature, in April 1925, established a joint commission made up of repre-

78. Massachusetts Department of Public Health, *Eleventh Annual Report* (1926), p. 6.

79. For an interesting description of support for the legislation, see Lombard, "The Massachusetts Cancer Program," pp. 7-11. For the major concerns of the Department in these years see Massachusetts Department of Public Health, *Eleventh Annual Report* (1926), pp. 73-74, and *Twelfth Annual Report* (1925), p. 3.

80. *BMSJ*, 192:371 (Feb. 19, 1925). The only item in the *Journal* relating to the legislative investigation is a request for cooperation with the Commission from Dr. Bigelow (193:465-466 [June 9, 1925]).

sentatives of the Departments of Public Health and Public Welfare to examine the services available for cancer patients. The commission's report, delivered in December, was admittedly "less specific than might be desired." The commission engaged Dr. Lombard to conduct the investigation and broadened its original mandate, which had stressed the need for facilities for inoperable cases, to include consideration of the adequacy of facilities for diagnosis, education, and all forms of therapy. The Health Department members of the commission did not even confine themselves to the question of cancer. They suggested instead that, if the state offered diagnosis and treatment to cancer patients, these services were equally applicable to other chronic diseases such as diabetes, nephritis, and heart disease.

The commission was unable to reach any agreement beyond the need to stimulate public education and to extend the existing private facilities. As a result, it submitted two separate and contradictory sets of recommendations: one endorsed by the members from the Department of Public Welfare advocated the construction of a 340-bed hospital as a minimum state commitment; the other, supported by Drs. Bigelow and Champion, agreed that "it is a settled principle in Massachusetts that public dependents who are sick should be cared for humanely and unhesitatingly." But, they insisted, this was "far from saying . . . that the State should enter the field of supplying medical care to the sick who are able to pay for it in whole or part." Their statement was a strong rejection of any right or obligation of the state to engage in medical practice which was not clearly preventive. There was no epidemiological evidence, they insisted, to sanction public care for chronic disease. Desirable as this might be from the viewpoint of social welfare, there was no evidence to justify medical intervention to promote such goals. This is "State medicine at its worst," they asserted, and it would have serious consequences since "sooner or later there would be erected such an army of dependents as would constitute far more of a menace to the State than does cancer itself."[81]

Drs. Bigelow, Champion, and Lombard believed that all aspects of treatment for the chronically ill should be left entirely in the hands of the private medical practitioner and that the special needs of the indigent should be met by the De-

81. "Resolve Providing for an Investigation Relative to the Prevalence of Cancer and to What Extent Further Hospital and Institutional Facilities are Necessary to Combat it," *Acts and Resolves 1925, Chapter 20* (April 16, 1925), pp. 458-459; "Special Report of the Departments of Public Health and Public Welfare Relative to the Prevalence of the Disease of Cancer Throughout the Commonwealth and Particularly the Disease in Its Inoperable Stage or Form," *Massachusetts Legislative Documents 1925, House 1200* (Dec. 15, 1925), pp. 91-98.

partment of Public Welfare. They were moved by the social problems faced by
the cancer patient, but it was clear to them that state-supported therapy, no
matter what its rationale, was the very issue that tended to keep the medical
profession from supporting public health measures. The legislature, meanwhile,
appeared entirely ready to forego the assistance of physicians; in 1926 it directed the Department of Public Health to establish cancer clinics throughout the
state without the support of local physicians if necessary. Such a stance was
entirely unacceptable to Dr. Bigelow and the majority of the Department of
Public Health, which identified itself first with the medical profession.[82]

Since the end of the nineteenth century, with the development of medical
prophylaxis, scientific preventive medicine had formed the acceptable framework for public health and for personal hygiene. Despite excursions into the
domain of education, efforts to convince the public of the need for self-reform
had not been notably successful. The legislature notwithstanding, the authority
of the Department of Public Health was substantially based on its medical and
scientific affiliation. Department spokesmen believed that it would be visionary
to mount a campaign against cancer without grounding it on medical authority.
Well aware of the lack of enthusiasm in the medical profession for this exercise
of state power, the Department was unable to find medical justification for a
tax-supported program designed to alleviate rather than prevent disease. The
legislature, on the other hand, felt that it was protected from the charge of
wielding excessive and arbitrary state power by subscribing to a scientific rather
than a humanitarian rationale. The legislation which established the first public
cancer hospital in the country and the first state-supported cancer clinics was
dedicated to a conception of the role of the state which was theoretically repugnant to both the public and the medical profession. Nonetheless, the Norfolk
State Hospital for alcoholics was renovated and the Pondville Hospital for cancer
opened in June 1926, with ninety beds and facilities for thirty ambulatory patients; the first cancer clinic opened in Newton in December 1927, with five
more to follow shortly.[83] Their success was a tribute not only to Dr. Bigelow's

82. "An Act to Promote the Prevention and Cure of Cancer and the Extension of
Resources for its Cure and Treatment," *Acts and Resolves 1926, Chapter 391* (May 28,
1926), p. 474. Lombard, "The Massachusetts Cancer Program," pp. 34-35; "Preliminary
and Final Reports of the Department of Public Health; Relative to the Care and Treatment of Persons Suffering from Cancer," *Massachusetts House Documents 1927, No.
400* (Dec. 15, 1926), pp. 27-37.

83. Massachusetts Department of Public Health, *Thirteenth Annual Report* (1928), pp.
6-7. At the dedication of the Pondville Hospital, Governor Fuller stated that the purpose
of the cancer program was to prevent the disease by making early treatment more available
and removing unnecessary fear; see address at the opening of the Pondville Cancer Hos-

obedience to legislative mandate, his tact, and his energy, but also to the emergence of public health as a profession.

The concept that public health work was a subspecialty of medicine, requiring training in the social sciences and biostatistics as well as the traditional physical sciences and clinical experience, was fostered by the development of schools of public health. The first program for the certification of health officers had not fully reflected this tendency; instead, it had integrated sanitary engineering and the environmental sciences within its prospectus. The School for Health Officers, sponsored jointly by Harvard and the Massachusetts Institute of Technology between 1913-1922, was intended to give postgraduate training to sanitary engineers and biologists, as well as to physicians.[84]

The director of the program, Dr. Milton J. Rosenau, who was also professor of preventive medicine and hygiene at the Harvard Medical School and a member of the Massachusetts State Board of Health, had published an important public health text in 1913. In this book Dr. Rosenau found it desirable to limit himself to the discussion of communicable disease since he believed this was the sole concern of preventive medicine. He implied that the contribution of a public health department to this effort was restricted to the verification of the etiology of infection and the scientific control of the transmission of pathogenic organisms. Even in the chapter on venereal disease, Rosenau emphasized the narrow scope of public health responsibility,[85] as did Dr. Allan J. McLaughlin

---

pital, June 21, 1927, in *Addresses and Messages to the General Court, Proclamations, Official Addresses, Correspondence and Statements of . . . Governor Alvan T. Fuller*, pp. 397-401. For an illuminating projection of the budgetary commitment required for state medical care of the chronically diseased in 1926, see Bigelow and Lombard, *Cancer and Other Chronic Diseases*, pp. 11-13.

84. Jean A. Curran, "The First School of Public Health," *Harvard Public Health Alumni Bulletin*, 23:2-5, 20 (Jan. 1966). While the school suggested that a medical degree was advisable for those who considered a career in public health, provisions were made for candidates with training in biology and engineering. The *Catalogue* for 1919 stated that students would be admitted "if they have satisfactorily completed two years work in a recognized medical school, or if they have received a bachelor's degree from a recognized college or technical school, or if they have had experience in public health work, provided they have pursued satisfactory courses in physics, chemistry, biology, and modern languages and the fundamental medical sciences." It was emphasized that employment possibilities were improved with a medical degree. Of the thirty-six men receiving certificates by 1919, eight had other than medical training. (*Circular of the School for Health Officers* [Sept. 1913]; *Catalogue of the School of Public Health* [May 1919], pp. 10, 27-31).

85. Rosenau, *Preventive Medicine and Hygiene*, pp. vii, 56-57. Milton J. Rosenau (1869-1946) received his M.D. at the University of Pennsylvania in 1889, and went on to a year of postgraduate work in Europe. From 1890 to 1909 he was director of the Hygienic

when he became Commissioner of the Massachusetts Department of Health a few years later.

The full differentiation of the medical from the engineering aspects of professional training in public health came with the establishment of schools of public health directly associated with schools of medicine. Johns Hopkins University opened its School of Hygiene in 1918 with the aid of an endowment from the Rockefeller Foundation, followed four years later by the Harvard School of Public Health, headed by Dean David L. Edsall of the Harvard Medical School.[86] The identification of professional training in public health with its medical origins tended to both narrow the area in which the public health official was competent to act and to make his judgments within this area decisive.

Although physicians had been placed in charge of the state's public health work since 1869, the prestige which they lent sanitary policy was not primarily the result of their training or reputation as general practitioners. During the years that Bowditch and Walcott chaired the State Board of Health, they had continued private practice, and they enjoyed a privileged position in the community especially because they were respected and responsible citizens of the Commonwealth. The advice of the Board was rarely challenged in these years, in part because of their status and in part because the regulatory role of state commissions and boards was consonant with state policy. Legislation had supported the social principle that the people must be protected from the selfish private interests or the wanton excesses which followed in the wake of rapid economic and social change. In this setting, the wisdom and judgment which Dr. Bowditch and Dr. Walcott freely contributed to the state gained as much from their worldly experience as from their proficiency as physicians.

With the establishment of the Department of Health in 1914, responsibility for protecting public health was delivered into the hands of another privileged group, physicians who devoted themselves exclusively to preventive medicine

---

Laboratory of the United States Public Health Service. He taught at Harvard Medical School from 1909-1935 and succeeded Theobald Smith as director of the Department of Health and the Biologics Laboratory from 1915 to 1920. Like Smith, he divided his time between the medical school and the laboratory. His successor, Benjamin White, was the first full-time director of the laboratory.

86. David L. Edsall, "The School of Public Health," in Samuel Eliot Morison, ed., *The Development of Harvard University Since the Inauguration of President Eliot, 1869-1929* (Cambridge, Mass.: Harvard University Press, 1930). Dr. Jean A. Curran, who has recently completed a history of the School of Public Health, found that Johns Hopkins received the original Rockefeller endowment at least in part because its program was fully integrated with the medical school, whereas Harvard's was not; from a interview in September 1967.

and served the state rather than the individual citizen. The changed outlook and status of the professional public health physicians were more important in determining the new role of the Department, than was public expectation that persons afflicted with cancer should receive additional assistance. Sensitive to the pejorative implications among physicians of their position as state employees, public health officials saw themselves rising above the conflicts that incriminated politicians, ascribed with dispassionate judgment that was founded in science. Salaried public health officials accepted their role as defenders of the state's "special interest" — the public's health.

The Commissioner and his staff came before the legislature annually with recommendations, marshaling medical experts, whenever possible, to testify in support of their briefs. In the 1920's public health officials played a newly combative role for which they sought allies mainly from the medical profession rather than from the nascent army of political and social reformers. They understood that success depended on the deference accorded their professional standing, and they spoke, in public at least, to this point.

Yet the physician who worked in public health had always voiced particular interest in the social benefits derived from good health. Until the last decades of the nineteenth century this was usually expressed in moral terms; intemperate personal behavior was linked with susceptibility to disease, and, consequently, the physician who, by example or guidance, fostered respect for the laws of nature and society made a significant contribution to the health of the body politic as well as the health of the patient.

With the development of knowledge about the specific etiology of contagious diseases, the relationship between scientific hygiene and social reform became more tangential. Yet benevolent concern for the underprivileged, whose ignorance of scientific law was no fault of his own, remained a compelling motive for the physician who often combined teaching or general practice with his duties as a health officer. Even when frustrated by the increasing inability to translate scientific knowledge into public practice, or by the intransigence of individuals who resisted hygienic advice, the public health official maintained a characteristically hopeful attitude. If the source of neglect could be determined with the same accuracy as the source of disease, and the measures of correction could be scientifically established and evaluated, then the bounty of preventive medicine could be made available to all. The new public health official was a multidisciplined scientist; this new guise not only altered his own appearance but, more significantly, it enabled him to re-enter the field of social reform under the banner of science.

In this setting the public health expert was a physician, drawing his early sustenance from medicine and establishing his competence and authority through the scientific training which gave both the general practitioner and the medical specialist the prerogative to judge that a given remedy was advisable or entailed unnecessary risks. In the 1920's both Dr. Lombard and Dr. Bigelow chose public health as their specialty and turned to Harvard for their postgraduate training.

Dr. Lombard was the first epidemiologist to work for the Massachusetts Department with the benefits of this background, and Dr. Bigelow the first, and only Commissioner until 1943 with a doctorate in public health. They saw themselves as buffers between the public and the medical profession and were convinced that the foundation of public health "must be sound medical direction." It was as physicians that they labored and warned their colleagues that "the medical revolution is imminent" and that the public believed the promotion of public health required a more active role for the Department. Evaluating the experiences of the Massachusetts cancer program seven years after its inception, Bigelow and Lombard came to ten conclusions, every one spelling out a proposal for marriage between the state and the medical profession to provide education, prophylaxis, therapy, and terminal care for any citizen who requested it.[87]

It was clearly not an acceptable proposal to many doctors, and hardly a contract between equal partners. One eminent physician deplored the degrading situation in which "the consulting room has deteriorated from a temple of health to an exchange in which business is transacted."[88]

But others responded more favorably; if not a marriage, at least an engagement was announced. Dr. Bigelow appointed a thirty-man advisory committee for the cancer program, on which many physicians as well as prominent laymen consented to serve. Physicians volunteered to act as consultants to the hospital and clinics, supplementing the paid professional staffs. When fifteen additional clinics were opened, they were sponsored jointly by the Department of Public

---

87. Bigelow and Lombard, *Cancer and Other Chronic Diseases*, pp. 15, 21, 71. Lombard received an M.P.H. in 1924. Bigelow did his postgraduate work at the Harvard Graduate School, receiving his Ph.D. in Public Health in 1921, the year before the School of Public Health was established.

88. William Dameshek, "Some Arguments Against State Medicine," *NEJM*, 204:1191 (June 4, 1931). For Bigelow's characteristically forthright position, see "Is the State's Cancer Program State Medicine?" *ibid*., 200:438-439 (Feb. 28, 1929).

Health and the local medical society, and clinics were not opened in the two communities where this cooperation was not forthcoming.[89]

Dr. Bigelow bound the medical profession as closely as he could to the Department of Public Health. In 1932 he announced that a "fine mutual understanding" existed so that the Public Relations Committee of the Massachusetts Medical Society and the Public Health Council held joint meetings. When physicians in some of the rural communities showed hostility to the development of district health services — reminiscent of their opposition to maternal and child care programs less than a decade before — Dr. Bigelow tried to smooth over the friction. With characteristic good faith he announced, somewhat prematurely, "Surely swords are being turned into plowshares."[90]

Dr. Bigelow's optimism and energy helped to gloss over the obstacles which beset his years in office. Each battle lost was but a temporary setback. His good humor and wit encouraged all his supporters and even seemed to turn the tide of stubborn resistance. His persistent struggle for mandatory pasteurization of milk failed. Yet to a large extent because of his personal campaign, 85 percent of all milk consumed in the state was being pasteurized by the time he left office in 1933.

Nevertheless, the problems that plagued his eight years as Commissioner loomed large. More than any of his predecessors, George Hoyt Bigelow was burdened by the discrepancy between available scientific information and its implementation. Bigelow, whose life was committed to the social use of medicine, often gave the impression that he regarded the usual measures of success in public health as somewhat spurious. For instance, when he cited annual figures indicating that more milk was pasteurized than in the previous year, he would simultaneously note how many years it would take for all milk to be pas-

89. Massachusetts Department of Public Health, *Twelfth Annual Report* (1927), pp. 2-3; Bigelow and Lombard, *Cancer and Other Chronic Diseases*, pp. 86-87.

90. Massachusetts Department of Public Health, *Eighteenth Annual Report* (1933), p. 4. The development of full-time professional services through the Nashoba and Southern Berkshire Health Districts was made possible through a substantial grant from the Commonwealth Fund of New York City. The stormy history of these "experiments" revealed opposition not only from local physicians, but from within the Department itself. The *Annual Reports* of the Department of Health show little of this controversy, and I am grateful to the Commonwealth Fund for the opportunity to examine their records of correspondence with members of the Department. Dr. Harold W. Stevens, medical officer of the Southern Berkshire District from September 1932 until 1935 and later district health officer, was particularly helpful. He described his experiences and shared his knowledge of the work and the people who led it during two interviews in the fall of 1968.

teurized at the current rate of progress. At other times he would remark in feigned amazement that in some areas milk "has become almost as emotional a fluid as liquor."[91]

Bigelow's brilliant career, following graduation from Harvard Medical School in 1916, took him to Haiti, to Antioch College, and to the Pay Clinic of Cornell Medical College before he was named Director of the Division of Communicable Disease in March 1924. His resignation from the Department in the summer of 1933, shortly after he had been reappointed Commissioner for the second time, took everyone by surprise. With characteristic energy he assumed his next job as medical director of the Massachusetts General Hospital, winning new friends and admirers.

His disappearance in December 1934 shocked all who had known him. Friends who gathered at Harvard's Memorial Chapel the following spring, after his body had been recovered in a Framingham reservoir, heard of his exuberance, his jokes, his impassioned pursuit of excellence in public health. Dr. Richard E. Cabot spoke of Bigelow's unwillingness to compromise integrity, his willingness to admit failure; finally, he likened his faith in the impossible to that of Peter Pan.[92] And perhaps it was this fantasy that sustained not only Bigelow but the work he had begun as well, for he had referred to the Department of Public Health as the Pied Piper of the state, invoking an image of children marching off to a somewhat illusory destination.

In many ways the state's cancer program, which Bigelow had guided, despite grave misgivings, was the single most impressive endeavor of the Department in the first part of the twentieth century. Despite the initial skepticism voiced by Lombard and Bigelow, the program, once implemented, reflected the several goals of public health: to prevent unnecessary disease; to bring together professional skill and public support; and to harness goodwill and science. Sophistica-

91. Massachusetts Department of Public Health, *Nineteenth Annual Report* (1934), p. 2; *Thirteenth Annual Report* (1928), p. 8, and *Sixteenth Annual Report* (1931), pp. 6, 18; *Commonhealth*, 16:3-4 (Jan.-Feb.-March 1929). Pasteurization became mandatory in Boston on January 1, 1929. Interviews with Dr. Harold W. Stevens, Dr. Harold L. Lombard, Dr. Robert E. Archibald, and Dr. Bigelow's personal physician, Dr. Paul Withington. Dr. Bigelow's daughter, Mrs. Joseph Allen, collected material which would not otherwise have been available. There were times when Bigelow's ability to make light over serious concerns may well have seemed inappropriate to some of his colleagues. For instance, see his remarks on the improvement of dietary habits as a consequence of the nutritional advice given by welfare agencies during the depression (Massachusetts Department of Public Health, *Eighteenth Annual Report*, [1933], pp. 2-3).

92. Bigelow's unexplained disappearance prompted a nationwide search which ended with the discovery of his body on March 23, 1935; see *NEJM*, 212 (March 28, 1935), 628-629. Memorial tribute, Richard Clarke Cabot, Memorial Church, Harvard University, May 12, 1935.

ted statistical analyses permitted careful evaluation of the program's achievements and failures. Patients had attended diagnostic clinics in greater numbers than envisioned at the outset. At Dr. Bigelow's insistence, the Pondville Hospital did not become a receptacle for terminal care of dying patients; instead, it became a first-rate treatment center encouraging fearful patients to seek medical assistance. And with the sponsorship of widely publicized Cured Cancer Clinics and well-attended professional training institutes throughout the state, the Department demonstrated its capacity as teacher of the layman and the physician.

However, another fact emerged which, although little noted, suggested a major issue left unresolved. Dr. Lombard's original investigations indicated that early diagnosis and prompt medical treatment, the sources of the major benefits projected by the cancer program, were least often sought by the poverty stricken and the uneducated. After seven years of work, he and Dr. Bigelow concluded that those who most regularly attended clinics were not the economically disadvantaged, but the middle class and the relatively well informed. The clinic population was drawn from those who already had access to medical assistance since 80 percent of all patients came as the result of a physician's referral rather than because of their own suspicion of incipient disease.

The Department faced a paradox and drew the logical conclusion: "It was then decided," wrote the Commissioner in 1936, "to have patients attending clinics referred by a physician as far as possible although persons would not be refused examination if they came of their own volition."[93] However much Dr. Bigelow, or his successor Dr. Henry D. Chadwick, might have wished to suggest some compelling basis for attracting the poor to attend cancer clinics, they found none. The Department of Health owed allegiance to two masters, and neither gave authority to do more than offer counsel. As state physicians there was no basis for constraining an individual to seek medical advice; as the servant of the Commonwealth the Department was only obliged to offer services commensurate with its estimation of the best public interest.

In the early years of state public health, when the source of disease was broadly defined, guidance for the prevention of disease necessarily included advice about behavior. Such advice was acceptable because men believed they

93. Lombard, "The Massachusetts Cancer Program," pp. 47-50; Bigelow and Lombard, *Cancer and Other Chronic Diseases*, pp. 86-89; Henry D. Chadwick and Lombard, "Progress in the Massachusetts Cancer Program," *Commonhealth*, 21:294-295 (Oct.-Nov.-Dec. 1934); Massachusetts Department of Public Health, *Twenty-second Annual Report* (1937), p. 15.

knew about behavior and its consequences. Now, circumscribed by a professional code which defined the state's preventive services in scientific terms, advice was acceptable because the expert who gave it had knowledge which could not be shared. The urge to seek advice must somehow be transferred to the skeptical.

No one in the Department believed that what was needed were additional powers for the enforcement of its professional judgement; nor did most physicians and laymen question the powers which had gradually accrued to state preventive medicine. Both within the Department and without, there was the consensus that professional evaluation of the efficacy of public health policy was the only basis for requesting additional authority.

It seemed possible now to objectively measure and describe the distance between sickness and health. Much of the population included those whose lives were affected by the improved quality of the environment, for which the Department could take a good part of the credit, and those whose contact with contagious disease was diminished, in which, again, the Department played a major role. It also included all those who acknowledged the value of science and sought medical assistance, facilitated frequently by the Department of Public Health. The remainder were those whose lives were foreshortened and burdened by an ignorance that seemed impervious to the gospel of scientific preventive medicine.

Epilogue

Ever since Lemuel Shattuck's recommendations for the promotion of public health in 1850, state sanitary policy in Massachusetts has been calculated to affect the ignorant as well as the enlightened. Shattuck assumed, as did exponents of state responsibility for public health who followed him, that the success of sanitary reform would depend upon the receptive temper of the community. These two principles were so entwined in the thought of public health reformers that they seldom occasioned any comment beyond affirmation.

Yet the formulation of state policy has also been contingent on two other factors: the ideas and practices which authorized government responsibility to regulate individual and corporate behavior; and beliefs about the origins and nature of threats to a harmonious life. The development of state responsibility for public health has, therefore, faced a dual task: of establishing objectives which meshed concepts of general welfare with specific definitions of health; and of elaborating methods to achieve goals consonant with acceptable social and scientific precepts. Within this context, the effectiveness of antidotes to disease and disorder has been largely measured by the espectation and satisfaction of reformers.

Public health reformers have assumed a continuity between the methods of preventing disease and the objective of good health. Recently social historians have noted the consequent confusion of "function" and "cause" which has accompanied the professionalization of reformers, implying that the expert hides social controls under the camouflage of interest in the public welfare.[1] While

1. Studies of professionalization in education, mental health and engineering have elaborated this theme, but Roy Lubove, in his *The Professional Altruist: The Emergence of Social Work as a Career* (Cambridge, Mass.: Harvard University Press, 1965), has most

it is true that the desire to prevent disease has generated support for measures which regulated what was considered socially undesirable behavior, the grounds for this elision of object and method were inherent in the definition of disease. The nature of the problems created by disease are determined by the character of social organization; preventive measures, therefore, incorporate the normative assumptions of the men who set society's goals.

In the eyes of the reformer the difference between nineteenth- and twentieth-century public health policy is not only the substitution of effective hygienic laws for exhortations to conscience and cleanliness, but the substitution of scientific for ethical objectives. Preventive method and purpose were closely aligned for the twentieth-century social critic, as well as the physician, who hoped to "completely eschew moral judgments" and shed the pejorative implications of benevolence to support his authority as the dispassionate spokesman for the public interest.[2]

Early public health reformers, on the other hand, invoked the harmony of nature and man as both the goal and the method of preventing disease. Humanitarian zeal, no less than scientific objectivity, permitted the formulation of the laws of health. Within the framework of state responsibility, the price of health was set, over a century ago as it is today, in conformity with the mores of society.

These were the assumptions which guided Massachusetts public health policy from the beginning, as its State Board of Health became the model for other states. So long as public policy for the prevention of disease could be assimilated within the context of state responsibility for the balancing of social tensions, the road ahead seemed clear. Shattuck identified the corrupting influence of society itself as the first threat to public health; his prescription for correction was to reduce the disruption caused by urbanization and immigration. He proposed that the sanitary survey would establish the components of disorder and reconstitute a unified law of God and man.

As the bacterial etiology of contagious disease was revealed, within the next

---

sharply directed attention to the resultant conflicting goals; see esp. chap. v, "In-Group and Out-Group: The Molding of a Professional Subculture." For a study of public health which derives from this analysis, see Lucy M. Candib, "A Social Study of the Health Center Movement: A New Approach to Public Health History" (unpub. Senior honors thesis, Radcliffe College, 1968).

2. Willard Waller, "Social Problems and the Mores," *American Sociological Review*, 1:933 (Dec. 1936). In the main body of this article Waller asks for recognition of the value judgments implicit in the identification of social problems; he concludes by calling for "scientific," i.e., objective sociology, freed from "the mazy interrelations of the humanitarian and the organizational mores."

fifty years the opportunity to shape public health policy in accord with nature's
rule seemed closer. State responsibility took on a new dimension with the production of diphtheria antitoxin and smallpox vaccine. There was little question
that the promotion of health must include the means to achieve it. As mortality
rates shrank, few doubted the wisdom of a policy which advanced public welfare at such a small cost to the taxpayer. The public interest was well served
when the state could dispense the benefits of science. In the first decades of
the new century, despite serious social and economic problems accentuated by
a heterogeneous population and the loss of markets for its agricultural and industrial products, Massachusetts retained its outstanding reputation for humanitarian and effective social welfare policies. The Department of Public Health
attracted distinguished public servants, and the quality and scope of its public
health work was emulated throughout the nation.

Over the years Massachusetts public health policy had hewed close to the restrictions imposed by the tenets of scientific hygiene and state politics. The
concept that health was equally available to all rested on assumptions to which
both the physician and the reformer subscribed. It permitted the Department
of Public Health to renounce controversy and advocate proven scientific methods, indirectly mediating the consequences of social and economic injustice.
Consequently, it was entirely consistent with established practice for the Department, in 1926, to insist that measures to mitigate social problems which
caused or resulted from chronic disease were outside its competence. The image
which the Department had built, and which it had been encouraged to maintain, prohibited the search for solutions to problems which originated from
society's inequities.

This explicit denial of responsibility for social reform marks the dividing line
between old and new public health ideology. There had been no such distinction for Lemuel Shattuck since the rules he sought fused public and personal
harmony and health. There had been no such distinction in public health measures to control contagious disease since mortality and morbidity rates could
be substantially reduced through sanitary engineering and immunization techniques, which obviated the alteration of personal behavior or the immediate environment. But as the control of contagious disease became less central to the
promotion of health it was both impossible to deny the relationship between
effective prevention and conduct and difficult to ignore the bond between the
social conditions surrounding the poor and their susceptibility to ill health.

Although the role cast for state-supported public health avoided engagement
with these issues, privately supported agencies accepted the challenge. At a

conference of the Milbank Memorial Fund in 1936, the evaluation of current public health measures led to a discussion of the criteria for new programs. Quantitative measures, so enthusiastically supported in the past, appeared to the participants to offer little basis for decisions about the "worthwhileness" of new programs. Dr. Wade Hampton Frost, from the Johns Hopkins School of Hygiene, went on to say that "activities directed purposefully toward the promotion of health cannot be separated, except in an artificial way, from the whole mass of human activities . . . and added to this is the difficulty that health itself is indefinable."

The conference appreciated the complexity of the issues raised by Dr. Frost and suggested that private foundations might lend public health administrators "technical assistance." Inferring that the prerequisite for more comprehensive state policies would depend on developing "a critical attitude" among responsible officials, the conference was ready to endorse such efforts but unable to initiate specific action.[3]

Although Massachusetts had a history of broadly conceived and innovative public policy, it seemed unlikely that there would be any reconsideration of the state's public health services at this time. At the urging of the Massachusetts Health Council, Governor James Michael Curley called for a commission to investigate the state's public health programs. A major objective of the inquiry was the coordination of various practices that had grown up over the years, frequently in response to an emergency rather than as the result of planning.[4]

The commission, established in 1935, was made up of leading public officials and private citizens who reflected the close tie of the medical profession with the state's public health work. Governor Curley appointed 12 men to the original commission, including 10 physicians, while 86 physicians contributed their services to the committee of 150 who conducted the painstaking investigations leading to the final report.[5] Their conclusions indicated that Massachusetts had failed to maintain the high standards of previous decades; for example, it was the only state in the Union without uniform quarantine regulations. Citing the inefficiency of conflicting practices and the disparity between state professional standards and partisan interests which vitiated the influence of local boards of

3. *The Next Steps in Public Health — Proceedings of the Fourteenth Annual Conference of the Milbank Memorial Fund* (New York: Milbank Memorial Fund, 1936), pp. 50-51.

4. "Resolve Providing for an Investigation by a Special Unpaid Commission of the Public Health Law and Policies in the Commonwealth" *Acts and Resolves 1935, Chapter 11* (May 10, 1935), p. 716.

5. "Report of the Special Commission to Study and Investigate Public Health Laws and Policies," *Massachusetts House Document, No. 1200* (Dec. 2, 1936), pp. 10-15.

health, the commission recommended greater centralization of authority and the delegation of additional powers to the Department of Public Health.

The report, however, suggested no basis for redirecting public health philosophy; on the contrary, it maintained that "the function of a state health department is that of a scientific technical bureau for the prevention of diseases and the promotion of the health of the people within its confines." This statement did not support any change in outlook; it continued a policy based on the assumption that health was equally available to all persons and that all were equally entitled to public health services as "in the case of police or fire protection."

Having described public health needs in "scientific technical" terms, the commission restricted itself to the consideration of appropriate solutions. Cognizant that economic considerations might limit the availability of medical assistance, the commission urged private physicians to give preventive advice as well as therapy and acknowledged state responsibility to provide such services until the public demanded better care and the physician reciprocated with comprehensive medical guidance. The commission also suggested that the state might share with the physician the economic burden of treating the indigent by adding such medications as digitalis and insulin to the prophylactics already provided free of charge. But, it added, "[T]he Commission does not believe in a system of state medicine which would render complete treatment facilities to all persons at public expense. Such a system would not be conducive to efficiency nor would it improve the general quality of medical services."[6]

Economic considerations complemented but did not determine the proper scope of state responsibility. The additional funds which the state would receive through federal Social Security legislation and the aid already provided by the Commonwealth Fund and the Rockefeller Foundation should be used to amplify existing programs and stimulate backward communities to raise their standards.[7] Financial aid would not alter the direction of public policy; it would, instead, smooth the way for those who lagged behind.

The commission appeared to address itself to the medical profession rather than to the public. It called upon physicians to make a greater commitment to the public welfare, to fill the gap between what the Department of Public Health would educate people to expect and what they now received. The commission accepted the medical definition of health and the medical-scientific model of prevention. In so doing, it left to the voluntary health agency and the

---

6. *Ibid.*, pp. 62, 33–50, 17, 25, 197, 243.
7. *Ibid.*, pp. 42-43, 52, 57-58, 84-85.

public foundation the broader concerns of health which had originally led to the assumption of state responsibility. Where the state was limited by legal or financial restrictions, the private agency could provide the extension of services.

The concluding sentence of the report suggested that the state should gradually retire from the field of preventive medicine. It proposed that the state had been forced to overstep the bounds of public responsibility, and it asked the physician to help reverse the tendency to increase state commitment to public welfare. The commission looked forward to the day when "the scope of public health [can] be limited to the regulation of the environment and the provision of technical aid to the physician."[8]

8. *Ibid.*, pp. 37-38, 245. Publications of the Milbank Memorial Fund, the Commonwealth Fund, and the Rockefeller Foundation indicate they shared this view of their role. It is not as clear that voluntary organizations such as the National Tuberculosis Association, which drew heavily on the services and contributions of the nonprofessional, were ready to tailor their activities to this dimension.

Appendixes
Note on Sources
Index

Appendix 1. Massachusetts State Health Organization, 1869–1969.

Since 1869 public health policy in Massachusetts has been supervised by a board or a council, appointed by the Governor of the Commonwealth, serving without salary, and responsible to the legislature. No explicit qualifications for membership existed until 1915, when legislation passed in the previous year stipulated that at least three members of the Public Health Council must be physicians; see Appendix V for required composition and terms of office for the Board and Council. From 1869 to 1879 one member of the Board was elected as the paid executive officer or secretary; after August 1914 the salaried Commissioner served as chairman of the Public Health Council. Aside from this, all members of the leading body responsible for public health in Massachusetts have served on a voluntary basis, many for terms lasting well over a decade.

1. 1869-1879 — Massachusetts State Board of Health

Henry I. Bowditch (Boston)	1869-1879, chairman	Physician
George Derby (Boston)	1869-1874, secretary	Physician
P. Emory Aldrich (Worcester)	1869-1872	Lawyer
William C. Chapin (Lawrence)	1869-1871	Manufacturer
Warren Sawyer (Boston)	1869-1873	Businessman
Richard Frothingham (Boston)	1869-1879	Historian
Robert T. Davis (Fall River)	1869-1879	Physician
George V. Fox (Lowell)	1872-1873	Lawyer
John C. Hoadley (Lawrence)	1874-1879	Civil engineer
Thomas B. Newhall (Lynn)	1874-1879	Businessman
David L. Webster (Boston)	1873-1879	Manufacturer
Charles F. Folsom (Boston)	1874-1879, secretary[a]	Physician

[a] After Derby's death, Charles F. Folsom, M.D., was appointed interim secretary to the Board from June to September, 1874, at a salary of eight hundred dollars. W. L. Richardson, M.D., was appointed as an additional executive officer to the Board from August-September 1875 to aid with the investigation of drainage and sewage ordered by the legislature; see Appendix VI.

2. (July) 1879-1886 — Health Committee of the Massachusetts State Board of Health, Lunacy, and Charity

Henry I. Bowditch (Boston)	1879-1880, chairman	Physician
Charles F. Folsom (Boston)	1880-1881[b]	Physician
Robert T. Davis (Fall River)	1879-1884	Physician
	1880-1881, chairman	
John C. Hoadley (Lawrence)	1879-1882	Civil engineer
Alfred Hosmer (Watertown)	1881-1882, chairman	Physician
Thomas Talbot (North Billerica)	1880-1884[c]	Lawyer
George P. Carter (Cambridgeport)	1880-1883	Businessman
Henry P. Walcott (Cambridge)	1882-1885, chairman	Physician
John Fallon (Lawrence)	1882-1886	Businessman
Edgar E. Dean (Brockton)	1883-1885	Physician
Charles E. Donnelly (Boston)	1883-1886[d]	Lawyer
Reuben Noble (Westfield)	1883-1885	Businessman
Samuel A. Green (Boston)	1885-1886, chairman	Physician
Edward Hitchcock (Amherst)	1884-1886	Physician

3. 1886-1914 — Massachusetts State Board of Health

Henry P. Walcott (Cambridge)	1886-1914, chairman	Physician
Elijah U. Jones (Taunton)	1886-1893	Physician
Hiram F. Mills (Lawrence)	1886-1914[e]	Civil engineer
Julius H. Appleton (Springfield)	1886-1890	Manufacturer
Frank W. Draper (Boston)	1886-1901	Physician
Thornton K. Lothrop (Beverly)	1886-1901	Lawyer
James White (Williamstown)	1886-1887	Businessman
Theodore C. Bates (Worcester)	1887-1888	Manufacturer
Joseph W. Hastings (Warren)	1889-1894	Physician
John M. Raymond (Salem)	1890-1892	Lawyer
Morris Schaff (Pittsfield)	1891-1892	Military
James W. Hull (Pittsfield)	1893-1911	Insurance
Gerard C. Tobey (Wareham)	1893-1911	Lawyer

[b]The Health Committee had three successive salaried health officers who were not members of the Committee during their service, but who performed the same functions as the secretary to the Board in the preceding decade: Charles F. Folsom, M.D., 1879-1880; Henry P. Walcott, M.D., 1880-1882; and Samuel W. Abbott, M.D., 1882-1886. Folsom and Walcott were subsequently appointed to the Board of Health, Lunacy, and Charity, and served on the Health Committee. Abbott continued as health officer to the re-established Board of Health. See Appendix II for salaried public health positions, 1886-1969.

[c]Talbot served on the Health Committee as chairman of the Board of Health, Lunacy, and Charity, from 1880-1882.

[d]Donnelly was chairman of the Board of Health, Lunacy, and Charity from 1883-1886.

[e]Throughout his twenty-eight years on the Board, Mills supervised the work at the Lawrence Experiment Station.

Charles H. Porter (Quincy)	1893-1911	Insurance
Julian A. Mead (Watertown)	1895-1914	Physician
John W. Bartol (Boston)	1902-1907	Physician
Robert W. Lovett (Boston)	1907-1914	Physician
Clement F. Coogan (Pittsfield)	1911-1914	Businessman
Joseph A. Plouff (Ware)	1911-1914	Lawyer
C. E. McGillicuddy (Worcester)	1911-1914	Lawyer
Milton J. Rosenau (Boston)	1913-1914	Physician

4. 1914-1969 — Massachusetts Department of Public Health[f]

Public Health Council:

William T. Sedgwick (Boston)	1914-1921	Biologist[g]
George C. Whipple (Cambridge)	1914-1923	Sanitary engineer[g]
Milton J. Rosenau (Brookline)	1914-1915	Physician[g]
William J. Gallivan (Boston)	1914-1919	Physician
David L. Edsall (Boston)	1914-1921	Physician[g,h]
Joseph E. Lamoureux (Lowell)	1914-1924	Physician
John T. Wheelwright (Boston)	1915-1919	Lawyer
Warren C. Jewett (Worcester)	1919-1925	Businessman
Sylvester E. Ryan (Springfield)	1920-1937	Physician
Roger I. Lee (Boston)	1921-1934	Physician
Richard P. Strong (Boston)	1921-1943	Physician
James L. Tighe (Holyoke)	1923-1947	Engineer
Francis H. Lally (Milford)	1924-1953	Physician
Gordon Hutchins (Concord)	1926-1937, 1944-1950	Engineer
Richard M. Smith (Boston)	1934-1949	Physician
Charles G. Lynch (Springfield)	1937-1940	Physician
George D. Dalton (Wollaston)	1937-1940	Physician
R. Nelson Hatt (Springfield)	1940-1942	Physician
Cecil K. Drinker (Brookline)	1943-1946	Physician[g,h]
Elmer S. Bagnall (Groveland)	1943-1945	Physician
George L. Schadt (Springfield)	1942-1943	Physician

[f]The Massachusetts Department of Health was established in August 1914; for legislation, see Appendix V. In 1920, when the Massachusetts state government went through a series of administrative reorganizations, the name was changed to the Department of Public Health. Because of the 1914 reorganization of public health work, the only significant additional change at this time resulted from assigning responsibility to this department for the Leper Hospital on Penikese Island, and the Tuberculosis Sanatoria at Lakeville, North Reading, Rutland, and Westfield.

[g]Although a number of physicians on previous Boards gave time to teaching, academic affiliation cannot have been considered a major professional identification, as it was for Sedgwick, Whipple, Rosenau, Leavell, Fair, and Berger.

[h]Drs. Edsall, Drinker, and Leavell were successively Deans at the Harvard School of Public Health; Edsall was a member of the Public Health Council until he became Dean in 1922, and Drinker came to the Council after retiring as Dean.

William H. Griffin (Boston)	1945-1957	Dentist
Charles F. Wilinsky (Brookline)	1946-1964	Physician
Raymond L. Mutter (Holyoke)	1947-1959	Engineer
Paul J. Jakmauh (Boston)	1949-1964	Physician
Paul F. Flaherty (Boston)	1950-1956	
Gordon M. Fair (Cambridge)	1956-1966	Engineer
Conrad Wesselhoeft (Boston)	1953-1960	Physician
Hugh R. Leavell (Cambridge)	1960-1963	Physician, Dr. P.H.[g,h]
Samuel Kovner (Brockton)	1960-	Businessman
Ralph E. Sirianni (Winthrop)	1963-	Lawyer
Allen S. Johnson (Longmeadow)	1964-1966	Physician
Frank B. Carroll (Jamaica Plain)	1964-1967	Physician, M.P.H.[i]
John H. Knowles (Boston)	1964-	Physician
Bernard B. Berger (Amherst)	1966-	Engineer[g]
John P. Rattigan (Newton)	1966-	Physician
Benjamin M. Banks (Brookline)	1967-	Physician

Commissioners:

William C. Hanson, M.D.	August-November 1914, Acting Commissioner
Allan J. McLaughlin, M.D.	1914-1918
Eugene R. Kelley, M.D.	1918-1925
George H. Bigelow, M.D. Ph.D.[i]	1925-1933
Henry D. Chadwick, M.D.	1933-1938
Paul K. Jakmauh, M.D.	1938-1943
Vlado A. Getting, M.D., Dr. P.H.[i]	1943-1953
Samuel B. Kirkwood, M.D.	1953-1958
Roy F. Feemster, M.D.	April 1958-December 1958, Acting Commissioner
Alfred L. Frechette, M.D., M.P.H.[i]	1959-

[i]With the development of postgraduate training in public health a number of physicians on the Council reflected this professional commitment in their postdoctoral degrees. Three of the ten commissioners, and an ever-increasing proportion of the salaried officers in the Department, received advanced degrees in public health.

Appendix II. Administration of State Authority for Public Health in Massachusetts, 1869–1936.

From 1869-1879 a member of the State Board of Health was elected by the Board as secretary, to serve as the salaried executive officer. In this decade the Board solicited assistance from experts outside the Board who submitted investigatory reports. In 1875 an additional executive officer was appointed for two months to aid with the investigation of the state's water supplies.

From 1880 to 1886 the Health Committee of the Board of Health, Lunacy, and Charity appointed a salaried Health Officer who was not a member of the Committee to carry out its executive functions.

After 1886 public health policy was elaborated through departments and later divisions. Directors of departments were chosen by the State Board of Health according to increasingly specific professional criteria, and until 1942 they were exempt from regulations of the Civil Service Commission (established in Massachusetts in 1884). All other positions came under civil service law, as well as meeting specific criteria set by the legislature and the State Board of Health.

1. 1891: Organization of departments and salaried personnel

Secretary to the Board[a]

Engineering

1 chief engineer
2 assistants
2 clerical

Water and Sewage

1 chief chemist
4 assistants
1 chief biologist
2 assistants
2 chemists
2 bacteriologists
5 assistants
} Lawrence Experiment Station[b]

Food and Drug[c]

3 chemists
3 inspectors

TOTAL: 29

[a]The secretary served as executive officer to the Board as a whole, with special responsibilities for the control of contagious diseases and contact with local boards of health; see Appendix V, 3, section 5. The chief engineer and the secretary were listed as "officers of the Board." After 1892 one of the chemists in the Food and Drug Department was listed as chief analyst and placed in charge of the work for the entire department.
[b]See Appendix VI, 1, section 6.
[c]See Appendix VI, 2.

2. 1913: Organization of departments and salaried personnel

Secretary to the Board

Assistant to the Secretary; 1 investigator; 5 clerical; 2 messengers; 11 health inspectors;[d] 4 clerical for district health work; 1 nurse

Engineering

1 chief engineer
11 assistants
4 rodmen
1 draftsman
6 clerical
1 messenger

Water and Sewage

1 chief chemist
8 assistants
1 lab assistant
2 clerical
2 assistant chemists ⎫
1 bacteriologist ⎬ Lawrence
1 lab assistant ⎭ Experiment
2 filtermen   Station
1 clerical
1 laborer

Food and Drug

1 analyst
3 assistant analysts
10 inspectors
4 clerical
1 messenger

Bacteriology[e]

1 pathologist
1 assistant
1 expert assistant
5 lab assistants
2 dieners
1 clerical
1 bacteriologist ⎫ Diagnostic
2 lab assistants ⎬ Laboratory
1 clerical ⎭

TOTAL: 104

[d]Health inspectors were first named in 1907; see Appendix V, 5.
[e]The Bacteriology Department was established in 1895, and it included both the Vaccine and Antitoxin Laboratory and the Diagnostic Laboratory. The pathologist served only part-time.

190

3. 1915: Organization of divisions and salaried personnel

Commissioner

Administration

6 clerical
2 messengers

Sanitary Engineers

1 chief engineer
12 assistants
5 clerical
1 messenger

Water and Sewage

1 chief chemist
5 assistants
1 biologist
1 assistant
2 clerical
1 chemist
1 bacteriologist   ⎫
1 assistant   ⎬ Lawrence Experiment Station
1 filter attendant   ⎭
1 laborer

Food and Drugs[f]

1 analyst
4 assistants
9 inspectors
3 clerical
1 messenger

Communicable Diseases

1 epidemiologist
1 assistant
8 district health officers
1 bacteriologist   ⎫
1 assistant   ⎬ Diagnostic Laboratory
2 lab assistants   ⎭
6 clerical

Biologic Laboratory[g]

1 pathologist[h]
2 assistants
1 biologist
5 lab assistants
3 other assistants
1 technician
1 clerical
1 janitor

Hygiene

1 director[i]
1 assistant
1 health educator
1 field worker
2 clerical

TOTAL: 102

[f] Arsphenamine for treatment of syphilis was produced by this division beginning in 1916.

[g] The pathologist, who also served as director of the laboratory, remained a part-time employee until 1920. The separation of the various laboratories indicated in this and the following chart continued until the establishment of the Institute of Laboratories in 1951.

[h] The Wasserman Laboratory was established in 1915. Although it was located at the Harvard Medical School, it remained under this division until 1944, when it was placed under the Division of Communicable Diseases where it remained until 1951.

[i] The first director of this division was a biologist with special training in public health, who served part-time. After 1918, as this division expanded its work, especially in the field of maternal and child health, the director was a physician working full-time.

4. 1935: Organization of divisions and salaried personnel[j]

Commissioner

Administration

1 secretary
1 epidemiologist
11 clerical

Sanitary Engineering[k]

1 chief engineer
15 assistants
12 clerical
1 lab coordinator
2 lab chiefs
10 chemists and
  bacteriologists } Water and Sewage Laboratory
1 lab assistant
1 handyman
1 laborer
1 watchman
3 clerical

Food and Drug

1 analyst
1 lab chief
5 chemists and
  bacteriologists
14 inspectors
2 lab helpers
1 laborer

Communicable Diseases

1 director
1 assistant
7 district health officers
8 clerical
5 bacteriologists
1 lab assistant } Diagnostic Laboratory
1 lab helper
1 laborer
2 clerical
1 assistant director
1 epidemiologist } Venereal Disease Subdivision[l]
1 health educator
3 clerical

Biologic Laboratory

1 pathologist
1 assistant director
11 chemists and bacteriologists
3 lab assistants
8 lab helpers
1 stable foreman
15 laborers
2 janitors
6 clerical

Adult Hygiene[m]

1 director
3 epidemiologists
3 social workers
2 education experts
15 clerical

Child Hygiene

1 director
2 pediatricians
1 epidemiologist
1 dental supervisor
4 nutritionists
2 education experts
6 nurses
15 clerical

1 chief
1 bacteriologist
1 lab technician
1 lab assistant
6 lab helpers
3 clerical
} Wasserman Laboratory

Tuberculosis[n]

1 director
1 assistant director
1 epidemiologist
1 supervisor construction
1 claims inspector
2 social workers
1 field nurse

1 supervisor
3 pediatricians
3 nurses
2 nutritionists
2 extra technicians
6 clerical
} Chadwick Clinics

TOTAL: 261

[j] With passage of the federal Social Security Act, a number of additional positions were created in 1936, especially in the Division of Child Hygiene.

[k] The Water and Sewage Laboratories were brought under the Division of Sanitary Engineering in 1930.

[l] The Venereal Disease subdivision was created in 1919. It became a separate division in 1937 and returned to the Division of Communicable Diseases in 1960.

[m] In 1929 the Division of Adult Hygiene was created from fifteen members of the cancer section of the Division of Hygiene. At the same time the Division of Hygiene was appropriately renamed the Division of Child Hygiene.

[n] With the assignment of responsibility for the four tuberculosis sanatoria to the Department of Public Health in 1920, a new division was established to take care of all work in prevention and treatment of tuberculosis. The first director was a member of the Public Health Council at the time of his appointment, but relinquished that role the next year. The Chadwick Clinics were established to undertake a special program for the prevention, diagnosis, and treatment of illness in school children, 1925-1935. Personnel listed here does not include the sanatoria.

Appendix III. Comparative Rating of the States in Public Health Work, 1915.

Charles V. Chapin's *A Report on State Public Health Work Based on a Survey of State Boards of Health* (Chicago: American Medical Association, n.d.) clarifies the rating code that appears on the following pages and identifies the criteria of "new public health" standards in the first decades of the twentieth century as follows:

Under supervision of local health officers is the subdivision "supervision" which means personal direction by some one from the central office. This appears to be the most important means of improving the local service and is given the highest rating . . . Under communicable diseases, completeness of notification is important. In a registration state the score depends on the ratio of cases to deaths. In a non-registration state it is a matter of judgment . . . Under the diagnostic laboratory credit of two is given for each additional disease if the laboratory is prepared to examine for diseases other than diphtheria, tuberculosis and typhoid fever. The score for amount of work depends on the ratio of the examinations for diphtheria, typhoid fever and tuberculosis to the deaths from these diseases but cities with local laboratories are deducted from the computation. If more than two vaccines or sera are distributed, credit of two is given for each additional one. The credit for the amount of serum distributed refers only to diphtheria antitoxin . . .

Under vital statistics a credit of forty is given for deaths if the state is in the registration area, and for births if it is probable that ninety per cent are reported. If the state has a good law, even if it is not as yet enforced, a credit for ten is given, but if the law is poor and less than ninety per cent of the deaths and births are reported, or if no data could be obtained from reports, or otherwise, no credit is allowed . . .

It is doubtless true, also, that many would give to sanitation a higher rating, yet if one compares it with matters of such preponderating importance as the control of communicable diseases and aggressive work against tuberculosis it will scarcely be maintained that the sanitation of schools and other public buildings and of hotels and camps is of more than one fourth the value of either.

In considering the control of water and sewage, it was thought that the investigation and approval of new projects, or the extension of old ones, is the most important duty of the engineer, while continued supervision of existing works and systematic surveys are each given an equal though slightly lesser credit.

Extra credits are given as follows: To Indiana, Kansas, Louisiana, North Carolina and Tennessee, ten each for fighting nostrums. To Maryland, Minnesota, New York, Pennsylvania, Vermont, Virginia, and Washington, ten, and Massachusetts fifty, for research. To Ohio twenty for the study of occupational disease, to Oregon twenty for social hygiene work and Pennsylvania twenty and Florida ten for school inspection. To Pennsylvania ten for housing control . . . [pp. 193-194].

195

RATING SHEET

State	Personal Supervision (60)	Conferences (20)	Bulletins (20)	Notification (30)	Direct Control (80)	Intensive Work (50)	Notification (20)	Sanatoria (20)	Hospitals (20)	Dispensaries (20)	General Education (30)	Intensive Work or Direct Control (30)	Scope of Work (10)	Amount (70)	Varieties (10)	Amount (40)	Deaths (40)	Births (40)	Tables (20)	Intensive Work (40)	Literature to Mothers (10)	Prevention of Ophthalmia (10)	Supervision of Midwives (10)	Newspapers (30)	Bulletins (30)	Exhibits (30)	Lectures (10)	Milk Supervision (40)	Sanitary Handling of Food (20)	School Construction (20)	Public Institutions (10)	Hotels and Camps (10)	Approval of Plans (40)	Surveys (30)	Supervision (30)	Extra Credits	Total (1000)
Alabama	0	0	0	7	0	0	10	10	0	0	0	0	10	10	0	8	0	0	0	0	0	0	0	0	10	0	0	0	0	10	0	0	10	0	0		105
Arizona	0	8	0	8	0	0	0	0	0	0	0	0	0	0	0	0	10	10	0	0	0	0	0	0	8	0	0	0	0	0	0	0	0	0	0		39
Arkansas	0	6	5	10	10	0	10	10	10	0	0	0	8	5	0	0	10	10	0	0	0	5	0	0	0	0	10	0	0	10	0	0	0	0	0		74
California	0	10	0	15	10	0	0	0	0	10	30	0	0	40	0	0	40	40	20	0	0	0	0	0	20	20	0	0	12	0	0	0	30	10	10		342
Colorado	0	10	5	23	10	0	10	10	15	0	0	0	0	15	6	0	40	10	0	0	0	0	0	0	0	0	0	0	8	0	0	8	20	0	0		106
Connecticut	0	10	0	19	0	0	0	0	0	0	10	0	8	60	0	30	40	10	0	0	0	5	0	0	10	0	0	30	0	0	0	0	20	20	0		393
Delaware	0	0	5	0	30	0	12	15	0	12	0	0	0	50	0	0	10	10	10	0	0	0	0	0	5	0	10	0	10	10	0	8	0	0	0		131
Florida	0	0	0	0	5	10	0	10	0	0	8	5	4	5	10	12	10	10	5	0	0	0	0	20	25	25	0	0	0	0	0	0	0	0	0		253
Georgia	0	0	0	0	0	0	0	0	0	0	0	0	0	10	0	10	10	10	0	0	0	0	0	10	8	0	0	5	5	5	0	0	0	0	0		156
Idaho	0	0	0	4	30	0	0	0	0	0	0	0	10	10	0	40	10	10	0	0	8	0	0	18	8	10	8	10	10	0	8	10	0	0	0	10	127
Illinois	5	0	10	17	20	0	0	0	0	0	10	0	4	10	0	0	10	10	10	0	0	10	0	24	25	20	10	10	12	5	0	10	30	30	30		346
Indiana	5	20	10	13	20	15	5	10	10	0	20	5	6	60	6	22	40	40	13	0	10	5	0	24	20	30	10	10	12	20	10	10	10	15	10	10	526

State	Total
Iowa	225
Kansas	499
Kentucky	385
Louisiana	315
Maine	280
Maryland	507
Massachusetts	745
Michigan	370
Minnesota	574
Mississippi	297
Missouri	152
Montana	246
Nebraska	66
Nevada	94
New Hampshire	320
New Jersey	555
New Mexico	0
New York	730
North Carolina	411
North Dakota	139
Ohio	462
Oklahoma	97
Oregon	227
Pennsylvania	716
Rhode Island	432
South Carolina	165
South Dakota	101
Tennessee	122
Texas	116
Utah	161
Vermont	486
Virginia	397
Washington	262
West Virginia	113
Wisconsin	392
Wyoming	10

Source: Charles V. Chapin, *A Report on State Public Health Work Based on a Survey of State Boards of Health* (Chicago: American Medical Association, n.d.), pp. 195-196. The table was based on data collected from 1914 to 1915.

Appendix IV. Registration of Vital Statistics: Selected Documents.

1. Memorial to the legislature from the American Academy of Arts and Sciences, February 1841. *First Annual Report . . . Relating to the Registry of Births, Marriages and Deaths in Massachusetts* (1843), pp. 25-27.

[Y]our memorialists, with a view to the interests of science, as well as of humanity, and the public health and morals, ask leave to call the attention of your honorable body to the expediency of providing, by law, for a more exact and efficient system of registering the deaths, births and marriages, within this Commonwealth; it having been found, by long experience, that the legal provisions already made are wholly insufficient to carry into effect the wise intentions of the Legislature.

In a measure of public policy, which has already been sanctioned by the Legislature, though with little practical effect, for a long series of years, it may seem to be superfluous to enter into a formal course of reasoning to prove its importance; yet it may not be altogether without use to advert to some of the practical considerations, which must doubtless have an influence on the question of adopting such further legal provisions as may be necessary to effect the purposes intended by the existing laws.

Among these considerations, that of affording more effectual means of promoting the public health, by ascertaining the causes of disease, deservedly holds the first place. Many of the causes of disease, as they affect different communities, engaged in a great variety of occupations, can be ascertained only by observations on an extensive scale, far beyond the reach of individual research; and an accurate return of deaths, from the different parts of the State, for a series of years, would greatly aid in the investigation of these causes. As an exemplification of this view of the subject, it is asserted that the relative prevalence of the disease of consumption is much greater in some places than in others; this prevalence is supposed by some to be counteracted, in a great degree, by that of certain other diseases; and the ascertaining of the truth in this case, would probably afford the means of lessening the number of those who would fall victims to this disease.

To the paramount considerations founded on the benefits which would result to the public health and morals, and the general advancement of science, more especially in the all-important department of political economy, as applicable to our own State, may be added others of scarcely inferior practical importance.

Among these, it may be observed that such an exact registration would afford the best means of determining, in a satisfactory manner, numberless questions of consanguinity, involving the legitimacy or illegitimacy of parties, and their rights of property, which are continually occurring in our courts of justice, as well between individuals as between the municipal corporations of this Commonwealth.

198

It is also a well-known fact, that the present *tables of mortality,* by which the expectation of human life is now calculated, in legal and other proceedings for the various purposes of annuities, of life estates in the various species of property, are extremely defective, and consequently too uncertain to be relied upon. Now an exact registration of the deaths, for a series of years, would furnish sufficient data for the construction of accurate tables, and when the vast amount of property depending on the accurate value, or expectation of human life, is duly considered, the high importance of such tables will be justly estimated.

Every married woman in the State has her right of dower, or life estate, in the real estate of her husband; and every married man (with very limited exceptions,) has an interest for life in the real estate of his wife. When such life estates are transferred, especially under compulsory process of law, it becomes highly necessary, for the purposes of justice, that the most ample means should be provided for making a correct estimate of property, both as respects the party holding the estate, and the party to whom it is so transferred, as well as those who may be entitled to the reversionary interest in such property. The same reasoning would be applicable to cases of estimating land held for life, which should be required by the public authorities for highways, or other public uses, or by towns or other corporations, for the like objects.

It often happens, also, that charitable institutions in this Commonwealth derive their funds from the bounty of philanthropic individuals, who frequently bequeath large amounts of property to such institutions, encumbered with the payment of annuities to certain individuals during their lives; but for want of correct data, such annuities cannot now be properly calculated. Now, by having exact tables, which can be obtained only by a long course of observations, and under some uniform system, sanctioned by legislative authority, all questions of the kinds above mentioned would be readily determined, and without the risk of doing injustice to any party interested.

Your memorialists would add, that the proposed system of registration, considered as a matter of political science, with particular reference to our own Commonwealth, as in integral portion of the United States, loses none of its importance, when we take into view the facilities which it will afford for ascertaining the ratio or law by which the native population increases from year to year, (as distinguished from the increase by emigration from other countries,) and for enabling us more justly to estimate the great interests, and the resources and means of the Commonwealth, in their relations to the public welfare of our common country.

Your memorialists, therefore, respectfully request that such measures may be adopted in the premises, as your honorable body, in its wisdom, shall deem the public interest to require.

2. Memorial to the legislature from the Massachusetts Medical Society, February 1841. *First Annual Report . . . Relating to the Registry of Births, Marriages and Deaths in Massachusetts* (1843), pp. 27-28.

The interest of humanity and science, as well as those of morals and the public health, would be essentially promoted by an efficient registration and return of deaths, births and marriages in all the towns of this Commonwealth. The law now requires a record of births and marriages; but the provision is not such, your memorialists are informed, as to secure any general or adequate attention being paid to it. No public record of deaths is made, except in a very few places. And no provision is made for any return of such records as are kept, so that their results may be rendered available for the purposes of general utility.

The census of successive periods shows a rapid rate of increase of our population, — exhibiting the remarkable fact, that the number of persons now living in this country is greater than that of all who have ever died in it since the first settlement of the country by Europeans. But in what degree this increase is the effect of causes naturally existing among us, or how far it is produced by immigration, there are at present no means of knowing. This, and many other questions of great importance in political economy and other branches of science, may be ascertained by an accurate comparison of the births and deaths with the existing population. The influence of the different employments and states of society on the public morals and the general welfare would be exhibited, and thus the means may be obtained of judging to what extent each should be fostered and encouraged.

But it is on account of its importance in promoting the public health, that your memorialists, as physicians, attach the strongest interest to this measure. Many of the causes of disease, as they affect different communities, engaged in a great variety of occupations, can only be ascertained by observations on an extensive scale, far beyond the reach of individual research. An accurate return of deaths from the different sections of the State, for a series of years, would greatly aid in the investigation of these causes, and would doubtless do much towards enabling us to find means for the removal of some of them. For example, the relative prevalence of consumption is much greater in some places than in others; and there are those who believe that its prevalence is in a great degree counteracted by that of certain other diseases. A full establishment of the truth in regard to this opinion, as it might be established by such returns as we propose, might do something at least to diminish the mortality of a disease, which now cuts off so many at the most interesting and useful period of life.

3. Legislation establishing the procedures for compulsory registration of births, marriages, and deaths. *Massachusetts Acts and Resolves 1842, Chapter 95* (March 3, 1842).

Section 1. The clerks of the several towns and cities in the Commonwealth shall, annually, in the month of May, transmit to the secretary of the Commonwealth a certified copy of their record of the births, marriages and deaths of all persons within their respective towns and cities, which may come to their knowledge; shall state the number of births and marriages, and the number of deaths, with the name, sex, age (and if an adult male, the occupation,) and the names of the diseases of which all persons have died, or are supposed to have died, together with the cause or causes of the death of all such deceased persons, so far as they may be able to obtain a knowledge of the same from physicians or others; and any clerk who shall neglect to make such return, shall be liable to a penalty of ten dollars, to be recovered, for the use of any town or city where such neglect shall be proved to have existed.

Section 2. The secretary of the Commonwealth, shall prepare and furnish to the clerks of the several towns and cities in this Commonwealth, blank forms of returns, as herein before specified, and shall accompany the same with such instructions and explanations as may be necessary and useful; and he shall receive said returns, and prepare therefrom such tabular results as will render them of practical utility, and shall make report thereof annually to the legislature, and generally shall do whatever may be required to carry into effect the objects of this act, and of the several provisions of the Revised Statutes not inconsistent with this act.

4. Selections from a report to the National Medical Convention (Philadelphia, May 1847) on "nomenclature of diseases adapted to the United States, having reference to the general registration of deaths," prepared by John H. Griscom, M.D. (New York City), Lemuel Shattuck (Boston), T. Romeyn Beck, M.D. (Albany), Edward Jarvis, M.D. (Dorchester, Mass.), G. Emerson,

Registration of Vital Statistics

M.D. (Philadelphia), Charles A. Lee, M.D. (Geneva, N.Y.). *Proceedings* of the National Medical Conventions (Philadelphia, 1847), pp. 133-138.

No subject is more intimately connected with the prosperity and happiness of a people than the degree of their public health. Some places and some circumstances are known to be more favourable than others to the development and prolongation of the vital energies of man; and it is a matter of great moment to the whole population collectively, and to each one individually, to know what facts exist in the place selected for residence, which influence its character in this respect. No subject which can claim public attention should excite greater interest than that of obtaining a knowledge of the diseases and causes of death in operation among us. It is of great consequence to all of us to know when, where, in what form, and under what circumstances, sickness and mortality take place; and whether they are uniform, or dissimilar in different places, or in the same place in different seasons, and under different circumstances. Wherever this knowledge is possessed, remedies for the amelioration or extinction of existing evils can be applied more intelligently, and with better hope of success.

Fortunately, there is a mode by which this information may be obtained, and by which the force of mortality pressing upon a people may be, in some respects, weighed and measured. This mode is, uniform and accurate registration of the causes and locality of death, and intelligible abstracts of those causes. This matter may be illustrated by the facts we already possess. Let the whole force with which mortality presses upon us be represented by 100. It appears by the Fourth Report of the Registration of Births, Marriages and Deaths, in Massachusetts, for 1845, page 55, that of 10,000 of all the deaths by known causes that year, 667 were by scarlatina. This disease, then, or this form or force of mortality, pressed upon us 6.67 per cent. of all forms or forces. It appears by the same Report, on page 82, that of 10,000 deaths 651 occurred in May and 1095 in September; showing that the proportional force of mortality was 68 per cent. less in the former than in the latter month. In 10,000 deaths in five different towns of the same population, 150 may occur in one and 300 in another, showing a different force in those places of 100 per cent. In this manner may this force be weighed and measured in all its details. The correctness of this measurement depends, however, upon the degree of accuracy by which the facts are registered and abstracted. A uniform and systematic plan of *registration* and *classification* is essential to secure this accuracy. From an extensive examination of the statements of deaths in different places in the United States, it appears that the same disease is sometimes given in one place, under a name different from that of the same disease in another place, and even in the same place, the same want of uniformity exists in regard to the names of diseases in different periods. This is a great evil, and it must be obvious that so long as it exists it will be difficult, if not impossible, to make a statistical abstract, on which to institute accurate comparisons of the prevalence of different diseases, or of the health of the people in different places or in different periods. To remedy this evil the plan of a nomenclature and classification of disease contained in the appendix is proposed. It is intended to apply uniformly to all sections of our country.

REGISTRATION. — The following rules should be observed in registering the cause of death.

I. Give causes of death the right names; and such as have the same meaning at all times, and in all places . . . [a]

II. Such names should be used as would give a clear definition of the cause of death . . .

III. A single word, or the least number of words possible, which would give this clear definition, should be preferred. Popular names may be used, but where no popular name in a single word is found, a technical or scientific term should be preferred . . .

IV. When more than one disease or causes have concurred in producing death, they may

[a]In the original text all headings are italicized.

be written under each other without being connected with other words or particles, and in the order of their appearance . . .

V. State as nearly as can be known by numbers, the duration of the disease or diseases, if more than one has concurred in producing the event, in years, months, or days . . .

VII [*sic*] In fatal cases of small-pox, measles, scarlatina, typhus, and the like diseases, state whether it was the second, third, &c. attack, wherein the patient has sustained more attacks than one. In ague, epilepsy, convulsive and other diseases which occur in fits and paroxysms, date the illness from the first fit, and add the duration of the last fit . . .

VIII. Surgeons in all cases of operations should return the primary disease, the operation, the secondary disease, and should state also the time from the commencement of the primary disease, the time from the operation, and the time from the appearance of secondary disease, reckoning in each instance to the death.

IX. In external causes of death, the nature of the injury and the circumstances of the death should be stated; and whether by accident or design . . .

X. When poison has been the cause of death, the time which elapses between its administration and the death should be registered as far as possible . . .

XI. The cause of the disease when clearly known, may be inserted . . .

XII. The cause of death should, if possible, be certified by a physician present during the last sickness; or, when no physician was present, by such other person as might be best qualified. These rules should be observed by coroners . . .

CLASSIFICATION. – There are many different causes of death, and many names to the same cause. Many vague, unmeaning, and incorrect terms are often used; and it would be difficult, if not impossible to make a statistical analysis embracing each in detail. It becomes necessary to group those that are synonymous, or nearly so, under one name, and those operating in a particular way or affecting a particular organ under one class. The advantages of such a classification are too obvious to require discussion. It has been well said, that "a nomenclature is of as much importance in this department of inquiry, as weight and measures are in the physical sciences."

The first question that presents itself is: How shall this classification be made? Various nosological arrangements of diseases have been proposed, possessing a greater or less degree of merit, but many of them appear better adapted to the general purpose of science than to statistical investigations. Those who study this subject will perceive that there are difficulties attending the details of any classification of diseases; and that it is not easy to make one that shall be entirely satisfactory, even to one's own mind. In making one, however, there are certain principles of known and acknowledged importance, which should be observed. Some diseases are known to have an epidemic and zymotic character, and the public health of a community is generally measured by the proportion to the whole deaths in which they prevail. Others are known not to have this character, but to be sporadic. Death is also produced by external causes without disease.

Here then are three classes of causes which it would seem might be separated. This division alone would, however, leave so large a portion among the sporadic, that some other subdivision becomes proper. To provide for this, a classification of diseases which affect a particular organ, has been adopted. Some special diseases, however (dysentery for instance,) belongs to the Zymotic, as others belong to the Sporadic class; and it has been suggested that the former should be divided as well as the latter. This might be useful for more minute analysis, but for general purposes too many subdivisions embarrass rather than simplify the information. In making investigations in which it is desirable to include all diseases of the digestive organs, it will be easy to separate the Zymotic diseases which affect these organs from the rest, and add them to those of the sporadic class.

The following rules should be observed in making a classification of diseases for statistical purpose.

I. All Zymotic diseases, or such as are known to be epidemic, endemic, or contagious under any circumstances, should be classed together.

II. All Sporadic disease, or such as are known not to be epidemic under any circumstances, should be separated into classes, according as they affect particular organs of the body; – such as are of uncertain or general seat, forming a distinct class.

III. Deaths by old age, or from external causes, should each form a class.

IV. For convenient reference, all the names in the classified causes of death, and others proposed to be used in the registers, and their synonyms, both popular and scientific, should be arranged alphabetically in a separate list, and accompanying each other, and opposite to each the synonym by which it is defined . . .

The report concluded with an analysis of the nomenclature and classification of disease prepared by William Farr, Registrar General of England, and a description of the accompanying Appendices; A, a model registration form; B, a proposed nosology; C, a list of names actually used in five major cities of the United States.

Appendix V. State Responsibility for Public Health: Selected Massachusetts Documents.

1. Selections from the introduction to the *Report of a General Plan for the Promotion of Public and Personal Health . . . Relating to a Sanitary Survey of the State* (1850). *The Shattuck Report,* facsimile ed., Cambridge, Mass.: Harvard University Press, 1948.

As the object of our commission is comparatively new, and may not be clearly understood by every person, we will state what we understand to be its intention. By a Sanitary Survey of the State is meant, an examination or survey of the different parts of the Commonwealth, — its counties, its towns, and its localities, — to ascertain the causes which favorably or unfavorably affect the health of its inhabitants. The word *sanitary* means *relating to health.*[a] When we speak of the sanitary condition of a town, we include a description of those circumstances which relate to, or have an effect upon, the health of its inhabitants. When applied to the inhabitants of a town or district, in their social capacity, it relates to public health; when to individuals, it relates to personal or private health.

The condition of perfect *public health* requires such laws and regulations, as will secure to man associated in society, the same sanitary enjoyments that he would have as an isolated individual; and as will protect him from injury from any influences connected with his locality; his dwelling-house, his occupation, or those of his associates or neighbors, or from any other social causes. It is under the control of public authority, and public administration; and life and health may be saved or lost, and they are actually saved or lost, as this authority is wisely or unwisely exercised.

The condition of perfect *personal health* requires the perfect formation of all the organs

[a]This word is derived from the Latin *sanitas,* meaning "soundness of body, health." It is sometimes written, erroneously, as we think, sanatory, sanotary, and sanitory. The most correct authors, however, now write, sanitary. *Hygiene* (from a Greek word, derived from Hygeia, the goddess of health, meaning to be well,) is defined "health, the preservation of health, that part of medicine which regards the preservation of health." *Hygiean* and *hygienic* have the same meaning as sanitary. These words are sometimes used as tehnical terms, especially by medical men; but we dislike, and see no good reason for substituting them for the more simple, proper, and comprehensive English words, health and sanitary, which are generally understood. We would divest our subject of all mystery and professional technicalities; and as it concerns every body, we would adapt it to universal comprehension, and universal application.

of the body, and the perfect performance of each of their functions, in harmony with all the others. Such a condition gives to its possessor, strength, energy, power, buoyancy or spirit, happiness. *Disease* may be an imperfection in some organ, or a derangement or improper action in some function, or both: and it may exist, and does actually exist, in all communities, in an infinite number of degrees, from the slightest deviation from a standard of perfect health, through all the varieties of sickness, to the lowest standard of vitality, just as the body is about to perform its last respiration. Such a condition gives to its possessor, weakness, lassitude, inability, depression, pain, misery, death. And one or the other of these conditions may be chosen, and is actually chosen, to a greater or less extent, by almost every human being.

WE BELIEVE *that the conditions of perfect health, either public or personal, are seldom or never attained, though attainable; — that the average length of human life may be very much extended, and its physical power greatly augmented; — that in every year, within this Commonwealth, thousands of lives are lost which might have been saved; — that tens of thousands of cases of sickness occur, which might have been prevented; — that a vast amount of unnecessarily impaired health, and physical debility exists among those not actually confined by sickness; — that these preventable evils require an enormous expenditure and loss of money, and impose upon the people unnumbered and immeasurable calamities, pecuniary, social, physical, mental, and moral, which might be avoided; — that means exist, within our reach, for their mitigation or removal; — and that measures for prevention will effect infinitely more, than remedies for the cure of disease . . .*

But whom does this great matter of public health concern? By who is this subject to be surveyed, analyzed, and practically applied? And who are to be benefited by this application? Some will answer, the physician, certainly. True, but only in a degree; but it will be infinitely more valuable to the whole people, to teach them how to prevent disease, and to live without being sick. This is a blessing which cannot be measured by money value. The people are principally concerned, and on them depend, in part, at least, the introduction and progess of sanitary measures . . .

2. Report of a Joint Special Committee of the Massachusetts General Court on the Expediency of establishing a State Board of Health. *Massachusetts Senate Documents 1869, No. 340* (May 22, 1869).

The importance of human life and health and of such care and watchfulness over them as properly belongs to government need not be enlarged upon. From the time of Moses, who added the sanction of divine authority to the wisdom of his sanitary rules, to the present day, no government has entirely neglected to assume control of such matters as seemed to affect the public health; all more or less imperfectly, but all according to their light. The want of wisdom of some of those measures — such, for instance, as the strict quarantines against plague enforced to countries where crowded humanity was suffered to fester in its own filth to afford fuel to be kindled by the accidental spark or to burst into the spontaneous combustion of open pestilence — has sometimes made hasty or impatient sceptics doubt the propriety of any interference or attempt to diminish the tendencies to disease. But the folly of quacks and the errors of honest but inaccurate observers ought not fairly to impeach the wisdom of more sincere or careful students of disease and health.

The great fact, established beyond controversy, that the average duration of human life has been steadily increasing ever since accurate tables of mortality have been kept, is most encouraging. That we have not yet reached perfection in our sanitary arrangements is yearly evinced by the immense amount of sickness and death from those classes of disease that are clearly traceable to removable causes.

John Simon, Esq., medical officer of the privy council of Great Britain, makes this remarkable statement in his report from 1858, which may undoubtedly be applied to Massachusetts "*mutatis mutandis*": – "That more than one-half of our annual mortality results from diseases which prevail with a very great range of difference in proportion as sanitary circumstances are good or bad; that according to the latest available evidence some of these diseases prevail twice or thrice, some of them ten or twenty times, some of them even forty or fifty times, as fatally in some districts as in other districts of England; that the result of their excessive partial development is to render the mortality of certain districts from 50 to 100 per cent. higher than the mortality of other districts, and to raise the death-rate of the whole country 33 per cent. above the death-rate of its healthiest parts."

To show that this statement might be made with equal truth of Massachusetts, take the following facts:–

The whole number of deaths in Massachusetts for 1867 was	22,719
The county showing the lowest death-rate, Barnstable, had deaths 1.38 to 100 persons living. Had this been the rate throughout the State the whole number would have been about	17,219
	5,500

less than actually occurred. The county of Suffolk had the highest death-rate, 2.26 per 100 living. Had this rate prevailed throughout the State the whole number would have been 28,796 an excess of 6,077 over the actual number, and of 11,577 over the number had the whole State been as healthy as Barnstable.

With such discrepancies as these there is certainly cause for investigation, and encouragement to hope for success in mastering the problems that are presented. Much has been already done – but much remains to be done. Men are ready who find sufficient reward for their own labors in the sense of public usefulness and the gratification of promoting the cause of social science. A small sum expended in giving them the necessary clerical and executive assistance will be all that seems immediately necessary.

It is the opinion of your Committee that a State Board of Health ought to be established, with such powers as will enable them thoroughly to investigate matters relating to public health, with a view to advise concerning it; but without any authoritative control or right or active interference . . .

3. Legislation establishing a State Board of Health. *Massachusetts Acts and Resolves 1869, Chapter 420* (June 21, 1869).

Section 1. The governor, with the advice and consent of the council, shall appoint seven persons, who shall constitute the board of health and vital statistics. The persons so appointed shall hold their offices for seven years: *provided,* that the terms of office of the seven first appointed shall be so arranged that the term of one shall expire each year, and the vacancies so created, as well as all vacancies occurring otherwise, shall be filled by the governor, with the advice and consent of the council; but any one may be reappointed.

Section 2. The board shall take cognizance of the interests of health and life among the citizens of this Commonwealth. They shall make sanitary investigations and inquiries in respect to the people, the causes of disease, and especially of epidemics and the sources of mortality and the effects of localities, employments, conditions and circumstances, on the public health; and they shall gather such information in respect to those matters as they may deem proper, for diffusion among the people. They shall advise the government in regard to the location of any public institutions. They shall, in the month of January, make report to the legislature of their doings, investigations and discoveries during the year ending December thirty-first, with such suggestions as to legislative action as they may deem necessary.

Section 3. The board shall meet at the state house once in three months, and as much oftener as they may deem expedient. No member except the secretary shall receive any compensation, but the actual   personal expenses of any member while engaged in the duties of the board shall be allowed and paid.

Section 4. It shall be the duty of the board, and they are hereby instructed, to examine into and report what, in their best judgment, is the effect of the use of intoxicating liquor, as a beverage, upon the industry, prosperity, happiness, health and lives of the citizens of the state. Also, what additional legislation, if any, is necessary in the premises.

Section 5. The board shall elect a secretary, either from their own number or otherwise; but when elected he shall be a member of the board and their executive officer. He shall perform and superintend the work prescribed in this law, and such other duties as the board may require. He shall receive from the treasury, in quarterly payments, an annual salary of twenty-five hundred dollars and his necessary travelling expenses incurred in the performance of official duties, after they have been audited by the board and approved by the governor and council, and all other necessary expenses arising in his office shall be paid out of the treasury in the same manner as those of the different departments of the government . . .

4. Selections from the opening address to the first meeting of the State Board of Health by Henry I. Bowditch (September 15, 1869). Massachusetts State Board of Health, *First Annual Report* (1870).

Gentlemen of the State Board of Health:

By the orders of the Governor of the Commonwealth, it devolves upon me to call you together. As the subject-matters for our discussion may be somewhat indefinite in all of our minds, I take the liberty of addressing a few words to you, in order that you may know not only what I consider the general nature of our duties, but may also understand how high I place these duties when I consider them in their relations to the present and future health of the citizens of the State. I may be mistaken in my estimate of the importance of the movement, the commencement of which to-day devolves upon us. I confess to you that I know of no higher office in the State than that which we now hold, viz., that of inaugurating the idea of "State Medicine" in Massachusetts. Upon our high or low appreciation of the position and of the duties resulting from that position, and upon our wise or foolish performance of these duties, depends the success of the object aimed at in the establishment of a State Board of Health. The last legislature, unconsciously, perhaps, on the part of many members thereof, has proposed a system that may be made by us capable of good to the citizens in all future time, or it may prove a perfect abortion. Our work is for the far future as well as for the present, and at this very opening of our labors we should try to place ourselves above the region of merely local or temporary excitement or of partisan warfare, in order that we may act wisely and for the ultimate good of the whole people.

In these introductory general remarks, as you will see, my object has been to impress upon you my views of the essential dignity of the offices we now hold, and that we should assume them with minds loyal to the truth and under a sense of individual responsibility in the premises.

I have used one expression about which I wish to enter into some detail, viz., "State Medicine in Massachusetts." What is the precise meaning of the expression? It is of very recent growth in our language. It has, in fact, arisen, I believe, within the last few years in England, where already it has become a great power for good. Its objects rank among the most important matters now discussed by the highest intellects and humanest hearts in Great Britain. It is, as I understand it, a special function of a state authority, which until these later days of scientific investigation has been left almost wholly unperformed or exercised only under the greatest incitements to its operation, such as the coming of the plague, cholera, smallpox, and some other equally malignant disease. By this function the authorities of a state are bound to take care of the public health, to investigate the causes of epidemic and of other diseases, in order that each citizen may not only have as long a life as nature would give him, but likewise as healthy a life as possible. As the chief object of the physician is the cure, if possible, of any ailment which is submitted to his care, so the far higher aim of State Medicine is, by its thorough and scientific investigations of the hidden causes of diseases that are constantly at work in an ignorant or debased community, to prevent the very origination of such diseases. Much has already been suggested in England towards the crushing out of fevers, etc. Still more recently one of the grandest results of State Medicine is its virtual recognition under international law by the appointment of joint governmental commissioners for the investigation and prevention of the spread of Asiatic cholera . . .

Dr. Bowditch continued with a "history of State Medicine in Great Britain" since 1848. He concluded:

The law requires us to diffuse among our people any already established laws of public health, and also whatever we may hereafter discover on that subject. I look upon this feature of the law with deep interest, for I believe by it we *may* do much service to the people.

How shall we diffuse this knowledge? Permit me to allude to a few evident methods.

(*a*). By lectures from our Secretary or from members of the Board on various special subjects connected with public hygiene – such as ventilating, and building, and location of houses; on various well-known diseases capable of partial or entire prevention on knowledge of causes being given. It may be a question, moreover, whether we should not authorize the Secretary to communicate with lecture committees of various towns and the American Literary Bureaus, and to make arrangements with physicians and others to deliver lectures relating to public health in various towns.

(*b*). By the Secretary holding meetings in the various parts of the State for discussions on the subject; meetings analogous to those now held on education, agriculture etc. He might invite the cooperation of local medical societies or special physicians. I have no doubt that such meetings, properly conducted, would attract the attention and interest of the public.

(*c*). By the publication in a compact form and the wide circulation of the pith, so to speak, of our general knowledge on public hygiene. How this should be done would remain an open question. If it could be done, there is no doubt of the good that would eventually result.

(*d*). By our annual reports to the legislature, which, I trust, will always be models of brevity and of compact learning – not a word too much or a word for effect merely – and so thoroughly indexed that even the busiest man on "change can in three minutes get at the essentials, and be prepared to study the details of any part or parts he may wish further to examine."

In conclusion, gentlemen, let me say that, while I feel alike our grave responsibilities and the dignity conferred on each one of us by His Excellency the Governor in his selection of us for these office, I have at the same time no misgivings; but on the contrary, the liveliest hope that this Board will faithfully and in an able manner perform its duties, and that thus it will become a real blessing to our State, not only at the present time, but long after every member of it has died. It will assuredly be such if we, the necessary originators of its various details, only look at our duties in the light of the broadest philanthropy and, as far as in us lies, the wisest statesmanship, and finally with all the knowledge that modern science can at present give us.

In making these introductory remarks, I have done only what seemed to be proper; but I hope that others will speak what seems to them good, so that starting on our new career with understanding minds and buoyant willing hearts, we may vigorously inaugurate State Medicine in Massachusetts

5. Legislation establishing health districts and inspectors. *Massachusetts Acts and Resolves 1907. Chapter 537* (July 19, 1907).

Section 1. The state board of health shall, as soon as may be after the passage of this act, divide the Commonwealth into not more than fifteen districts, to be known as health districts, in such manner as it may deem necessary or proper for carrying out the purposes of this act.

Section 2. After the division aforesaid has been made, the governor, with the advice and consent of the council, shall appoint in each health district one practical and discreet person, learned in the science of medicine and hygiene, to be state inspector of health in that district. Every nomination for such office shall be made at least seven days prior to the appointment. The said state inspectors of health shall hold their offices for a period of five years from the time of their respective appointments, but shall be liable to removal from office by the governor and council at any time.

Section 3. Every state inspector of health shall inform himself respecting the sanitary condition of his district and concerning all influences dangerous to the public health or threatening to affect the same; he shall gather all information possible concerning the prevalence of tuberculosis and other diseases dangerous to the public health within his district, shall disseminate knowledge as to the best methods of preventing the spread of such diseases, and shall take such steps as, after consultation with the state board of health and the local state authorities, shall be deemed advisable for their eradication; he shall inform himself concerning the health of all minors employed in factories within his district, and, whenever he may deem it advisable or necessary, he shall call the ill health or physical unfitness of any minor to the attention of his or her parents or employers or the state board of health.

Section 4. The state inspectors of health shall be under the general supervision of the state board of health and shall perform such duties other than those hereby imposed upon them as the said board from time to time shall determine. They shall keep a record of their proceedings and observations, shall annually make a report of the same to said board on or before the thirty-first day on October, shall from time to time furnish said board with such information as it may require touching circumstances affecting the public health in their respective districts, and shall in every instance where written suggestions are made by them to the local authorities send copies of such suggestions to said board.

Section 5. The state inspectors of health shall, under the direction of the state board of health and in place of the inspection department of the district police, enforce the provisions of . . . chapter one hundred and four of the Revised Laws so far as said section provides that factories shall be well ventilated and kept clean . . . and the powers and duties heretofore conferred and imposed upon . . . the district police . . . are hereby conferred and imposed upon state inspectors of health or such other officers as the state board of health may from time to time appoint: *provided, however,* that neither said board of health nor any inspector thereof shall have authority to require structural alterations to be made in buildings, but shall report the necessity therefor to the inspection department of the district police . . .

Section 6. The governor, with the advice and consent of the council, shall establish the salaries of said state inspectors of health, having regard in each district to the extent of territory, the number of inhabitants, the character of the business there carried on, and the amount of time likely to be required for the proper discharge of the duties. The salaries thus established shall be paid from the treasury of the Commonwealth monthly.

Section 7. There may be expended out of the treasury of the Commonwealth annually, for the purposes specified in this act, for salaries, and for other expenses, a sum not exceeding five thousand dollars.

Section 8. For the purpose of carrying out the provisions of this act the state board of health may employ from time to time experts in sanitation . . .

6. Legislation establishing a full Department of Health, *Massachusetts Acts and Resolves 1914, Chapter 792* (July 7, 1914).

Section 1. There is hereby created a State Department of Health which shall exercise all the powers and perform the duties now conferred and imposed by law upon the state board of health. The state department of health shall consist of a commissioner of health and a public health council. There shall also be directors of divisions, district health officers and other employees as hereinafter provided.

Section 2. The commissioner of health shall be appointed by the governor, with the advice and consent of the council, and he shall be a physician skilled in sanitary science and experienced in public health administration. The term of office of the commissioner of health shall be five years. He shall receive an annual salary of seventy-five hundred dollars and shall devote his entire time to his official duties. The commissioner of health shall be the administrative head of the state department of health. His powers and duties shall be to administer the laws relative to health and sanitation and the regulations of the department; to prepare rules and regulations for the consideration of the public health council; and, with the approval of the public health council, to appoint and remove directors of divisions, district health officers, inspectors and other necessary employees, and to fix their compensation, subject to the approval of the governor and council, within the limitations of appropriations therefor. Directors of divisions and district health officers shall be exempt from civil service regulations. The commissioner of health shall submit annually to the public health council a report containing recommendations in regard to health legislation; and he shall perform all executive duties now required by law of the state board of health and such other duties as are incident to his position as chief executive officer. He may direct any executive officer or employee of the state department of health to assist in the study, suppression or prevention of disease in any part of the commonwealth.

Section 3. The public health council shall consist of the commissioner of health and six members, hereinafter called the appointive members, at least three of whom shall be physicians, and who shall be appointed by the governor, with the advice and consent of the council. Of the members first appointed, two shall hold office until the first day of May in the year nineteen hundred and fifteen, two until the first day of May in the year nineteen hundred and sixteen, and two until the first day of May in the year nineteen hundred and seventeen, and the terms of office of the said members thereafter appointed, except to fill vacancies, shall be three years. Vacancies shall be filled by appointment of the governor, with the advice and consent of the council, for the unexpired term. The public health council shall meet at least once in each month, and at such other times as they shall determine by their rules, or upon the request of any four members, or upon the request of the commissioner of health. The appointive members shall receive ten dollars a day while in conference, and their necessary travelling expenses while in the performance of their official duties. It shall be the duty of the public health council to make and promulgate rules and regulations; to take evidence in appeals; to consider plans and appointments required by law; to hold hearings; to submit annually to the general court, through the governor, a report, including recommendations as to needed health legislation; and to discharge other duties required by law; but it shall have no administrative or executive functions.

Section 4. There shall be in the state department of health such divisions as the commissioner of health may, with the approval of the public health council, from time to time determine. The commissioner of health shall appoint and may remove, with the approval of the public health council, a director to take charge of each division, and shall prescribe the duties of such division. The compensation of directors of divisions shall be fixed by the commissioner of health, within the limits of appropriations therefor, and subject to the approval of the governor and council.

Section 5. The commissioner of health, with the approval of the public health council shall, from time to time, divide the state into eight health districts and shall appoint and may remove a district health officer for each district, with the approval of the public health council, at a compensation, subject to the approval of the governor and council, not exceeding thirty-five hundred dollars a year. The district health officers shall not engage in any any other occupation and shall give their entire time to the performance of their duties. The commissioner of health may, from time to time, order two or more of said district health officers to work in one district in order to study, suppress or prevent disease. Each district health officer shall have all the powers and perform the duties now provided by law for inspectors of health and further shall, under the direction of the commissioner of health, perform such duties as may be prescribed by, and shall act as the representative of the commissioner of health and under his directors shall secure the enforcement within his district of the public health laws and regulations. Said district health officers shall be graduates of an incorporated medical school, admitted to practice in the commonwealth, or shall have had at least five years' experience in public health duties and sanitary science.

Section 6. For carrying out the purposes of this act there shall be appropriated for the purposes of the state department of health, over and above the amount already appropriated for the state board of health for the year nineteen hundred and fourteen, the sum of ten thousand dollars.

Section 7. Present employees shall be continued in office until their successors are appointed and qualified, or until removed by the commissioner: *provided, however,* that no employee shall be removed who was appointed, or is now employed, under the provisions of the civil service laws and regulations, other than for cause, except division heads and district health officers who shall be appointed as hereinbefore provided . . .

Appendix VI. Extension of State Authority for Public Health: Selected Massachusetts Documents.

1. Protection of public water supplies.

   A. Legislation to prevent the pollution of the water supply. *Massachusetts Acts and Resolves 1878, Chapter 183* (April 26, 1878).[a]

Section 1. No person or persons, or corporation public or private, shall discharge directly or cause to be discharged directly, human excrement into any pond in this Commonwealth used as a source of water supply by any city or town therein, or upon whose banks any filter basin so used is situated, or into any river or stream so used or upon whose bank such filter basin is situated within twenty miles above the point where such supply is taken, or into any feeders of such pond, river or stream within such twenty miles.

Section 2. No person or persons, or corporation public or private, shall discharge or cause to be discharged into any pond in this Commonwealth used as a source of water supply by any city or town therein, or upon whose banks any filter basin so used is situated, or into any river or stream so used or upon whose banks such filter basin is situated, within twenty miles above the point where such supply is taken, or into any feeders of such pond, river or stream within such twenty miles, any sewage, drainage, refuse or polluting matter of such quality and amount as either by itself, or in connection with other matter shall corrupt, or impair the quality of the water for domestic use, or render it deleterious to health.

Section 3. The prohibitions contained in the two previous sections shall not be construed to destroy or impair rights already acquired by legislative grants, or to destroy or impair prescriptive rights of drainage or discharge, to the extent to which they lawfully exist at the date of the passage of this act; and nothing in this act contained shall be construed to authorize the pollution of any waters in this Commonwealth, in any manner now contrary to law.

This act shall not be applicable to the Merrimac or Connecticut Rivers, nor to so much of the Concord River as lies within the limits of the city of Lowell.

Section 4. The state board of health shall have the general supervision of all rivers, streams and ponds in this Commonwealth which are or shall be used by any city or town

[a]Three years before the board was authorized to investigage and report to the legislature on "a system or method by which . . . cities or towns may be properly drained . . . rivers, estuaries and ponds may be protected against pollution . . . with the view to the preservation of the health of the inhabitants . . . securing a proper system of drainage and sewerage, without injury to the rights and health of others; also . . . how far said sewage may be utilized and disposed of" (*Acts and Resolves 1875, Chapter 192* [May 8, 1875]).

as sources of water supply, with reference to their purity, together with the waters feeding the same, except the Merrimac, Connecticut and Concord Rivers. It shall be the duty of said board to examine the same from time to time and to inquire what pollutions exist and their causes. Whenever a violation of any of the provisions of this act is committed the said board may, if in its judgment the public health shall require, order any person or persons, or corporation public or private, to cease and desist from such violation and to remedy the pollution or to cleanse or purify the polluting substances in such a manner and to such a degree that they shall be no longer deleterious to the public health before being cast or allowed to flow into the waters thereby polluted: *provided,* that before making such order the said board shall assign a time and place for hearing the party or parties to be affected, and shall give him or them an opportunity of being heard thereon, and after such notice and hearing, and *provided, also,* that upon the application of any city or town to said board alleging the violation of any of the provisions of this act, and the pollution of its water supply thereby, it shall be the duty of said board to grant a hearing upon due notification of the party or parties to be affected as aforesaid, and upon proof of such violation to issue the order or orders already mentioned in this section.

Section 5. The supreme judicial court or any one of its justices in term time or vacation shall have power to issue an injunction to enforce the orders of the said board of health.

Section 6. The orders of the said board of health shall be served upon the party or parties found to have violated any of the provisions of this act, and such party or parties if aggrieved thereby shall have the right of appeal to a jury . . . of the laws of eighteen hundred and sixty-five. During the pendency of the appeal the pollution against which the order has issued shall not be continued contrary to the order of the said board.

    B. Legislation to permit the State Board of Health to conduct experiments for the purification of water, leading to the establishment, in 1887, of the Lawrence Experiment Station. *Acts and Resolves 1886, Chapter 274* (June 9, 1886).

Section 1. The state board of health shall have the general oversight and care of all inland waters and shall be furnished with maps, plans and documents suitable for this purpose, and records of all its doings in relation thereto shall be kept. It may employ such engineers and clerks and other assistants as it may deem necessary – provided, that no contracts or other acts which involve the payment of money from the treasury of the Commonwealth shall be made or done without an appropriation expressly made therefor by the general court. It shall annually on or before the tenth day of January report to the general court its doings in the preceding year, and at the same time submit estimates of the sums required to meet the expenses of said board in relation to the care and oversight of inland waters for the ensuing year; and it shall also recommend legislation and suitable plans for such systems of main sewers as it may deem necessary for the preservation of the public health and for the purification and prevention of pollution of the ponds, streams, and inland waters of the Commonwealth.

Section 2. Said board shall from time to time as it may deem expedient, cause examinations of the said waters to be made for the purpose of ascertaining whether the same are adapted for use as sources of domestic water supplies or are in a condition likely to impair the interests of the public or persons lawfully using the same, or imperil the public health. It shall recommend measures for prevention of the pollution of such waters and for removal of substances and causes of every kind which may be liable to cause pollution thereof, in order to protect and develop the rights and property of the Commonwealth therein and to protect the public health. It shall have authority to conduct experiments to determine the best practicable methods of purification of drainage or disposal of refuse arising from manufacturing and other industrial establishments. For the purposes aforesaid it may employ such expert assistance as may be necessary.

Section 3. It shall from time to time consult with and advise the authorities of cities and towns, or with corporations, firms or individuals either already having or intending to introduce systems of water supply or sewerage, as to the most appropriate source of supply, the best practicable method of assuring the purity thereof or of disposing of their sewage, having regard to the present and prospective needs and interests of other cities, towns, corporations, firms or individuals which may be affected thereby. It shall also from time to time consult with and advise persons or corporations engaged or intending to engage in any manufacturing or other business, drainage or refuse from which may tend to cause the pollution of any inland water, as to the best practicable method of preventing such pollution by the interception, disposal or purification of such drainage or refuse: *provided,* that no person shall be compelled to bear the expense of such consultation or advice, or of experiments made for the purposes of this act. All such authorities, corporations, firms and individuals are hereby required to give notice to said board of their intentions in the premises, and to submit for its advice outlines of their proposed plans or schemes in relation to water supply and disposal of drainage and refuse. Said board shall bring to the notice of the attorney-general all instances which may come to its knowledge of omission to comply with existing laws respecting the pollution of water supplies and inland waters and shall annually report to the legislature any specific cases not covered by the provisions of existing laws, which in its opinion call for further legislation.

2. Protection of food and drugs.

Legislation to prevent the sale of adulterated food and drugs. *Acts and Resolves 1882, Chapter 263* (May 26, 1882).[a]

Section 1. No person shall, within this Commonwealth, manufacture for sale, offer for sale or sell any drug or article of food which is adulterated within the meaning of this act.

Section 2. The term "drug" as used in this act shall include all medicines for internal or external use, antiseptics, disinfectants and cosmetics. The term "food" as used herein shall include all articles used for food or drink by man.

Section 3. An article shall be deemed to be adulterated within the meaning of this act, —

(*a.*) In the case of drugs, — (1.) If, when sold under or by a name recognized in the United States pharmacopoeia, it differs from the standard of strength, quality or purity laid down therein; (2.) If, when sold under or by a name not recognized in the United States pharmacopoeia but which is found in some other pharmacopoeia, or other standard work on *materia medica,* it differes materially from the standard of strength, quality or purity laid down in such work; (3.) If its strength or purity falls below the professed standard under which it is sold:

(*b.*) In the case of food, — (1.) If any substance or substances have been mixed with it so as to reduce, or lower, or injuriously affect its quality or strength; (2.) If any inferior or cheaper substance or substances have been substituted wholly or in part for it; (3.) If any valuable constituent has been wholly or in part abstracted from it; (4.) If it is an imitation of, or is sold under the name of, another article; (5.) If it consists wholly or in part of a diseased, decomposed, putrid, or rotten animal or vegetable substance, whether manufactured or not; or, in the case of milk, if it is the produce of a diseased animal; (6.) If it is colored, coated, polished, or powdered, whereby damage is concealed, or if it is made to appear better or of greater value than it really is; (7.) If it contains any added poisonous ingredient, or any ingredient which may render it injurious to the health of a person consuming it.

[a]Two years later the legislature provided that not less than 3/5 of the annual appropriation under this Act must be spent protecting milk and milk products; see *Acts and Resolves, 1884, Chapter 289.*

The state board of health, lunacy and charity may from time to time declare certain articles or preparations to be exempt from the provisions of this act; and the provisions hereof shall not apply to mixtures or compounds recognized as ordinary articles of food, provided that the same are not injurious to health, and are distinctly labelled as mixtures or compounds.

Section 4. The state board of health, lunacy and charity shall prepare and publish from time to time lists of the articles, mixtures or compounds declared to be exempt from the provisions of this act, in accordance with the preceding section. The said board shall also from time to time fix the limits of variability permissible in any article of food, or any drug, or compound, the standard of which is not established by any national pharmacopoeia.

Section 5. The state board of health, lunacy and charity shall take cognizance of the interests of the public health relating to the sale of drugs and food and the adulteration of the same, and shall make all necessary investigations and inquiries in reference thereto, and for these purposes may appoint inspectors, analysts and chemists, who shall be subject to its supervision and removal.

Within thirty days after the passage of this act the said board shall adopt such measures as it may deem necessary to facilitate the enforcement hereof, and shall prepare rules and regulations with regard to the proper methods of collecting and examining drugs and articles of food. Said board may expend annually an amount not exceeding three thousand dollars for the purposes of carrying out the provisions of this act.

Section 6. Every person offering or exposing for sale, or delivering to a purchaser, any drug or article of food included in the provisions of this act, shall furnish to any analyst or other officer or agent appointed hereunder, who shall apply to him for the purpose and shall tender him the value of the same, a sample sufficient for the purpose of the analysis of any such drug or article of food which is in his possession.

Section 7. Whoever hinders, obstructs, or in any way interferes with any inspector, analyst, or other officer appointed hereunder in the performance of his duty, and whoever violates any of the provisions of this act, shall be punished by a fine not exceeding fifty dollars for the first offence and not exceeding one hundred dollars for each subsequent offence . . .

3. Control of contagious disease.

A. Legislation to require notification of the local board of health; see *Acts and Resolves 1884, Chapter 98* (March 21, 1884).[a]

Section 1. When a householder knows that a person within his family is sick with small pox, diphtheria, scarlet fever or any other disease dangerous to the public health, he shall immediately give notice thereof to the selectmen or board of health of the town in which

[a]Legislation to restrict the spread of smallpox was enacted in 1701, and from time to time thereafter as enforcement became a problem. In 1809 the towns were required to insure vaccination; later this became discretionary. In 1883 local boards of health were required to notify the State Board of Health, Lunacy, and Charity of all cases of smallpox (*Acts and Resolves 1883, Chapter 138*). A year later school committees were made responsible for imposing quarantine in cases of smallpox, scarlet fever, or diphtheria (*Acts and Resolves 1884, Chapter 64*). Nine years later local boards were required to notify the State Board of Health within twenty-four hours in all cases of disease "dangerous to the public health," however the specific diseases were not identified (*Acts and Resolves 1893, Chapter 302*). The Board named the following diseases reportable: smallpox, scarlet fever, measles, typhoid, diphtheria, membranous croup, cholera, yellow fever, cerebro-spinal meningitis, hydrophobia, malignant pustule (anthrax), leprosy, and trichinosis.

215

he dwells, and upon the death, recovery or removal of such person, the rooms occupied and the articles used by him shall be disinfected by such householder in a manner approved by the board of health. Any person neglecting or refusing to comply with either of the above provisions shall forfeit a sum not exceeding one hundred dollars.

Section 2. When a physician knows that a person whom he is called to visit is infected with small pox, diphtheria, scarlet fever or any other disease dangerous to the public health, he shall immediately give notice thereof to the selectmen or board of health of the town; and if he refuses or neglects to give such notice he shall forfeit for each offence not less than fifty nor more than two hundred dollars.

Section 3. The boards of health in the several cities and towns shall cause a record to be kept of all reports received in pursuance of the preceding sections and such record shall contain the names of all persons who are sick, the localities in which they live, the diseases with which they are affected, together with the date and the names of the persons reporting any such cases. The boards of health shall give the school committee immediate information of all cases of contagious diseases reported to them according to the provisions of this act.

Section 4. The secretary of the Commonwealth shall furnish the boards of health with blank books for the record of cases of contagious disease as above provided.

B. Circular from the State Board of Health giving information and advice on the prevention of tuberculosis, January 1895.[a]

The object of the State Board of Health in issuing the following circular is to furnish information (1) as to the nature of pulmonary consumption, (2) the conditions which favor its spread, and (3) the best methods of preventing it.

1. – As to the Nature of Consumption.

Consumption is the most destructive disease of New England, the number of persons annually dying from this cause in Massachusetts amounting to nearly six thousand. Modern research places it among infectious diseases.

The specific virus or poison of the disease consists of a minute germ, the "bacillus of tuberculosis," which exists in the tissues and expectoration of the sick, and which may in various ways enter the bodies of the well and reproduce the disease in them. In the proper care and disposal of the expectoration of the sick, it is probable, lies one of the chief methods of preventing the spread of the disease.

2. – Conditions which favor the Spread of Consumption among Human Beings.

Defective ventilation. One of the chief conditions which is favorable to the production of consumption is the continuous and habitual breathing of unrenewed air. Consequently, in workshops, factories, school rooms, public buildings, halls, churches, and the inhabited apartments of dwellings and tenement-houses the absence of adequate means of ventilation favors the spread of consumption.

Dampness of soil on which the house stands, and dampness of the immediate neighborhood are favorable conditions for the production of consumption. The occupancy as living or sleeping rooms of apartments which are constantly damp or are partly or wholly underground, undoubtedly has a similar effect.

Overcrowding in dwellings, in factories, and in workshops where men and women work for several hours each day, is also a favorable condition for spreading the disease. Density of population increases the liability to this disease. Observations in Massachusetts extending over a period of twenty years (1871-90) show that the deaths from consumption in densely settled districts, as compared with those in sparsely settled districts of the State stood in the ratio of 1,000 deaths in the former to 727 in the latter.

[a]Tuberculosis was made reportable in 1907.

216

Another factor which favors the spread of this disease is the presence of dust in the air of apartments, factories, mills, and workshops. Hence occupations or trades in which men, women or children are exposed to the inhalation of irritating dust increase the liability to contract the disease among such operatives. An examination of the reports of the Registrar General of England for several successive years shows that fishermen, who are of all classes the least exposed to dust inhalation, are also comparatively exempt fron consumption.

Insufficient and badly selected food. While the influence of improper and insufficient feeding upon the predisposition to consumption is not so directly proven as are the effects of certain other conditions, there is yet sufficient evidence to show that a restricted diet or one composed exclusively of single elementary constituents, as for example, the starches alone, and these in too limited quantities, probably predisposes to consumption.

Intemperance in the use of alcoholic stimulants has also been shown to act in the same direction.

Undue physical or mental strain, overwork, worry and anxiety, and the prolonged suckling of infants (beyond ten to twelve months) are conditions contributing to the same end.

3. – Preventive Measures.

Having the foregoing predisposing conditions in view, the measures which are essential for the prevention of this disease may be clearly understood.

1. *The prevention of overcrowding.* In tenements and in dwelling-houses the prevention of overcrowding diminishes the liability to contract tubercular disease among the occupants.

Hence the adoption of measures which shall counteract the effect of overcrowding is desirable. Ventilation is one of the most efficient of such measures. Adequate ventilation should be provided in all factories, halls, school-houses and other buildings in which people assemble in considerable numbers. Simple of methods of ventilation in the living and sleeping rooms of dwellings are also essential to healthy living. Open fireplaces, movable transoms in sleeping rooms, provision for admitting fresh air at the windows by special means are all useful precautions.

2. *Household as well as personal cleanliness* is essential to the prevention of consumption. The removal of dust from floors should be practised and care should be taken that such dust is removed by such means as will insure the least diffusion through the air of rooms during their occupancy.

3. *Occupations.* The selection of a healthy occupation is a matter of no small importance. Sedentary occupations in ill-ventilated apartments and those which expose the workman to the inhalation of dust should be avoided. Different sorts of dust vary in harmful effects. The sharp dust produced in the grinding of needles and steel tools and in the mining of metals is especially irritating, and the mortality from consumption among operatives in such industries is high. Operatives engaged in such occupations may diminish the liability to harm by wearing "respirators" over the mouth and nose, while at work.

In several factories where consumption had made serious inroads upon the operatives, the adoption of measures for the prevention of a dusty atmosphere secured a marked diminution of the prevalence of this disease among the workmen employed in them.

Regular daily exercise in the open air is of the first importance for all persons who are engaged in sedentary occupations.

The owners and superintendents of *factories, mills* and *workshops* can accomplish much toward the prevention of tuberculosis among the operatives by the introduction of adequate systems of ventilation and heating, and by the use of hard, smooth floors without cracks or crevices.

The dust should be removed from the floors at night, after working hours, and not during the occupancy of the workrooms. The use of moisture in the removal of dust, and careful wiping with damp cloths is preferable to sweeping up the dust when dry. Spitting upon the floor should be forbidden.

4. *Food.* As an essential requisite to the prevention of consumption, a diet of sound, wholesome food, in which the chief elementary forms of nutriment are harmoniously combined (the fats, starches, and proteins) is necessary. Such a diet should consist mainly of

bread and the various cereals with butter and other fats in generous measure, together with meat, fish and fruits. This does not imply a luxurious or expensive diet, but rather one that is nutritious and easily digested.

The question of the effect of the use of the *meat* and *milk* of *tuberculous animals* does not yet appear to be so well settled as to admit an unqualified conclusion.

In the absence of absolute and definite evidence, it is therefore desirable that the *meat* of all suspected animals should be cooked thoroughly before using it as food. The *milk* of such animals should be entirely excluded from the food supply.

5. *Overwork, anxiety, worry* and *exhaustion* should be avoided. Mothers should be advised to *wean suckling infants* by the end of the first year.

6. *Disposal of Sputa.* With reference to those who are sick with consumption or tuberculosis, and especially with reference to the possibility that their presence among other human beings may prove a source of danger on account of infection, the following recommendation as to the disposal of the expectoration of consumptives should be especially noted.

Observation and experiments have demonstrated the fact that in this expectoration (especially when dried) lies the chief danger of infection, and hence its proper disposal becomes a matter of prime importance. Therefore, sputa should never be allowed *to become dry,* and should be destroyed as quickly as possible. Consumptives should be instructed not to expectorate about rooms, in streets or highways, in railway or street cars, or in vehicles of any sort, but should spit into rags which can be burned, or into cups or other receptacles containing a little water or other material which may be thoroughly disinfected before the same is allowed to pass into the drain or sewer. Such receptacles should be cleansed with boiling water.

A healthy person should not sleep in the same room with a consumptive.

7. *Disinfection.* Sputa may best be burned when deposited upon pieces of cloth or rags; and when put into cups or receptacles holding water the whole should be disinfected with a saturated solution of carbolic acid, which may be obtained of any reliable druggist.

Disinfection should be practised in the case of rooms or apartments which have been vacated by consumptives or those in which such persons have died. There is a growing belief, supported by observation, that rooms which have been inhabited by consumptive families may become permanently infected, and ought not to be occupied until radical measures have been taken to cleanse and disinfect them. Each room vacated by a tuberculosis patient should be disinfected and especially the floor and lower parts of the walls. For this purpose washing the floor and all woodwork with a corrosive sublimate solution, one part to one thousand (about one teaspoonful to a gallon of water) should be practised, and the bed and clothing of the last occupant should be submitted to steam disinfection or to boiling water. Strong soapsuds also have efficient disinfecting power, and may be used for washing floors and woodwork. The disinfection should be thoroughly done, but especially so in cases where the habits of the consumptive in regard to disposal of his sputa have been careless.

As a means of spreading information upon this important subject, local boards of health can undoubtedly accomplish much toward the prevention of a consumption, by issuing a circular like the following:–

The Prevention of Consumption

Consumption is the most destructive disease of New England, the number of persons dying annually from this cause in Massachusetts amounting to nearly six thousand.

The disease is infectious, and can be communicated from one person to another. The chief danger exists in the expectoration of the sick, and if this expectoration is carefully destroyed little danger need be feared.

Consumptives should be instructed not to spit upon the floors of rooms, public halls, street and railway cars, and other vehicles, nor in the streets, but into pieces of cloth, or receptacles made for the purpose, containing water, or a saturated solution of carbolic acid (one part carbolic acid crystals to about fifteen parts of water). Such bits of cloth should be destroyed by fire, before the sputa become dry, and other receptacles should be cleansed with scalding water, their contents having been destroyed or otherwise carefully disposed of. Handkerchiefs which may have been used from necessity should be boiled half an hour before washing.

A healthy person should not sleep in the same room with a consumptive.

Remember that sputa must never be allowed to become dry.

4. Identification of noncontagious diseases as a public health problem.

A. Resolution to investigate the prevalence of cancer and the need for public facilities. *Acts and Resolves 1925, Chapter 20* (April 16, 1925).

Resolved, That the departments of public health and public welfare, acting jointly for the purpose of this resolve, are hereby directed to make a study and investigation of the prevalence of the disease of cancer throughout the commonwealth, and particularly of the disease in its inoperable stage or form.

They shall also determine as nearly as may be practicable all the existing bed facilities in hospitals and institutions now available for persons suffering from this disease, and more particularly bed facilities available for persons suffering from the disease in its inoperable stage or form.

Following such study and investigation the two departments, acting jointly, shall report to the general court their findings and recommendations, if any, together with drafts for such legislation as may be necessary to carry their recommendations into effect, by filing the same with the clerk of the house of representatives not later than December fifteenth of the current year.

In case the result of such investigation shall in the joint opinion of the two departments indicate that additional hospital facilities are needed for the care of persons suffering from cancer, the departments shall carefully consider and submit as part of their legislative recommendations such method or plan as in their judgment will best serve the needs of the commonwealth, whether by the creation by the commonwealth, of a new institution for the purpose or by the enlargement of existing state, county or municipal institutions or private charitable institutions, or of any of them, and in what manner if any, the commonwealth can best stimulate and assist in making available such additional facilities for care and treatment of persons suffering from cancer.

For the purpose of this study and investigation, the two departments acting jointly, in addition to such service as may be furnished by their permanent staffs, may employ additional clerical, medical and other expert assistance and may expend therefor from such amount, not exceeding four thousand dollars, as may be appropriated by the general court such sums as may be approved by the governor and council.

B. Legislation to authorize medical care of cancer patients through the Department of Public Health, *Acts and Resolves 1926, Chapter 391* (May 29, 1926).

Whereas, It is important for the protection of the public health that immediate steps be taken for the further prevention of cancer and the cure and treatment of persons afflicted with cancer, therefore this act is hereby declared to be an emergency law, necessary for the immediate preservation of the public health.

Be it enacted, etc., as follows:

Section 1. The department of public health, hereinafter called the department, is hereby authorized and directed to formulate a plan for the care and treatment of persons suffering from cancer, with a view to taking any necessary initial steps toward the establishment of necessary hospital facilities for such care and treatment by the use of existing buildings or by additions to existing buildings. The department shall, from time to time, submit such plan to the governor and council and to the budget commissioner, and shall report its final plan to the general court not later than October fifteenth in the current year, with drafts of such legislation as may be necessary to carry the same into effect, and shall at the same time file copies thereof with the said budget commissioner.

Section 2. The department shall establish and organize cancer clinics in such parts of the commonwealth as it may deem most advantageous to the public health and shall conduct such clinics with or without co-operation on the part of municipalities, local physicians and other agencies.

Section 3. Subject to appropriation, the department may expend during the current fiscal year for the purposes of sections one and two a sum not exceeding fifteen thousand dollars.

Section 4. For the purpose of providing immediate care and treatment for persons suffering from cancer, the department is hereby authorized to make use of the Norfolk state hospital and may suitably condition and equip the same. Subject to appropriation, there may be expended for the purposes of this section during the current fiscal year a sum not exceeding one hundred thousand dollars.

Appendix VII. Mortality in Massachusetts, 1865–1940: Number of Deaths per 1,000 Living.

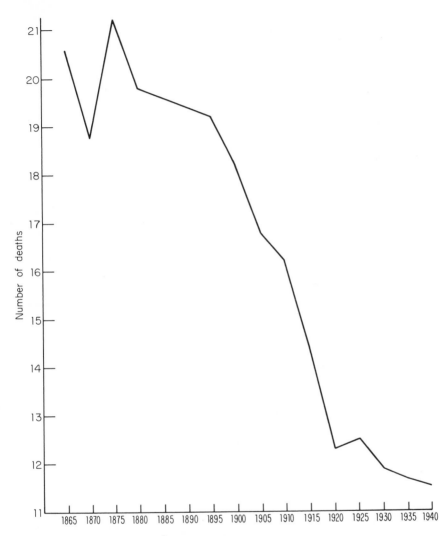

Sources: *77th Annual Report on the Vital Statistics of Massachusetts . . . 1918,* for the years 1815-1918; *Annual Reports on the Vital Statistics of Massachusetts,* for the years thereafter. "The crude death rate obtained by estimating the ratio of the number of deaths to the living population has been employed for many years as an index of the sanitary condition with that of other communities," Massachusetts State Board of Health, *Twenty-fifth Annual Report* (1894), p. xliii.

Appendix VIII. Life Expectancy in Massachusetts, 1855–1941. Expectation in years at birth and at age 20, by sex.

Years	At birth		At age 20	
	Male	Female	Male	Female
1855	39	41	60	60
1878-1882	42	44	62	63
1890	43	44	60	62
1893-1897	44	47	61	63
1900-1902	46	49	63	64
1909-1911	49	53	62	65
1919-1920	54	57	65	66
1925-1931	59	63	66	69
1939-1941	63	68	67	71

Source: *Statistical History of the United States from Colonial Times to the Present* (Stamford, Conn.: Fairfield Publishers, 1965), Ser. B 76-91. Data for 1919-1931 are for white population only.

Appendix IX. Mortality from Certain Contagious Diseases in Massachusetts, 1865–1940. Number of deaths per 1000,000 population occurring in Massachusetts from smallpox, tuberculosis of the respiratory system, typhoid and paratyphoid, and diphtheria.

Year	Smallpox	Tuberculosis	Typhoid	Diphtheria
1865	17	368	134	93
1870	9	343	91	46
1875	2	347	64	114
1880	2	308	50	134
1885	1	307	40	78
1890	0	259	37	73
1895	0	223	27	71
1900	<1	190	22	53
1905	<1	164	18	52
1910	0	138	13	21
1915	<1	117	7	20
1920	<1	97	2	15
1925	0	71	2	8
1930	0	57	1	4
1935	0	43	<1	1
1940	0	35	<1	<1

Source: *Statistical History of the United States,* Ser. B 155-162. The accuracy of these data are of course subject to more than problems arising from failure to report, since diagnosis was based on changing criteria.

223

Appendix X. Reporting Certain Contagious Diseases in Massachusetts, 1916–1940. Number of cases of selected diseases designated as "dangerous to the public health," and therefore reported to the Massachusetts Department of Public Health; see Appendix VI, 3, n. 1.

Year	Population	Smallpox	Pulmonary tuberculosis	Typhoid and Paratyphoid	Diphtheria
1916	3,657,980	32	7878	1515	7282
1917	3,706,574	65	8365	1546	10,322
1918	3,802,132	27	7833	1067	6922
1919	3,835,615	40	6977	938	7929
1920	3,880,153	29	6696	935	7513
1921	3,935,743	37	6168	917	9100
1922	3,991,333	2	5562	693	8826
1923	4,046,923	6	5356	622	9018
1924	4,102,513	12	5376	566	7290
1925	4,158,103	3	5385	592	4482
1926	4,110,556	4	5444	547	3401
1927	4,191,638	2	5049	466	4750
1928	4,212,720	19	4873	310	4052
1929	4,233,802	273	4538	307	4255
1930	4,254,884	2	4696	318	3322
1931	4,275,566	6	4421	256	2381
1932	4,297,050	43	3994	225	1811
1933	4,318,130	0	3541	172	1041
1934	4,339,210	0	3585	140	629
1935	4,361,570	0	3592	117	390
1936	4,382,900	0	3208	142	307
1937	4,404,220	0	3534	382	175
1938	4,425,545	0	3220	147	159
1939	4,446,870	0	2959	111	197
1940	4,316,725	0	2816	191	144

Source: Records of the Massachusetts Department of Public Health, Division of Communicable Diseases. The population was extrapolated from Massachusetts State Census (1925, 1935) and the United States Census (1920, 1930).

Note on Sources

Before getting into a substantive discussion of the sources used for this study, I should like to explain my bibliographic organization. In some ways it would have been desirable to group the material topically, dealing in turn with social statistics, sanitary science, prevention of contagious disease, and the etiology and epidemiology of noncontagious disease, in order to demonstrate conceptual changes taking place between 1842 and 1936. I have rejected this arrangement in favor of a plan which indicates where the primary sources I consulted may be found. I made this choice because these collections invite extended examination by scholars working from diverse points of view. Social and urban historians, historians of medicine, and demographers, for example, will find in these same documents, journals, and manuscripts evidence of the discrete events too often covered only by the aphorisms associated with urbanization and industrialization.

My notes will, I hope, serve as a guide to new sources as well as define the limits of my research. Since the footnotes include complete reference to all the secondary works I have drawn upon, this essay is restricted to a discussion of those interpretations which have proved most helpful in my research, or of those which have not been specifically cited.

This essay reflects my belief that changing views of public health can be identified in three ways: through findings reported by individuals and institutions assuming responsibility for public health; through an understanding of the social and political milieu which made explicit scientific methods of preventing disease acceptable in a given period; and through a study of the roles of both advocate and recipient of these preventive and therapeutic measures.

The annual *Reports of the State Board of Health* are the foundation for any history of public health in Massachusetts over the past century. These *Reports,* issued regularly but under slightly varying titles since 1870, are available in the *Public Documents of Massachusetts* series, as well as in single copies. Complete runs of these records are readily available since they were sent to the members of the General Court and to city and town councils throughout the Commonwealth; they were also distributed freely to other states and to interested individuals in the United States and abroad.

Between January 1870 and July 1879 the state published eleven *Reports of the State Board of Health*. For the next seven years it was the obligation of the Board of Health, Lunacy, and Charity to protect the health of the citizens of the Commonwealth. The six annual *Reports* issued by this Board from January 1880 to July 1886 included a "Health Supplement" for each volume except the third, published in 1882. When the State Board of Health was re-established as a separate body in 1886, it resumed publication of the *Report of the State Board of Health* series, number eighteen appearing in 1887 and continuing through number forty-six in 1915. At the close of 1916, after reorganization of the administration of public health services, the first *Report of the State Department of Health* appeared; subsequent numbers were published annually until 1941, after 1920 as the *Report of the Department of Public Health*. Because of the exigencies of World War II, a *Consolidated Report* was issued for the years 1942-1949 and repeated for 1950-1956. Since then, there have been annual *Reports*.

The early volumes include studies of such questions as housing, alcoholism, and slaughtering as well as investigations of water supplies, crowding, and disease. Members of the academic and professional community around Boston contracted to conduct these investigations which yield the kind of material traditionally sought by the social historian. In addition, the more technical and statistical data which dominate the *Reports* after 1886 provide a rich resource to illuminate the social attitudes and political expression which accompanied new knowledge about the etiology of disease. Reports from local boards of health, from the departments and divisions which were created to assume new responsibilities, detailed accounts of specific epidemics, and proposals for new legislation — all support historical inquiry into the social and scientific assumptions which guided and reflected the elaboration of preventive techniques.

The annual reports of the other investigative and regulatory commissions and boards which flourished in Massachusetts are informative. I have consulted those published by the Massachusetts Board of State Charities for the years 1865-1879 and those of the Massachusetts Bureau of Statistics of Labor for 1870-1871. Single or serial reports of legislative committees have been indicated in the footnotes. Generally these reports can be found in the *Massachusetts House Documents* or the *Massachusetts Senate Documents* published regularly after 1826, or in the *Massachusetts Public Documents* series, published intermittently from 1846 to 1858 and annually thereafter. Occasionally, as in the case of the *Report of a Commission Appointed to Consider a General Drainage System for the Valleys of the Mystic, Blackstone, and Charles Rivers* (1886) or the *Report of the Special Commission to Study and Investigate Public Health Laws and Policies* (1936), an important study is not in the bound *Documents* series. These reports, usually of single extended investigations, can be found at the Massachusetts State Library. Another useful collection of single reports, especially those having to do with water policy from 1886 to 1914, is George Chandler Whipple, *State Sanitation: A Review of the Work of the Massachusetts State Board of Health*, Vol. II, (Cambridge, Mass.: Harvard University Press, 1917).

The *Report of the Sanitary Commission of Massachusetts* (1850) deserves special attention. Better known as *The Shattuck Report,* facsimile ed. (Cambridge, Mass.: Harvard University Press, 1948), this survey is frequently cited as the first comprehensive work on public health to be published in the United States. In addition to a compendium of Massachusetts health statutes from 1660 to 1849, and proposals for the future, *The Shattuck Report* includes an estimate of health conditions in English cities and on the continent and provides information about what were viewed as the major threats to health in an urbanizing society. Unfortunately the appendixes, which include detailed information on four Massachusetts towns, were not included in the facsimile edition; they provide additional insight into urban and rural life in antebellum Massachusetts.

The Shattuck Report received very brief but favorable notices upon publication. Only three, however, examined the report in depth. These included: E. H. Clarke, "Sanitary Reform," *North American Review,* 73:117-135 (July 1851); Edward Jarvis, "Review of the Report of the Massachusetts Sanitary Commission," *American Journal of Medical Sciences,* n. s., 21:391-409 (April 1851); and *Buffalo Medical Journal,* 6:596-610 (1850-1851).

For the three decades preceding the establishment of the State Board of Health, the most detailed information about health in Massachusetts is found in the annual *Report of the Secretary of the Commonwealth to the Legislature under the Act of March, 1842, Relating to the Registry of Births, Marriages and Deaths in Massachusetts.* This was first published in 1843 and regularly thereafter. Although these records are clearly incomplete until after a second revision of the law in May 1849 and therefore especially subject to misleading interpretation, the data provide useful information on the causes of "premature mortality" before 1869. After the establishment of the State Board of Health, the collection and publication of vital statistics remained the responsibility of the Secretary of the Commonwealth, appearing after 1917 as the annual *Report on the Vital Statistics of Massachusetts.* Since 1964 responsibility for gathering these records has been transferred to the Department of Public Health.

The inadequacy of *Registration Reports* before 1849 is in large part due to the failure of Boston's city clerks to submit records. Two important documents by Lemuel Shattuck supply much of the missing information: *The Vital Statistics of Boston: Containing an Abstract of the Bills of Mortality for the Last Twenty-Nine Years, and a General View of the Population and Health of the City at Other Periods of its History,* originally published in the *American Journal of the Medical Sciences,* n.s., 1:369-401 (1841), and reprinted by the Boston Registry Department in 1893 as *Bills of Mortality, 1810-1849, With an Essay on the Vital Statistics of Boston from 1810-1841;* and Shattuck's *Report to the Committee of the City Council Appointed to Obtain the Census of Boston for the Year 1845, Embracing Collateral Facts and Statistical Researches Illustrating the History and Condition of the Population and Their Means of Progress and Prosperity* (Boston, 1846).

The early *Registration Reports* include tables of "Diseases Nosologically Arranged" which give evidence of the movement to develop a more useful and standard system of disease classification in the years when state and professional regulation of medical practice was virtually nonexistent. Changes in naming and grouping diseases continued to be recorded over the next century. These tables suggest that the interesting conceptual and practical problems which accompanied the identification of disease by specific etiology rather than symptom can be followed in the *Registration Reports* as well as in the lists of dangerous diseases published by the Board of Health and articles in the medical journals.

In addition, the second and fourth *Registration Reports* (1843, 1845) include letters from Lemuel Shattuck urging methods to improve the collection of vital statistics. The seventh *Report* (1848) carried a statement by the Secretary of the Commonwealth that there was no need for special interpretation of the collected statistics "because the design appears very distinctly on the face of them, and their importance cannot be heightened by any analysis." However, with the eighth *Report* (1851) which covered a twenty-month period, there appeared extended "Analytical Observations" by a prominent physician, Dr. Josiah Curtis. This practice continued until 1916 when the responsibility for analysis was assumed by a statistician. The physicians who were appointed to the task, especially in the early years, were among the most ardent advocates of public health measures, and their comments indicate the nature of medical support for state control of sanitary measures.

A useful guide to Massachusetts state papers is Adelaide R. Hasse, *Index of Economic Material in Documents of the States of the United States: Massachusetts, 1789-1904* (Baltimore: Carnegie Institution of Washington, Lord Baltimore Press, 1908). As indicated in the introduction, the term "economic" is broadly interpreted, and the alphabetically arranged headings include information on health and related topics. Within each category the citations are listed chronologically and divided into serial and nonserial publications, with an indication of where the obscure items may be found. Under the heading "public health" there is a useful listing of *Manuals* issued by the State Board at irregular intervals for the local boards, which include the statutes in force at the time of publication. The *Massachusetts Inventory of Published Statistical Series* (Boston: Commonwealth of Mass., Office of Planning and Program Coordination, 1970), was published after I completed my work. These listings do not include all the data available, especially for the earliest periods. When used as a guide, however, this *Inventory* should greatly facilitate future work.

In contrast to the wealth of material available in the Massachusetts *Documents,* it is difficult to find satisfactory reporting of legislative debate. The *Journal of the House of Representatives of the Commonwealth of Massachusetts* was published after 1864, and the *Journal of the Senate* after 1868, but they are abbreviated and disappointing. Manuscript "Journals" are available at the Massachusetts State Library for the earlier period covered in this study. Boston newspapers are a better source of information on the sessions of the General Court, and I have consulted the *Daily* and *Semi-Weekly Advertiser* for the years 1842-1869, the *Herald* from 1851-1900, the *Globe* after 1872, and the *Evening Transcript* between 1869-1899. The formal statutes appeared in the *Acts and Resolves,* published in one volume from 1839-1915, and separately thereafter.

Manuscript minutes of the State Board of Health meetings from its inception are located in the Commissioner's office of the Massachusetts Department of Public Health, but my research did not show that they differed in any substantial way from the published *Reports.* Few health boards were established outside Boston until late in the nineteenth century, and even these did not publish an elaborate annual report. The notes from the towns and cities which are found in the annual *Reports of the State Board of Health* indicate that the minutes of the existing boards of health or records of the selectmen meeting to consider matters of public health might clarify the complex relationship between local and state authorities and the role of the medical profession in establishing public health standards. I did examine the manuscript minutes for the Worcester Board of Health for the years 1885-1900; they showed that this local group was more responsive to public and professional requests for diagnostic and therapeutic services than would otherwise have been suspected.

Manuscript material relating to the Southern Berkshire Health District for 1932-1939, provided by Dr. Harold Stevens, and the files of correspondence which I received permission to consult at the Commonwealth Fund indicate the need for additional research on the relationship between private foundations and state public health service in the twentieth century.

In addition to its *Annual Report,* numerous broadsides, and special pamphlets, the Massachusetts State Board of Health published a *Weekly Bulletin* from 1883-1905, listing outbreaks of disease. From January 1906-July 1914 this was superseded by a *Monthly Bulletin* which included articles and reports primarily directed to local boards of health and health officers. In August 1914 the name was changed to the *Public Health Bulletin,* with articles of more general interest and professional reports reflecting the reorganization of public health services in the state. The slogan, "The Commonhealth of the Commonwealth," taken from Governor David I. Walsh's address to a convention of the Association of Massachusetts Boards of Health appeared on the masthead in May 1915, and in July 1918 the name of the publication was changed to the *Commonhealth.* The *Commonhealth* became a bimonthly in 1919 and a quarterly in 1923. For the years 1918-1936 in particular, this journal is an invaluable source of information about the proliferation of public health programs and the rapid inclusion of paramedical personnel in the professional status previously accorded to physicians and sanitary engineers.

There is a wide range of professional journals for the entire period of my work. The position of the medical profession can be followed in part through the *Medical Communications of the Massachusetts Medical Society,* published annually from 1790 to 1914. These volumes include the annual address to the Massachusetts Medical Society as well as numerous articles concerning medical theory and practice. There is a useful *Index of Medical Communications,* *Library of Practical Medicine and Publications of the Massachusetts Medical*

Society, 1790-1901 (Boston: David Clapp and Son, 1903). After 1914, the *Boston Medical and Surgical Journal* became the official voice of the Massachusetts Medical Society.

The *Boston Medical and Surgical Journal,* first published in 1828, has the longest run of any weekly medical publication in the United States. For the years covered by this study it was possibly the most influential medical journal in the East, attracting many contributions and subscribers from outside Massachusetts. After 1914 it became the *New England Medical Journal.* Joseph Garland, first editor of the reorganized publication wrote a comprehensive history of this weekly, "The Boston Medical and Surgical Journal, 1828-1928," *NEJM,* 198:1-13 (Feb. 23, 1928).

Other journals, some rather short lived, were consulted on specific issues or for a limited time; the *American Journal of Medical Sciences* (Philadelphia), a quarterly journal of wide influence first published in 1827, was especially useful for the years before the Civil War, as was the *Journal of Medical Inquiry* (Philadelphia). The *American Medical Times,* a weekly series edited by Drs. Stephen Smith and Elisha Harris from 1860 to 1864, reflected the concerns of New York physicians who led the public health movement later.

On the national level interest in public health is recorded in the *Proceedings of the National Medical Conventions* (Philadelphia, 1847), held in New York in May 1846 and in Philadelphia in May 1847. Following these meetings the *Transactions of the American Medical Association* commenced publication.

Massachusetts made a significant contribution to the publication of public health periodicals with the *Journal of the Massachusetts Association of Boards of Health,* a quarterly which appeared first in January 1891, eight months after the organization of the Association. The Association, a relatively informal group, consisted of public health workers, members of the better-organized local boards of health, and Dr. Charles V. Chapin of the Providence, Rhode Island, Board of Health. The name of the publication was changed to the *American Journal of Public Hygiene and the Journal of the Massachusetts Boards of Health* and continued to publish a second series under this formidable title for three years beginning in November 1904. In November 1907 a third series began under the shortened title *American Journal of Public Hygiene,* but the publication remained the official organ of the Massachusetts Association as well as speaking for the Laboratory Section of the American Public Health Association. In November 1908 this journal became the publication of the American Public Health Association and was distributed nationally. Two years later, when the APHA decided to finance a new journal, the *American Journal of Public Hygiene* came to an abrupt halt, and the monthly *Journal of the American Public Health Association* appeared in 1911. The next year the name was changed to the *American Journal of Public Health,* which continued until 1928, when Volume 18 appeared with a new format and name, the *American Journal of Public Health and the Nation's Health.*

Another source for reconstructing the past of serial publications is *Public*

Health: Reports and Papers of the American Public Health Association, published annually from 1875-1908 and containing the major addresses delivered at national meetings from 1873 to 1907. Volumes 30-33 of this series appear in two parts. Part 2 of the years 1905-1907 is a supplement to the *Journal of Infectious Diseases,* published for the Laboratory Section of the APHA; the entire volume for 1905 is taken up by the "Report of the Committee on Standard Methods of Water Analysis . . . " The final volume (1908) is a republication of the November 1907 issue of the new *American Journal of Public Hygiene,* mentioned above.

This account should facilitate study of the diversity in public health publication activity on a state and national level. I would also be pleased if this information saves others from searching, as I did, for the *Papers and Reports of the American Public Health Association* for the years 1908-1912; apparently they were not published, although they are listed in the *Union List of Serials* and other reliable guides.

A number of other journals were consulted for information on attitudes toward social welfare and public health from the end of the nineteenth century through the first four decades of the twentieth century: *Publications of the American Statistical Association,* first published in 1888, appeared as *Quarterly Publications of the American Statistical Association* after 1920; *Social Hygiene,* first published in 1914, appeared as the *Journal of Social Hygiene* after 1921; *Charities,* 1897-1901, and *Charities and Commons,* 1905-1909; *Survey,* 1897-1932, and *Survey Graphic* after 1933. The *Milbank Memorial Fund Quarterly,* first published in 1923, and the various publications of the Commonwealth Fund after 1918 are a largely untapped source of detailed information, especially on local health services and programs directed to special problems.

References to reports resulting from special investigations or congresses are indicated in the footnotes, but there are three instances where these reports particularly suggest the need for further study. The antebellum *Proceedings* of the National Quarantine and Sanitary Conventions have been briefly described by Harold M. Cavins, "The National Quarantine and Sanitary Conventions of 1857 to 1860 and the Beginnings of the American Public Health Association," *BHM,* 13:404-426 (April 1943). However, the verbatim reports of these meetings require much more detailed examination since the protagonists represent the two major facets of contemporary thought about the etiology of disease. In addition, because all major cities in the United States were represented at these meetings, the reports constitute a source for mid-nineteenth-century urban history.

The *Transactions* of the 15th International Congress of Hygiene and Demography which took place in Washington, D.C., in 1912 contain a number of significant papers by Massachusetts public health leaders. The first congress took place in Brussels in 1852, and subsequent meetings were called irregularly. American participation began in 1891, when Dr. Samuel W. Abbott of the Massachusetts State Board of Health was among the delegates discussing the epidemiology of diphtheria. Study of American participation in succeeding meetings (1894, 1898, 1903) would be of interest.

And finally, the report of the President's Research Committee on Social Trends, *Recent Social Trends,* 2 vols. (New York: McGraw-Hill, 1933), contains a range of papers on public health and related issues. Henry F. May, "Shifting Perspectives on the 1920's," *Mississippi Valley Historical Review,* 43:405-427 (Dec. 1956), indicates the importance of these studies which were first commissioned by President Hoover in 1929. The social historian will find in these two volumes both data and declarations of intent to enrich his understanding of the complex events taking place in the years between the two world wars.

The surviving manuscript collections of individuals who played key roles in the Massachusetts public health movement tend to vary sharply in quality and quantity. I was unable to consult the private papers of Theobold Smith for the years he was associated with the Board of Health because I was not given access to the collection. A fascinating study of Smith's years at the Bureau of Animal Industry was brought to my attention after this manuscript was completed. Claude E. Dolman, "Texas Cattle Fever: A Commemorative Tribute to Theobald Smith," *Clio Medica* (London), 4:1-31 (1969), corroborates my impression of Smith's professional stature and personal style in an article that can serve as a model for historians of medicine. William T. Sedgwick apparently left no personal papers of any kind, but his published papers facilitate an appreciation of his broad influence. A laudatory biography, *A Pioneer in Public Health: William Thompson Sedgwick* (New Haven, Conn.: Yale University Press, 1924), written by three of his students, E. O. Jordan, G. C. Whipple, and C.-E. A. Winslow, is an aid in following his early training and his rejection of a medical career. Letters or unpublished papers of individuals such as Walcott or Bigelow were studied through the courtesy of their families.

The Lemuel Shattuck Papers at the Massachusetts Historical Society include correspondence and journals of great interest, not only for this study, but also as an indication of Shattuck's extensive correspondence abroad with such men as Chadwick, Farr, and Quetelet.

The letterbooks, journals, and casebooks of Henry I. Bowditch are at the Francis A. Countway Library of Medicine (Boston), as are three letterbooks of Edward Jarvis. Much of the Bowditch material was published by his son, Vincent Y. Bowditch, *Life and Correspondence of Henry Ingersoll Bowditch,* 2 vols., (Cambridge, Mass.: Harvard University Press, 1902).

The manuscript "Autobiography," of Edward Jarvis, located at Harvard's Houghton Library, deserves attention by students of social statistics. It contains a wealth of information about Jarvis' frustrated endeavors in various careers, and, among other assets, it is entirely legible since it was dictated to a professional secretary.

There is no comprehensive collection of papers and letters left by Henry P. Walcott. The letters gathered at the Clendening Medical Library in Kansas City, Kansas, are, for the most part, formal acknowledgments of invitations which reveal little about Walcott although they do suggest a good deal about the kind of sociability enjoyed by a Cambridge widower at the turn of the century. The occasional letters found at the Harvard University Archives are more interesting. This is particularly true of the letters included in the Charles William Eliot Correspondence Books. The Countway Library also has a few Walcott letters.

Harvard University Archives has files of manuscript material mixed with newspaper clippings, published papers, and other memorablia for George Derby, Theobald Smith, and George H. Bigelow, and the Countway Library has an interesting scrapbook from a dinner held in Smith's honor in 1914.

The Charles V. Chapin Papers at the Rhode Island Historical Society have already been carefully examined by James H. Cassedy for his book *Charles V. Chapin and the Public Health Movement* (Cambridge, Mass.: Harvard University Press, 1962). However, I turned to the Chapin Papers because I found no record of his early evaluation of the Massachusetts State Board of Health. The typescript carbon of Chapin's 1911 letter to Governor Foss proved helpful.

Two other collections were consulted for supporting material. The David I. Walsh Papers, including his correspondence and the typescript copies of all his public addresses, are located at the Dinand Library of the College of the Holy Cross in Worcester, Massachusetts. Walsh's papers have received little attention; a worthwhile exception is John H. Flannagan, Jr., "The Disillusionment of a Progressive: U.S. Senator David I. Walsh and the League of Nation's Issue, 1918-1920," *New England Quarterly,* 41:483-504 (Dec. 1968). William J. Grattan's thorough and sympathetic treatment of Walsh's early life and political career, "David I. Walsh and His Associates: A Study in Political Theory," (unpub. diss., Harvard University, 1957), lays the groundwork for extending Richard M. Abrams' provocative interpretation, *Massachusetts Politics 1900-1912: Conservatism in a Progressive Era* (Cambridge, Mass.: Harvard University Press, 1964), further into the twentieth century. Walsh is but one of the new breed of politicians emerging in this period to substantially change the relationship between political activism and social reform.

Similarly, the Alexander Lincoln Papers at the Schlesinger Library, Radcliffe College, Cambridge, Massachusetts, indicate a shift in the ideology and role of groups and individuals who had traditionally advocated public support for social welfare measures. The Lincoln Papers are a source of information on one focus of resistance to new federal welfare commitment in the 1920's, and they provided most of the evidence to guide my search for a rationale behind Massachusetts opposition to the Sheppard-Towner Act.

The remainder of this essay indicates some of the published books and articles which supported my research. I have not separated primary from secondary material in any rigid way since such an organizaton would infer an arbitrary distinction I have sought to avoid in the study itself.

Physicians and laymen contrasting sanitary problems of the past with contemporary conditions have both criticized outmoded practice and provided insights about their own assumptions. Measures for the promotion of public health depend at least in part upon theories of the etiology and transmission of disease. Among the early medical books and papers I consulted were: Elisha Bartlett's address to the American Physiological Society in Boston, January 30, 1838, "Obedience to the Laws of Health, a Moral Duty" (Boston, 1838), and *The History, Diagnosis and Treatment of the Fevers of the United States* (Philadelphia, 1847). Alfred Stillé, *Elements of General Pathology: A Practical Treatise of the Causes, Forms, Symptoms, and Results of Disease* (Philadelphia, 1848); Jacob Bigelow, *Nature in Disease* (Boston, 1854); Bigelow's 1835 address to the Massachusetts Medical Society, "On Self-limited Diseases," *Medical Communications of the Massachusetts Medical Society*, 5:319-358 (1830-1836); and Morrill Wyman's 1863 address, "The Reality and Certainty of Medicine," *Medical Communications of the Massachusetts Medical Society*, 10:215-255 (1861-1866). The use of "pathology" in Stillé's text is interesting at a time when "physiology" was the more common expression in this context. This volume, like the others mentioned here, went through several editions, but for obvious reasons I have indicated the earliest date of publication.

Because Henry I. Bowditch played such a critical role in the first decade of the State Board of Health, his studies were particularly important; see *Consumption in New England: Or Locality One of Its Chief Causes* (Boston, 1862); *Is Consumption Ever Contagious or Communicated From One Person to Another in Any Manner?* (Boston, 1864); and "Topographical Distribution and Local Origins of Consumption in Massachusetts," *Medical Communications of the Massachusetts Medical Society*, 10:59-138 (1861-1866). More than a decade later Bowditch delivered an evaluation of obstacles to improved public health in his address as the chairman of the State Medicine and Public Hygiene section of the American Medical Association; see *Transactions of the American Medical Association*, 26:301-317 (1875), and *Public Hygiene in America* (Boston, 1877), which is an expanded version of an address to the 1876 International Medical Congress meeting in Philadelphia on the centennial of the American Revolution. Albert H. Buck, ed., *A Treatise on Hygiene and Public Health*, 2 vols. (New York, 1879), includes articles on all aspects of individual and public hygiene by Bowditch's contemporaries, including some of his colleagues in Massachusetts.

Phyllis Allen, (Richmond), "Etiological Theory in America Prior to the Civil War," "Some Variant Theories in Opposition to the Germ Theory of Disease," *JHMAS*, 2:489-520 (August 1947), and 9:290-303 (July 1954), and "Early American Animalicular Hypotheses," *BHM*, 24:734-743 (Sept.-Oct. 1947), are scholarly considerations of American ideas about disease. Erwin H. Ackerknecht, "Anticontagionism Between 1821-1867," *BHM*, 22:562-593 (Sept.-Oct. 1948), is a comprehensive treatment of European anticontagionism including theories about the transmission of the major diseases with which Americans were concerned during this period. Ackerknecht's article, "Elisha Bartlett and the Philosophy of the Paris School," *BHM*, 24:43-60 (Jan.-Feb. 1960), describes the influence of French medicine and Louis in particular on the generation of American students preceding Bowditch. I found George H. Daniels, "Finalism and Positivism in Nineteenth-Century American Physiological Thought," *BHM*, 38:343-363 (July-Aug. 1964), enlightening although he is concerned with intellectual problems that were virtually ignored by the men I studied.

The physician's own view of his responsibility and competence to prevent disease and promote health is recorded in part through his attitude toward the role of his profession and its organizations. Some of this can be found in papers published in the *Medical Communications of the Massachusetts Medical Society*, such as Josiah Bartlett, "A Dissertation on the Progress of Medical Science in the Commonwealth of Massachusetts," 2:235-270 (1813); Zadok Howe, "On Quackery," 5:295-318 (1830-1836); and John R. Bronson, "A Review of Medicine: Its Worth and Work," 12:101-136 (1881).

Public statements of physicians associated with state health work throughout the period are of particular interest. See, for instance, a speech by Henry I. Bowditch to the graduating class of the Harvard Medical School, *An Apology for the Medical Profession as a Means for Developing the Whole Nature of Man* (Boston, 1863), and an address to the Rhode Island Medical Society two decades later, *Past, Present and Future Treatment of Homeopathy, Eclecticism and Kindred Delusions* (Boston, 1887). Henry P. Walcott was less given to making general statements on the position of medicine in society, but his speech to a graduating class of the Yale Medical School, *The Physician, the College, and the Commonwealth* (New Haven, Conn., 1893), is a noteworthy exception. In the twentieth century public health measures tended to evoke heated arguments on the relationship between medical practice and public policy, with implications beyond the specific program at issue. Among the articles consulted were George H. Bigelow, "Is the State's Cancer Program State Medicine?" *NEJM*, 200:438-439 (Feb. 28, 1929), and "Relation of Clinics and Health Associations to the Medical Profession," *NEJM*, 202:949-951 (May 15, 1930); G. W. Haigh, "In Defense of State Medicine," *NEJM*, 202:1078-1083 (May 29, 1930); Walter Dameshek, "Some Arguments Against State Medicine," *NEJM*, 204:1187-1193 (June 4, 1931). More recently, Alfred L. Frechette, "The Massachusetts Medical Society and the Organization of Public Health Services — Retrospect and Prospect," *NEJM* 265:153-159 (July 27, 1961), and Roy L. Cleere and others, "Physicians' Attitudes Toward Venereal Disease Reporting," *JAMA*, 202:941-946 (Dec. 4, 1967) indicate some concerns of physicians currently directing the work of the Massachusetts Department of Public Health.

For a more general introduction into the history of medical practice in Massachusetts, Henry R. Viets, *A Brief History of Medicine in Massachusetts* (Boston: Houghton, Mifflin, 1930), and Walter L. Burrage, *A History of the Massachusetts Medical Society, With Brief Biographies of the Founders and Chief Officers, 1791-1922* (Norwood, Mass.: privately published, Plimpton Press, 1923), are helpful. John B. Blake, "The Medical Profession and Public Health in Boston," *BHM*, 26:218-230 (May-June 1952), "The Origins of Public Health in the United States," *AJPH*, 38:1534-1550 (Nov. 1948), and *Public Health in the Town of Boston 1630-1822* (Cambridge, Mass.: Harvard University Press, 1959), are more scholarly and interpretative, and of far greater interest to the general reader and the historian with a special interest in the development of public health.

Blake's many publications on the history of medicine and public health, like those of Richard H. Shryock and George Rosen, helped shape my study in countless ways, and selection of the most significant of their contributions is virtually impossible. See, especially, Shryock, *The Development of Modern Medicine: An Interpretation of the Social and Scientific Factors Involved*, rev. ed. (New York: Alfred A. Knopf, 1957), *Medicine and Society in America, 1660-1860* (New York: New York University Press, 1960), and *The National Tuberculosis Association 1904-1954: A Study of the Voluntary Health Movement in the United States* (New York: National Tuberculosis Association, 1957). Among Shryock's articles, see "The Interplay of Social and Internal Factors in the History of Modern Medicine," *Scientific Monthly*, 76:221-230 (April 1952), "Public Relations of the Medical Profession in Great Britain and the United States, 1600-1870," *Annals of Medical History*, n.s., 2:308-339 (May 1930), and "The Origins and Significance of the Public Health Movement in the United States," *Annals of Medical History*, n.s., 1:644-665 (Nov. 1929).

George Rosen's *A History of Public Health* (New York: M. D. Publications, 1958), covers more ground with less possibility for interpretation than the work cited above, but his many articles develop specific themes along dimensions that few other scholars have attempted. See, for instance, "Approaches to a Concept of Social Medicine: An Historical Survey," *MMFQ*, 26:7-21 (Jan. 1948), "Economic and Social Policy in the Development of Public Health," *JHMAS*, 8:406-430 (Oct. 1953), and "Public Health Problems in New York City During the Nineteenth Century," *New York State Journal of Medicine*, 50:73-78 (Jan. 1, 1950).

Very much in the same league is Charles E. Rosenberg's *The Cholera Years: The United States in 1832, 1849 and 1866* (Chicago: Chicago University Press, 1962), an enlightening treatment of ideas about the etiology of disease and preventive measures focusing primarily on New York City. His article, with Carroll S. Rosenberg, "Pietism and the Origins of the American Public Health Movement: A Note on John H. Griscom and Robert H. Hartley," *JHMAS*, 23:16-35 (Jan. 1968), provides information about two contemporaries of Shattuck, an interesting contrast to the first major figure in this study.

Frances R. Packard, *History of Medicine in the United States* (New York: Paul B. Hoeber, 1931) and William Norwood, *Medical Education in the United States Before the Civil War* (Philadelphia: University of Pennsylvania Press, 1944), are more parochial studies. Henry B. Shafer, *The American Medical Profession, 1783-1850* (New York: Columbia University Press, 1936) is far less useful than Joseph F. Kett, *The Formation of the American Medical Profession, 1780-1860* (New Haven, Conn.: Yale University Press, 1968). Howard D. Kramer has written a series of articles on the early public health movement: "Effect of the Civil War on the Public Health Movement," *Mississippi Valley Historical Review*, 35:449-462 (Dec. 1948); "The Germ Theory of Disease and the Early Public Health Program in the United States," *BHM,* 22:233-247 (May-June 1948); "The Beginnings of the Public Health Movement in the United States," *BHM,* 21:352-376 (May-June 1947); "Agitation for Public Health Reform in the 1870's," *JHMAS,* 3:473-488 (Autumn 1948); "The National Board of Health," *JHMAS,* 4:75-79 (Winter 1949); "Early Municipal and State Boards of Health," *BHM,* 24:503-529 (Nov.-Dec. 1950).

Unfortunately there is no comprehensive study of American medicine since the Civil War, but James G. Burrow, *AMA: Voice of American Medicine* (Baltimore: Johns Hopkins Press, 1963), covers some aspects of professional growth and organization. Charles Rosenberg, "The American Medical Profession: Mid-Nineteenth Century," *Mid-America,* 44:163-171 (July 1962), describes the background for later developments. Two articles by George H. Daniels on the professionalization of science and its social role served to focus my consideration of late nineteenth- and early twentieth-century medicine and public health; see "The Process of Professionalization in American Science: The Emergent Period 1820-1860," *Isis,* 58:151-166 (Summer 1966), and "The Pure Science Ideal and Democratic Culture," *Science,* 156:1699-1705 (June 30, 1967). William P. Shepard, "The Professionalization of Public Health," *AJPH,* 38:145-153 (Jan. 1948), indicates the changes in function and organization which emerged with new criteria of proficiency. Far more suggestive are descriptions of curriculum and listings of instructors in the Harvard-Massachusetts Institute of Technology *Circular of the School for Health Officers* (Boston, 1913) and the *Catalogue* of the joint School of Public Health (1914-1921), as well as the early publications of the Harvard School of Public Health organized in 1922. See also George C. Whipple, "The School for Health Officers," *Harvard Alumni Bulletin* 19:188-190 (Nov. 1916); Jean A. Curran, "The First School of Public Health," *Harvard Public Health Alumni Bulletin,* 23:2-5, 20 (Jan. 1966), and *Founders of the Harvard School of Public Health, With Biographical Notes, 1909-1946* (New York: Josiah Macy, Jr., Foundation, n.p., 1970). Although Roy Lubove, *The Professional Altruist: The Emergence of Social Work as a Career* (Cambridge, Mass.: Harvard University Press, 1965), tends to emphasize the social control implicit in social reform, I found this study useful.

Professional identity of the physician specializing in public health work was in part responsible for new literature about the nature of disease and the history of preventive measures, written by men who were themselves leaders in the field. Outstanding among these were Charles V. Chapin, *Sources and Modes of Infection* (New York: John Wiley, 1912), and "The Evolution of Preventive Medicine," *JAMA,* 76:215-216 (Jan. 1921); Theobald Smith, *Parasitism and Disease* Princeton, N.J.: Princeton University Press, 1934); Charles-Edward Amory Winslow, *The Conquest of Epidemic Disease: A Chapter in the History of Ideas* (Princeton, N.J.: Princeton University Press, 1944). Wilson G. Smillie wrote a number of highly optimistic volumes which provide information placed in a rather narrow perspective; see *Public Health: Its Promise for the Future: A Chronicle of the Development of Public Health in the United States, 1607-1914*

(New York: Macmillan, 1955). Ralph C. Williams, *The United States Public Health Service,* 1798-1950 (Washington, D.C.: Government Printing Office, 1951), is straightforward and useful. I found *Preventive Medicine and Hygiene* (New York: D. Appleton, 1913) a popular textbook by Milton J. Rosenau, Professor of Hygiene at Harvard Medical School and director of the state's Vaccine and Antitoxin Laboratory, an aid in understanding both the aspirations and recommendations of early twentiety-century public health practice.

Considering how rich the resources, it is surprising how little has been written on the history of state public health organization. Philip D. Jordan, *The People's Health: A History of Public Health in Minnesota to 1948* (St. Paul: Minnesota Historical Society, 1953), is a noteworthy exception. More recently, with the support of the Louisiana Department of Public Health, the first of a two-volume history of that state's pioneering institution has appeared; see Gordon E. Gillson, *The Louisiana State Board of Health: The Formative Years* (Baton Rouge: n.p., 1966). Dr. Ben Freedman, of the Department of Public Health in Louisiana celebrates the founding of the first state public health organization in "The Louisiana State Board of Health, Established 1855," *AJPH*, 41:1279-1285 (Oct. 1951). There are a number of monographs providing useful comparative information about different state organizations; see, for instance, Susan Wade Peabody, "Historical Study of Legislation Regarding Public Health in the States of New York and Massachusetts," *Journal of Infectious Diseases,* suppl. 4 (1909); James Wallace, *The State Health Departments of Massachusetts, Michigan and Illinois, With a Summary of Activities and Accomplishments, 1927-1928* (New York: Commonwealth Fund, 1930). In addition almost every state health department has published a volume describing its achievements on the occasion of an appropriate anniversary; most of these include a brief, laudatory history.

Men and women associated with the Massachusetts Department of Public Health have provided brief historical surveys concentrating on outstanding events and personalities; see Eleanor J. MacDonald, "A History of the Massachusetts Department of Public Health," *Commonhealth,* 23:83-124 (April-May-June 1936); Merrill E. Champion, "Seventy-five Years of Public Health in Massachusetts," *NEJM,* 232:241-247 (March 1, 1945). A special anniversary issue of *Commonhealth* (1947), "Seventy-fifth Anniversary of the Massachusetts Department of Public Health, 1869-1944," by Mary Carr Baker and Raymond S. Patterson, describes the highlights of state action focusing on five critical periods beginning with Lemuel Shattuck. A number of Departmental histories prepared to aid this last study are available in the files of the division of Health Education; manuscripts from the Institute of Laboratories and the Rutland Tuberculosis Sanatorium are of unusual interest. *State Sanitation: A Review of the Work of the Massachusetts State Board of Health,* 2 vols. (Cambridge, Mass.: Harvard University Press, 1917), by George C. Whipple, Professor of Sanitary Engineering at MIT and Harvard is a useful traditional institutional history with emphasis on control of water-borne diseases.

Municipal health departments have received even less attention, although an occasional biography such as Cassedy's study of Chapin, cited before, are very informative. Colonial urban health has fared best, largely because of John B. Blake's history of public health in Boston to 1820, mentioned above, and John Duffy, *Epidemics in Colonial America* (Baton Rouge: Louisiana State University Press, 1953). More recently the first of two volumes by John Duffy on New York City has appeared; *A History of Public Health in New York City, 1625-1866* (New York: Russell Sage Foundation, 1968). Histories of nineteenth-century urban development on the whole have neglected the area of health; see, for instance, the otherwise excellent history of an important Massachusetts industrial community, Donald B. Cole, *Immigrant City: Lawrence, Massachusetts 1845-1921* (Chapel Hill: University of North Carolina Press, 1963). There is no published work to continue Blake's history; Dorothy Therese Scanlon, "The Public Health Movement in Boston, 1870-1910," (unpub. diss., Boston University Graduate School, 1956) serves as an introduction to some of the sources for the more recent period. For a title that is more informative than the article itself, see the transcript of a speech delivered by Boston's Health Commissioner to the City Federation of Women's Clubs: Stephan L. Maloney, "The Evolution of the Present Boston Health Department; Its Early Development and Association with Boston's Historical Characters, and the Organization, Activities, Budgets and Functions of the Health Department as it is Today, 1620-1923."

Mazyck P. Ravenel, ed., *A Half Century of Public Health* (New York: American Public Health Association, 1921), describes the breadth of public health concern after fifty years and includes an interesting introductory article by Dr. Stephen Smith, one of the founding members of the American Public Health Association. C.-E. A. Winslow, "A Half Century of the Massachusetts Public Health Association," *AJPH*, 30:325-335 (April 1940), and Frances Denny, Roy F. Feemster, and Samuel C. Prescott, *Fifty Years of Public Health in Massachusetts: A Brief History of the Massachusetts Association of Boards of Health, 1890-1936, and Its Successor the Massachusetts Public Health Association, 1936-1940*, (n.p.:n.d.), are less impressive despite the extraordinary history of this group.

Among the vast number of books and articles published in the first decades of the twentieth century which evaluated past efforts and exhorted vigilance and expanded activity in the future, the following are especially informative: Samuel W. Abbott, "The Past and Present Condition of Public Hygiene and State Medicine in the United States," in Herbert B. Adams, ed., *Monographs in American Social Economics*, XIX (1900); Lee K. Frankel, "Science and Public Health," *AJPH*, 5:281-289 (April 1915): Charles W. Eliot, "The Main Points of Attack in the Campaign for Public Health," *AJPH*, 5:619-625 (July 1915); William T. Sedgwick, "American Achievements and Failures in Public Health Work," *AJPH*, 5:1103-1108 (Nov. 1915); Charles V. Chapin, *A Report on State Public Health Work Based on a Survey of State Boards of Health* (Chicago: American Medical Association, 1915); Alice Hamilton and Gertrude Seymour, "The New Public Health," *Survey*, 37:166-169 (Nov. 18, 1916), 37:356-359 (Jan. 20, 1917), 38:59-62 (April 21, 1917); Ellen H. Richards, *Sanitation in Daily Life*

(Boston: Whitcomb and Barrows, 1917); E. O. Jordan, "The Relations of Bacteriology to the Public Health Movement Since 1872," *AJPH,* 11:1042-1047 (Dec. 1921); Edward G. Huber, "The Control of Communicable Diseases Prevalent in Massachusetts With a Study of the Mortality Due to Them in the Past Seventy-five Years," *BMSJ,* nineteen installments from July 8, 1926-Nov. 11, 1926.

In conclusion it is appropriate to list briefly a few of the books and articles which have been consulted for direction and information on specific aspects of sanitary reform and serve as ballast for publications cited elsewhere in this essay. James H. Cassedy, "The Registration Area and American Vital Statistics: Development of a Health Research Resource, 1885-1915," *BHM,* 39:221-232 (May-June 1965), is conceptually a prelude to his book *Demography in Early America: Beginnings of the Statistical Mind, 1600-1800* (Cambridge, Mass.: Harvard University Press, 1969). The volume brings together material that was not readily available before and provides an interpretive framework. What remains to be done is likely to be even more rewarding — a full-scale study of ideas about the use and meaning of vital statistics in the first three-quarters of the nineteenth century. Massachusetts data have provided the material for a number of excellent articles; see John B. Blake, "The Early History of Vital Statistics in Massachusetts," *BHM,* 29:46-98 (Jan.-Feb. 1955); Robert Gutman, "The Birth Statistics of Massachusetts during the Nineteenth Century," *Population Studies,* 10:69-94 (July 1956), and "Birth and Death Registration in Massachusetts: I, The Colonial Background, 1639-1800," *MMFQ,* 36:57-74 (Jan. 1958), "II. The Inauguration of a Modern System, 1800-1849," 36:373-402 (Oct. 1958), "III, The System Achieves a Form, 1849-1869," 37:297-326 (July 1959). Although other states collected far less substantial data than Massachusetts until much later in the century, a number of different approaches to "the statistical mind" and its accomplishments should provide the basis for illuminating comparative studies of the nineteenth century. Dr. Cassedy's final chapter, as well as some of the recent demographic studies from seventeenth- and eighteenth-century France, England, and colonial America suggest a new approach to studies of health and disease in the formative period of state public health organizations. For two stimulating papers to whet the appetite, see Thomas McKeown and R. G. Brown, "Medical Evidence Related to English Population Changes in the Eighteenth Century," *Population Studies,* 9:119-141 (Nov. 1955); and George Rosen, "Problems in the Application of Statistical Analysis to Questions of Health: 1700-1880," *BHM,* 28:27-45 (Jan.-Feb. 1955). For a suggestion that the study of vital statistics in twentieth-century public health would raise old questions in a new light, see George H. Bigelow and Angelina Hamblen, "Changing Causes of Death," *NEJM,* 202:215-217 (Jan. 30, 1930); Bigelow, "What are Death Rates in Massachusetts Doing?" *NEJM,* 208:1313-1316 (June 22, 1933); Greer Williams, "Needed: A New Strategy for Health Promotion," *NEJM,* 279:1031-1035 (Nov. 7, 1968).

Part of the background for the most widely acknowledged health issue of today is presented in Nelson M. Blake, *Water for the Cities: A History of the Urban Water Supply Problem in the United States* (Syracuse, N.Y.: Syracuse University Press, 1956). Recognition of need did not dissolve the paradox of conflicting solutions 170 years ago any more than it does today; see Lemuel Shattuck, *Letter . . . in Answer to Interrogatories of J. Preston, in Relation to the Introduction of Water into the City of Boston* (Boston, 1845). John B. Blake, "Lemuel Shattuck and the Boston Water Supply," *BHM*, 29:554-562 (Nov.-Dec. 1955), uses this opportunity to take a much-needed second look at Shattuck himself and places the father of Massachusetts sanitary reform in reasonable perspective. C. F. Chandler, "Water Supply of Cities: Report Upon the Sanitary Chemistry of Waters, and Suggestions with Regard to the Selection of the Water Supply of Towns and Cities," *Public Health: Reports and Papers of the American Public Health Association*, 1:533-563 (1875), and John S. Billings, "Sewage Disposal in Cities," *Harper's New Monthly*, 71:577-584 (Sept. 1885), are representative of technical knowledge in the years just prior to the establishment of filtration systems for public water supplies. And Duane D. Baumann, *The Recreational Use of Domestic Water Supply Reservoirs: Perception and Choice* (Chicago: University of Chicago Department of Geography Research Paper No. 121, 1969), is a masterful presentation of the persistence of conflicting assumptions in this area of public policy, drawing heavily on Massachusetts experience which is, historically, both of long duration and unique.

Information on the development of Massachusetts public health laboratories came largely from the records published annually in the *Report* of the State Board of Health. Interviews with Dr. James A. McComb, who retired in 1967 after forty years service in the State Laboratories, and with Dr. Geoffrey Edsall, the present Director of the Institute of Laboratories, were supplemented by a number of valuable short manuscript histories tracing aspects of the laboratory work since 1894. The following published articles were of interest because they represented different points of view held by scientists who played a role in the work they described: Theobald Smith, "The New Laboratory of the Massachusetts State Board of Health for the Preparation of Diphtheria Antitoxin and Vaccine," *Journal of the Massachusetts Association of Boards of Health*, 14:231-236 (Nov. 1904), and "Public Health Laboratories," *BMSJ*, 143:491-493 (Nov. 8, 1900); James O. Wails, "The First Bacteriologic Laboratory in Massachusetts," *NEJM*, 234:391 (March 14, 1946); Edwin J. Cohn, "The University and the Biologic Laboratories of the State of Massachusetts," *Harvard Medical School Alumni Bulletin*, 24:75-79 (April 1950); Geoffrey Edsall, "Public Health and the Laboratory," *AJPH*, 40:1368-1371 (Nov. 1950).

Although this study examines infant and chronic disease as two foci of changing public health practice, there is little published to indicate that other historians of public health have identified these as critical areas of changing policy. Quite recently the history of childhood in the sixteenth and seventeenth centuries has claimed the attention of demographers and social historians both here and abroad, and it will, I hope, encourage further investigation. Henri Siebert, "The

Progress of Ideas Regarding the Causation and Control of Infant Mortality,"
BHM, 8:546-598 (April 1940); and John B. Blake, *Origins of Maternal and
Child Health Programs* (New Haven, Conn.: Yale University School of Medicine,
1953), suggest two possible approaches to this important subject. More recently
two articles discuss one important phase of federal legislation in this area, but
my research indicates a different complexion to the controversy; see Edward R.
Schlesinger, "The Sheppard-Towner Era: A Prototype Case Study in Federal-
State Relationships," *AJPH*, 57:1034-1040 (June 1967); Stanley J. Lemons,
"The Sheppard-Towner Act: Progressivism in the 1920's," *Journal of American
History*, 55:776-786 (March 1969). The Children's Bureau Publications are a
largely untapped source for further research in this area. Grace Abbott, *Ten
Years' Work for Children* (Washington, D.C.: Government Printing Office,
1923), and Dorothy E. Bradbury, *Four Decades of Action for Children: A
Short History of the Children's Bureau* (Washington, D.C.: Government Printing
Office, 1956), are abbreviated, institutional accounts. The four articles listed
below indicate the kinds of resources on child health that are amenable to under-
standing changing criteria of legitimacy in public health work: James P. Lynde,
"Infant Mortality: Its Causes and Prevention," *BMSJ*, 107: 49-54 (July 13,
1882); Josephine S. Baker, "Future Lines of Progress in Child Hygiene Work,"
New York Medical Journal, 101:1169-1171 (June 5, 1915); Louis I. Dublin,
"Infant Mortality in Fall River, Massachusetts: A Survey of the Mortality
Among 833 Infants Born in June, July, and August, 1913," *Publications of the
American Statistical Association*, 14:505-520 (June 1915); Merrill Champion,
"The Maternity Benefit Movement in Massachusetts," *Survey*, 45:864-865
(March 12, 1921).

I am not aware of any historical study of changes in ideas or policy relating to
chronic diseases, although this is clearly subject to such treatment. My limited
work in this areas was stimulated by a provocative investigation conducted by
the two men who cautiously guided this work in Massachusetts; see George H.
Bigelow and Herbert L. Lombard, *Cancer and Other Chronic Diseases in
Massachusetts* (Cambridge, Mass.: Houghton, Mifflin, 1933); Bigelow, "The
Massachusetts Cancer Program,"; and Lombard, "The Care of Chronic Diseases,"
in *Proceedings of the National Conference of Social Work*, 57th Annual Session
(Chicago: University of Chicago Press, 1931).

Finally, the multitude of ways in which public health is closely identified with
state responsibility for the dependent deserves a separate bibliographic essay.
The titles listed below are a sample of the sources which guided my work and
are in no sense inclusive. Paul Goodman, "Ethics and Enterprise: The Values of a
Boston Elite, 1800-1860," *American Quarterly*, 18:437-451 (Fall 1966); Robert
H. Bremner, *From The Depths: The Discovery of Poverty in the United States*
(New York: New York University Press, 1956), and "The Impact of the Civil
War on Philanthropy and Social Welfare," *Civil War History*, 12:292-303 (Dec.
1966); Sidney Fine, *Laissez Faire and the General Welfare State: A Study of
Conflict in American Thought, 1865-1901* (Ann Arbor: University of Michigan

Press, 1956); Albert Deutsch, "Medicine and Social Welfare," *BHM*, 11:485-502 (May 1942); Samuel Mencher, *Poor Law to Poverty Program: Economic Security Policy in Britain and the United States* (Pittsburgh, Pa.: University of Pittsburgh Press, 1967). George Rosen, "The Medical Aspects of the Controversy Over Factory Conditions in New England, 1840-1850," *BHM*, 15:483-497 (May 1944); Homer Folks, "Disease and Dependence," *Charities*, 11:297-300 (Nov. 14, 1903), and "The Case of Public Health vs. Public Welfare," *AJPH*, 28:917-918 (Aug. 1938); Robert W. Kelso, *The History of Public Poor Relief in Massachusetts, 1620-1920* (Boston: Houghton, Mifflin, 1922), and "The Transition from Charities to Public Welfare," *Annals of the American Academy of Political and Social Science*, 105:21-25 (Jan. 1923); George E. Vincent, "Public Welfare and Public Health," *Annals of the American Academy of Political and Social Science*, 105:36-41 (Jan. 1923); Alton A. Linford, *Old Age Assistance in Massachusetts* (Chicago: University of Chicago Press, 1949).

Students in the history of public health are fortunate to have three excellent current bibliographies in the history of medicine to facilitate their work; The Wellcome Historical Medical Library publishes a quarterly *Current Work in the History of Medicine* which began in 1954; a "Bibliography of the History of Medicine in the United States and Canada," has been published annually by the *Bulletin of the History of Medicine* since 1940; most recently, the National Library of Medicine has published an annual *Bibliography of the History of Medicine* (Vol. I, 1965–). The section on the "History of Medicine" in John B. Blake and Charles Roos, eds., *Medical Reference Works, 1679-1966: A Selected Bibliography* (Chicago: Medical Library Association, 1967) should be consulted. These excellent guides underscore the need for a comprehensive bibliography in the history of social welfare.

Index